MOTIVATING
HEALTH
BEHAVIOR

Motivating Health Behavior

John P. Elder
E. Scott Geller
Melbourne F. Hovell
Joni A. Mayer

Delmar Publishers Inc.™

I(T)P™

NOTICE TO THE READER

Publisher does not warrant or guarantee any of the products described herein or perform any independent analysis in connection with any of the product information contained herein. Publisher does not assume, and expressly disclaims, any obligation to obtain and include information other than that provided to it by the manufacturer.

The reader is expressly warned to consider and adopt all safety precautions that might be indicated by the activities described herein and to avoid all potential hazards. By following the instructions contained herein, the reader willingly assumes all risks in connection with such instructions.

The publisher makes no representations or warranties of any kind, including but not limited to, the warranties of fitness for particular purpose or merchantability, nor are any such representations implied with respect to the material set forth herein, and the publisher takes no responsibility with respect to such material. The publisher shall not be liable for any special, consequential or exemplary damages resulting, in whole or in part, from the readers' use of, or reliance upon, this material.

Cover design by Timothy J. Conners

Delmar Staff
Senior Acquisitions Editor: William Burgower
Senior Editorial Assistant: Debra Flis
Project Editor: Carol Micheli
Production Coordinator: Jennifer L. Gaines
Senior Design Supervisor: Susan C. Mathews
Art/Design Coordinator: Timothy J. Conners

For information, address Delmar Publishers Inc.
3 Columbia Circle, Box 15-015
Albany, New York 12212

Copyright © 1994
by Delmar Publishers Inc.
The trademark ITP is used under license.

printed in the United States of America
published simultaneously in Canada
by Nelson Canada,
a division of The Thomson Corporation

2 3 4 5 6 7 8 9 10 XXX 00 99 98 97 96 95 94

Library of Congress Cataloging-in-Publication Data

Motivating health behavior / John P. Elder . . . [et al.].
      p.   cm.
   Includes index.
   ISBN 0-8273-4963-7
   1. Health promotion. 2. Health behavior. I. Elder, John P.
   [DNLM: 1. Health Promotion. 2. Health Behavior. WA 590 M918
1994]
RA427.8.M68   1994
613 — dc20
DNLM/DLC
for Library of Congress   93-12430
                                                                          CIP

Contents

Preface

Motivating Health Behavior presents a basic how-to guide for future or current health professionals and others conducting health promotion programs. Therefore, *MHB* emphasizes specific behavior change technologies: "behavior modification," marketing, training, and education, because we consider behavior change to be the core of this emerging field. Our treatment of the topic of "education" is limited to a brief chapter on how to set educational objectives. We feel that the field has gone past the realm of knowledge change; moreover, there are many high quality texts currently on the market on how to conduct health education in its more traditional form. However, as it is neither feasible nor ethical simply to "jump in" and change someone's health behavior, the reader will also receive a healthy dose of content in community organization, planning, research, and evaluation integrated with intervention strategies in what we call our **ONPRIME** model.

The authors of this book are behavioral psychologists who work in public health promotion. Hopefully, this commonality among us will contribute to the logic and coherence of our writing. We will nevertheless not pretend to represent the premier discipline among the behavioral sciences; anthropology, sociology, political science, and economics all contribute greatly to the understanding of health and illness. Nor do we assume that, within psychology, behaviorism has beaten back all competitors; cognitively-oriented theories continue to hold their own and perhaps have even increased in popularity in the past decade. (Witness the burgeoning popularity of social marketing and its cognitive basis, as discussed in Chapter 10). Hopefully, we have presented a balanced view with respect to our sister disciplines and theories.

The behaviorism theme of *MHB* stems from (a) our own training and experience, (b) our belief that behavior analysis and modification is the most precise and specific theory of the many which have been applied to changing health behavior, and (c) a corresponding lack of working knowledge of "behavior mod" among health promoters, at least relative to other intervention approaches. This text should serve either as a central focus for students in health psychology or behaviorally-oriented health promotion classes, or as a complement to orientations represented among professionals and students more thoroughly immersed in other health education or health communications theoretical systems. In any case, the behavior change approach presented herein will hopefully prove as user-friendly to our readers as it has to our past students.

The specific intervention topics selected for in-depth exploration — tobacco use, injury control, nutrition, sexually transmitted diseases (STDs) and teen pregnancy prevention, child survival, and environmental protection — have been selected for three reasons. First, they comprise major health issues facing the planet's population. Second, they represent the spectrum of issues and technologies which mold the field of health promotion. Third, they range in health promotion targets and content from the typical (e.g., nutrition) to the atypical (e.g., environmental protection). Space limitations prevented the inclusion of chapters on other important topics, such as alcohol and drug control, heart disease prevention, health promotion among the elderly, the prevention of violence and abuse, and others. We regret that these important issues haven't gotten their just attention. We have attempted to subsume these topics in other chapters so that readers can generalize from our principles and targeted topics to problems with which they have to work.

Throughout the world, millions of people from infancy to old age die each year from behaviorally-related causes. Hundreds of thousands of these have been exploited by tobacco, alcohol and other illness industries. Health promotion is a serious business. It is also arguably the most reinforcing health discipline for those of us lucky enough to have health promotion jobs, which in turn helps explain why health promoters are upbeat people. Therefore, *MHB* presents material in an occasionally light-hearted fashion: We want the reader to learn — and have fun.

Acknowledgments

It may prove impossible to name all individuals who have contributed by word or deed to the development of this book, given the length of time over which it has been written. Nevertheless, we shall attempt to thank at least some of the more conspicuous contributors.

Jenny Offner word processed most of the manuscript, cheerfully and tirelessly tracking taped and stapled pages, partially crossed-out words, and a half dozen different reference styles. Amelia Arroyo and Anna Morghen skillfully coordinated communication with publishers and even among authors. Diane Evans, Mary Perl, and Cynthia Wright also provided valuable clerical assistance.

Many health promotion projects have been used as examples in various parts of this text. Several have been invoked in key passages throughout, reflecting their overriding importance in formulating the conceptual and experiential basis for the book. Among this group is the Pawtucket Heart Health Program, headed by Dick Carleton and Tom Lasater. Formerly with PHHP was Dave Abrams, with whom a conversation in the Countways Library led to the framework presented in Section III. Current and ongoing projects whose components are referred to frequently include Project SHOUT (whose project director is Marianne Wildey), Proyecto Salsa (led by Nadia Campbell, Jeanette Candelaria, and Carmen Moreno), the California Statewide Tobacco Control Program Independent Evaluation (with Erin Kenney heading the team of Chris Edwards, Deborah Parra-Medina, Cathy Crooks, and others), and other health promotion programs staffed largely by our former students. Also, the HEALTHCOM Project (led by Mark Rasmuson, Will Shaw, and Bill Smith) focused and stimulated much of our thinking on international health and social marketing. Moshe Engleberg gave some much needed polish to the latter chapter. We initially talked about writing this book before having had a chance to work with all of these talented people; fortunately, we were delayed.

Betsy Clapp put her creative attentions into photography for the book and helped finish objectives and other last-minute details. Susan Peplinski and Lisa Ware Duke also contributed to its editing. Cathy Crooks and Terry Conway provided suggestions for its classroom use, as they tolerated its rough draft format in their health promotion classes.

We are indebted to Si Osgrove for his journalistic skills and efforts. He diligently edited the book twice for content, grammar, and spelling, and suggested adding the glossary, which he compiled. Erica Bennett carried the editing task across the finish line.

Finally, we would all like to express our thanks to our students, past and present, who have challenged and shaped our thinking about health promotion. Particularly, we would like to thank the students in a course at SDSU entitled "Motivating Health Behavior" who have endured crude drafts of this text in its previous incarnations, and through shaping, differential reinforcement, and even occasional negative reinforcement, did much to help improve it.

List of Tables

Section I:

The Basics

Chapter 1

Introduction

OBJECTIVES

After finishing this chapter, the reader should be able to:

1. Define health promotion.
2. Describe reasons for the recent emergence of this public health specialty.
3. List seven steps in health promotion planning, intervention and evaluation.

A PUBLIC HEALTH RETROSPECTIVE

In 1854, an English anesthetist named John Snow was determined to seek the end to a cholera epidemic taking the lives of thousands of Londoners. With some inspired epidemiological research, he discovered that households obtaining their water from a Southwark and Vauxhall Company pump in the St. James Parish district of London experienced a high rate of cholera, whereas those who obtained water from Lambeth Water Company's pump were generally healthier. He convinced authorities to shut off the pump in the Southwark and Vauxhall Company district, which immediately resulted in a major reduction in the cholera infection rate.

But Sir John was not content. To promote acceptance of this shut-off and the resulting inconvenience, he distributed leaflets at the entry to St. Paul's Cathedral and had gaslamp lighters shout out clean water information during their nightly rounds (the British Broadcasting Corporation was not yet on the air in those days). "OK, so we got the dirty water shut off," he thought, "and people haven't rioted. But how long will the pump in St. James Parish stay clean? I've started to teach Londoners what dirty water is, but how do I teach them to clean it up? Or to keep it clean? If they *do*

1

get sick, how can they be trained to deal with the illness? How do I work with people? How can I best communicate this information?''

The first part of this historical fiction is true. John Snow did actually identify the source of the London cholera epidemic by analyzing which pump was making people sick. By shutting this pump down, he protected thousands of residents not yet infected by this deadly disease. He did not promote acceptance of this intervention; however, we can assume that the Smyth family simply had to walk much farther to get a bucket of water for their daily use. He did not teach people how to boil and disinfect dirty water, nor, more importantly, about the importance of not using the source of drinking water as a toilet. He did not study how best to communicate his public hygiene strategy —in fact, it's safe to assume he did not even think about involving the public in any active way. Although John Snow is a public health hero, other groups who concurrently grappled with major health and social issues — such as child labor, industrially-based air pollution, and slavery — stood to learn little from this scientific breakthrough and technological solution.

In the succeeding century, general social welfare and the technology of public health (or at least as applied in industrialized countries) witnessed astonishing advances. Madame Curie discovered radium, Louis Pasteur developed the germ theory of fermentation, and Sir Alexander Fleming discovered penicillin. Malnutrition was virtually erased from Europe. Slavery was gradually abolished in the 19th century, first in European colonies and finally in the U.S. Access to public education was greatly expanded and illiteracy sharply reduced. Women obtained the right to vote. In 1982, smallpox was declared vanquished through the worldwide campaign called ''Operation Smallpox Zero.'' Public health challenges continued to be met through increasingly sophisticated technology backed by ever more comprehensive policies and enforcement.

Yet one aspect of public health remained virtually static in the century between John Snow's discovery of the contaminated London pump and the eradication of smallpox. The beneficiaries of these changes — the families who now got clean water to drink, the babies who were vaccinated, and the poor who were employed on public work projects — were treated more as passive consumers rather than active collaborators in this

social and medical progress. Knowledge and behavior change was left to educational and religious institutions. The hallmarks of public health were the protection of health and the prevention of illness through technological and policy changes developed by the intellectually and politically powerful.

ENTER HEALTH PROMOTION

In the past two decades, health promotion has exploded onto the scene and changed all of the rules. The technology of behavior change has achieved a status equal to that of medical technology or policy approaches to public health improvement. In many public health campaigns, health promotion is the primary or even the only approach employed. Why such a sudden and dramatic change? A variety of social and economic forces undoubtedly contributed to the rapid emergence of health promotion, including the following:

1. The traditional approach to the practice of medicine — the ''Medical Model'' — came under attack from consumer groups, allied health professionals, and even physicians themselves. The term **''medical model'' denotes the passive compliance of a patient to clinical procedures, which the physician or other clinician directs, as though it were neither necessary nor even possible for the patient to understand and participate in the treatment regimen.** Other than answering questions during diagnosis, the patient with a brain tumor does not participate in the surgery needed to remove it. Although this is an extreme case, **the Medical Model generally implies that illnesses need to be treated rather than prevented,** and the intervention ends when the treatment has been completed rather than with the maintenance of good health or ''wellness.''

Just as the Medical Model defined clinical medicine, a modified version of this same model was the basis for the philosophy of public health, which, in turn, was largely dominated by medicine. However, clinicians and the public alike found this approach to be often ineffective. Even sophisticated treatments required compliance from the patient. For example, patients had to understand when to take their medicine and return for their next appointment, and to agree with the physician's directions. The importance of behavior change — coinciding with the emergence of the specialties of Psychosomatic, Preventive, and Behavioral Medicine — was gradually recognized in the medical field. At the extreme, treatment procedures which did not actively involve the patient were seen as potentially harmful. Such procedures confuse or debase patients, making them likely to avoid both the treatment recommendations and the person making them. Also, failure to maximize a patient's expectations of success precludes taking advantage of all potentially necessary treatment elements. That the Medical Model at times violated the dictum, *primum non nocere* (the first thing is to do no harm), was recognized in widely read books such as Ivan Illyich's *The Medical Nemesis*. While the survival of the Medical Model was not (and is not) threatened, the arrival of health promotion marked a diminishing of its influence on public health.

2. Not only were patients taking charge of their own lives, the political scene also witnessed a rapid transition, especially during the era of the "60s." The process of decolonization set in full motion by World War II was being completed in Asia and Africa. Street demonstrations speeded the end of U.S. involvement in Vietnam. The civil rights movements championed by Martin Luther King, Jr., Malcolm X, and Cesar Chavez opened doors to opportunities which were previously the nearly exclusive domain of white males. Women organized to take control over their own lives and bodies. Encouraged by the rapid transmission of news through the electronic media which depicted the potential, or at least the necessity for action, people all over were assuming ever larger roles in their own lives as well as in the political processes of their communities and nations.

3. Technological breakthroughs accompanying the control of polio, the eradication of smallpox, and the development of the x-ray and the electrocardiogram were reaching their points of diminishing return. Life expectancy was not extended by expanding the availability of increasingly "high-tech" medical services. While heart transplants and even artificial hearts grabbed headlines and shed rays of hope into the lives of a few unfortunate families desperate to hold onto a loved one, costs of such "heroic" medical procedures were simply astronomical. Families of average means could never hope to pay such medical bills, even assuming the (unlikely) full recovery of their afflicted relative, stemming from such extraordinary interventions. In the meantime, children of both the urban and rural poor were threatened by inadequate perinatal care, endemic drug and alcohol abuse, malnutrition, and violence. They did not need *better* medical care; they just needed *some* medical care.

4. There has also been increasing recognition that human behavior was largely responsible for illness and premature mortality and, conversely, for the maintenance of health. In the late 1940s, the Framingham Study began tracking the health and related behaviors of residents of this suburban Boston-area town, seeking to identify what risk factors for heart disease could be identified in this initially healthy population. Using a "prospective cohort design" (see chapter 6), the researchers demonstrated that the development of high blood pressure and high serum cholesterol resulted in higher rates of heart attacks. For the first time, however, there was documentation that specific behaviors — not just physiological results of these behaviors — were the erstwhile culprits in the chain of events leading up to the industrialized world's number one cause of death. Not only cigarette smoking, but also diets high in sodium, fat, and cholesterol were identified as behavioral risk factors for heart disease. At the same time, Doll and Hill in England and Wynder in the U.S. drew the first scientific link between smoking and lung cancer. The behavior that perhaps most Americans knew had killed Babe Ruth and would soon claim such Hollywood notables as Humphrey Bogart, Clark Gable, and Gary Cooper had finally been fingered, although it would take over a decade for a national health official to integrate this finding into policy (see chapter 17).

Epidemiological research of this nature continued for a period of time, while health professionals began to study whether behaviors such as excessive eating, smoking, and exercising were modifiable in small groups of high risk individuals. Finally, in the early 1970s, researchers in North Karelia, Finland, and Stanford, California, launched efforts to reduce the risk for heart disease in targeted communities by increasing exercise and reducing smoking and unhealthy eating in entire populations (see chapters 16 and 18). For the first time, changing health behaviors to prevent diseases had been attempted on a public health scale. The rest, as they say, has been history. Health promotion became a fully accepted public health technology. Public health education emphasizing behavior change had been adjudged as not only as effective as, but also cheaper than, technology development or policy change.

5. Finally, even those specializing in technological or policy aspects of public health—such as environmental health or health services administration—began to recognize the role of behavior change in their specialties. Environmental and Occupational Health now involves anything from getting consumers to reduce their amount of household garbage to promoting worker safety, while administrators emphasize how to increase worker efficiency and morale (see chapters 15 and 22). All of these activities require some expertise in the technology of behavior change, whether by direct or indirect means. The role of "health promotion" is moving well past its original borders and into the realms of policy and behavioral technology, and protection and prevention.

HEALTH PROMOTION AND INTERVENTION DEFINED

Our definition of health promotion is as follows: **"the modification of human behavior and environmental factors related to that behavior which directly or indirectly promotes health, prevents illness, or protects individuals from harm."** This definition reflects the emphases of this book:

- Our focus is on health behavior and how to change it. It is not on attitude or knowledge change except as these relate to behavior change.
- We will be examining strategies which have either a direct or indirect effect on health. Although the building blocks of health promotion

are related to individual behavior (such as exercise), public health promotion requires that we look at changing target individuals (including policymakers, gatekeepers, health care providers, work supervisors, and media personalities) who can influence large numbers of people. These individuals can also assist us in making structural changes (e.g., in policies, regulations, laws, socioeconomic factors, and the physical environment) which will support and maintain health gains. This book uses examples from small group and individual behavior change, but stresses the need to move beyond this narrow focus.

- We will extend the concept of health promotion into the realms of activism, policy, and technology; beyond "promotion" *per se* and into prevention and protection. In all cases, however, we will continue to relate the subject matter back to human behavior and how to change it.

Intervention is a health promotion aimed at a target audience which alters a preexisting condition related to that target audience's behavior. The purpose of the intervention is to create healthful behavior(s).

WHY A BEHAVIORAL EMPHASIS?

A complete education in public health includes a broad understanding of the social and behavioral sciences as well as the various theoretical orientations most closely associated with the field of health promotion. As we examine the next two chapters, however, health and illness can generally be defined in terms of healthy and harmful behaviors. Therefore, the most appropriate technologies for changing these behaviors are those most closely associated with the specialty of behavioral psychology, including behavior modification, social learning theory and related fields. We do not mean to imply that other theoretical formulations, such as the Health Belief Model or the Theory of Reasoned Action, are inadequate planning or implementation frameworks. As discussed in chapter 3, these and other theories explain health promotion with different semantics which, when translated, say many of the same things that are central to behavioral psychology.

Nor do we pretend that psychology alone holds

the only key to understanding individual behavior. On the contrary, psychology's individual orientation is inadequate for examining the cultural and social forces explaining much of human behavior and society's problems. For understanding these broader perspectives, anthropologists, sociologists, economists, and political scientists are better equipped and avoid "blaming the individual" for illnesses based in poverty or ignorance. However, even social change begins with individual behavior — whether it be voting, volunteering, exercising economic power by purchasing certain consumer items and avoiding others, or organizing a community coalition to tackle a health-related problem. We integrate techniques such as motivation, education, training, social marketing, and community organization (detailed in Section II) into a cohesive whole within the framework of behavioral psychology and the coinciding health promotion model presented in this book.

AN EMPIRICAL ORIENTATION

Health promotion has both applied and research roots (just as do preventive medicine and epidemiology, respectively). Often, one hears well-trained health promotion professionals complain, "We don't have the time, resources, or expertise to do research. We just have to get out there and change things." In chapters 5, 6, and 11 we argue that:

a. Research is an integral part of health promotion; without it, we run a variety of risks, including discontinuing an effective program or spending precious resources on an ineffective one;

b. Thorough needs assessment research not only helps us plan a more effective program, but consistent with the philosophical foundation of health promotion, it also initiates the process of community involvement; and

c. Health promotion research may benefit skills in statistics, computer programming, or research design. However, such basic skills as collecting and graphing objective data, understanding the logic of controlled studies, and being able to write and present in a clear and concise fashion allow us to function as field researchers even when sophisticated technical assistance is not available.

Once basic health promotion intervention and evaluation approaches are described in Section II, we go on to examine their applications in Sections III and IV.

A CULTURAL PERSPECTIVE

The authors and most readers of this book grew up, live, and work in an industrialized society. And, much of the conceptual and empirical foundation of health promotion referred to in *Motivating Health Behavior* was accomplished by our colleagues or others with a similar cultural grounding. Therefore, this book is largely based on a perspective on health issues in the developed world. In this regard, three assertions are relevant:

First, maintain that the laws of behavior and change are universal. People around the world act in some ways and not in others because they have been taught and reinforced for doing (or not doing) so. Clearly, the form and content of this learning will vary dramatically among the world's diverse cultures — or for that matter, among subgroups of single, multicultural nations. However, a basic understanding of the processes of education, motivation, and communication can be generalized across cultures.

Second, whereas most of the published research in epidemiology, health behavior, and health promotion (as in medicine) deals with subject matters more relevant to the developed than underdeveloped world, the bulk of the world's suffering and dying occurs in the latter. In Guatemala, one in twenty-five of all children will die before the age of five, twice as many as in the U.S. It is estimated that ten times as many adults in Kenya are infected with HIV compared to Swedish adults. Yet, all of these infamous killers of people in the developing world have behavioral causes and antidotes — breastfeeding and oral rehydration, family planning and safe birthing practices, and safer sex. While poverty and related structural factors are the universal common denominator for illness and premature death, the links between health and behavior have no frontiers; neither do health problems and solutions.

Third, although the spread of HIV infection has been our most recent example of how a disease crosses borders with impunity, the spread and control of infectious diseases has always had international implications. We can never really be safe from such threats until everyone in the world is safe. Also, the tobacco industry in Western nations, particularly the U.S., is increasingly ogling markets in the underdeveloped world to take up the slack in demand created by the successes of health promotion efforts on the domestic scene. And tobacco interests continue to prosper (see chapter 17). Yet those involved in anti-tobacco efforts implicitly boast of the successes achieved since the 1964 Surgeon General's Report. Are we really succeeding—or are we just spreading the problem around? Your answer may depend on whether your focus is individual or true public health. *Motivating Health Behavior* emphasizes ways in which we can "think globally and act locally."

THE ONPRIME MODEL

This book is organized around a seven-step sequence of planning, intervention, and evaluation procedures represented by the acronym **ONPRIME. ONPRIME stands for organizing, needs resources assessment, priority-setting, research, intervention, monitoring, and evaluation.** To get started, we complete this introductory section

with a description of the basic conceptual issues involved in defining "health" and "behavior." In the second section, we launch into issues involved in planning health promotion programs, the first part of the **ONPRIME** model shown in Figure 1–1. Specifically, issues of working within existing organizational structures or creating new ones are addressed. Particular attention is given to Rothman's categories of social planning, social action, and locality development **(PAL)**. Next, needs/resource assessment techniques, represented by the acronym **KARS** (Key informant interviews, Archival research, Rates-under-treatment assessment, and Surveys), will be described.

Once the needs/resources assessment data are in, we go back to the target population or organizational leadership and set program priorities. This, in turn, defines the intervention-oriented research fine-tuning our intervention planning.

Now we're ready for the heart of the book, the specific intervention techniques which typify health promotion. One chapter each will be devoted to skills training, education, motivation, and social marketing. (This is represented, in a different sequence, by **STEM**, and we promise this is our last acronym.) Finally, we describe techniques for monitoring the progress of health promotion programs and evaluating the results, completing

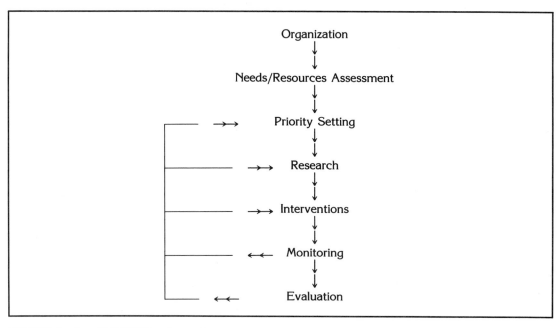

FIGURE 1–1. ONPRIME's elements

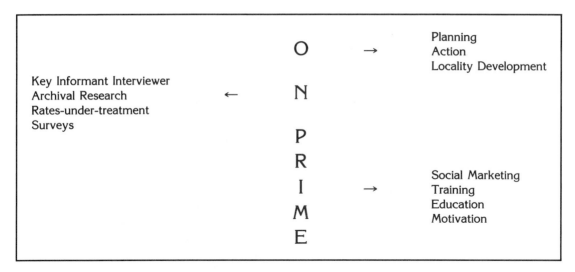

FIGURE 1–2.   Detailed elements of ONPRIME

the **ONPRIME** sequence. **ONPRIME's** constituent acronyms are presented in Figure 1–2.

The third section of this book considers all elements of the **ONPRIME** process and especially the **STEM** interventions at four different levels (individual, group, organizational, and community). The final section examines special topics and examples in health promotion, describing and critiquing programs conducted in special settings (e.g., at the worksite), with special problems (e.g., sexually transmitted diseases), and with specific populations (e.g., women aged 14–25). Finally, we discuss the application of behavior change techniques to ever-broader problem areas (e.g., protecting the environment) and the future of health promotion.

Each chapter begins with a list of objectives to guide your reading. Some chapters end with exercises relevant for individuals or with group discussions to expand your understanding of that content area.

Finally, there is no better way to understand research and intervention techniques than to apply them, even if only to oneself. A self-change project which will "walk you through" the various techniques described in the **ONPRIME** sequence is recommended for every student of health promotion. Hopefully, not only will this help you understand how better to motivate health behavior, but will also improve your own health!

SUMMARY

While the field of public health has developed rapidly over the past century and a half, health promotion is a relatively recent arrival on the scene. The decline of the Medical Model, the realization of the limits of medical technology, the successes of efforts to empower people and communities, and the recognition of the role of human behavior in illness and health have all contributed to health promotion's recently acquired status. The **ONPRIME** model of planning, implementation, and evaluation integrates the diverse conceptual and applied contributions to this quickly changing and expanding public health field. Before presenting this model, however, we will examine in detail definitions of health and behavior.

EXERCISES

1. Interview individuals from different generations—perhaps a parent or a grandparent and a primary school student. What was their initial concept of health and illness? How was it learned? Has it changed over time?
2. Self-Change Project: Begin thinking about a personal health behavior that you would like to change. More details will be forthcoming at the end of each of the following chapters.

Chapter 2

Definitions of Health

OBJECTIVES

By the end of this chapter, the reader should be able to:

1. Describe the three main goals of *Healthy People 2000*.
2. Identify general trends in U.S. infant and adult mortality today in contrast to the trends twenty-five years ago.
3. Distinguish among promotion, protection, and prevention as described in *Healthy People 2000*.
4. List the criteria for the development of the objectives specified in *Healthy People 2000*.
5. Define the "measures for better health" as stated in *Healthy People 2000*.
6. Describe the major threats to the health of children in underdeveloped countries.
7. State the purpose of the Alma Ata Declaration and identify the ten components describing "health care" within the document.

INTRODUCTION

Our subject is neither "motivation" nor "motivating behavior," but motivating *health* behavior. We now come to the critical focus of this book, namely, the concept of "health." Before we actually review definitions, let's examine the health in the U.S., other industrialized countries, and underdeveloped nations.

We have come to take the seemingly miraculous cures of modern medicine almost for granted. And we tend to forget that our improved health has come more from preventing disease than from treating it once it strikes. Our fascination with the more glamorous "pound of cure" has tended to dazzle us into ignoring the often more effective "ounce of prevention" as well as continual warnings that more needs to be done, such as that from President Jimmy Carter's foreword to *Healthy People* more than a decade ago:

"We are killing ourselves by our own careless habits. We are killing ourselves by carelessly polluting the environment. We are killing ourselves by permitting harmful social conditions to persist —conditions like poverty, hunger and ignorance —which destroy health, especially for infants and children."[1]

HEALTHY PEOPLE 2000

The year 1991 marked the publication of the U.S. Department of Health and Human Services' *Healthy People 2000*, an update of the landmark *Healthy People* published twelve years earlier. This 700 page tome sets out the prospects and problems before us in the remaining years of the millennium, basking for a moment in the satisfaction about progress made in some areas since the late 1970s, yet stating concern about other more stubborn obstacles to reducing morbidity and mortality further. More alarming still is the widening disparity between the nation's "haves" and "have nots," manifested perhaps more clearly in health than in any other arena.

This disparity is giving the U.S. something of a reputation. Among industrialized countries, our health status is actually slipping: Americans are currently twenty-fourth among the world's wealthier nations in terms of infant mortality—the lowest standing ever recorded. We have slipped nearly that low in life expectancy, as well.

Nevertheless, in the decade from 1977 to 1987, substantial progress was realized on a number of fronts for controlling the major killers of Americans. Of the four leading causes of death in the U.S., only cancer-related mortality showed no decrease in this time span. Death from heart disease, injuries, and stroke dropped 10 percent or greater.[2]

Table 2–1 shows the progress made in reducing mortality among individuals from birth through adulthood and in reducing the incapacity among the oldest age group in the period from 1977 to 1987. These data are placed in the context of the actual targeted reductions set forth in the original *Healthy People* for the year 1990. As depicted, progress was on target for children, adults, and older adults, while lagging for infants and adolescents/young adults.

The increasing national attention toward reaching these targets is by no means attributable solely to a governmental desire to "do good." Prevention simply makes good economic sense. Here are some of the illness bills we Americans run up every year:

- 284,000 coronary bypass procedures @ $30,000;

TABLE 2–1
Progress Toward Health for Each Age Group, 1977–1987*

Age Group	Targeted Death Rate Reduction* for 1990	Actual 1987 Status	Amount of Change Needed to Reach Goal
Infants	35%	28%	7%
Children	20%	21%	1% or over
Adolescents and young adults	20%	13%	7%
Adults	25%	21%	4%
Older Adults	20% fewer days of restricted activity	17%	3%

*except for older adults, where restricted activity was targeted.
SOURCE: *Health, United States, 1989 and Prevention Profile*, Centers for Disease Control, National Center for Health Statistics

- 600,000 stroke patients treated and rehabilitated @ $22,000;
- Neonatal intensive care for 260,000 low birth weight babies @ $10,000;
- Treatment for 118,000 new AIDS cases @ $75,000 over the remaining lifetime: $2,600,000,000.

Add the costs of treatment and rehabilitation for cancer, injuries, alcoholism, drug abuse, and vaccine-preventable diseases and we reach the astronomical total of billions of dollars spent needlessly in this country each year. This total does not include the loss of economic productivity realized when we fail to prevent illness or disability in our workforce.[3]

Healthy People 2000 established the following goals for the decade of the '90s:

I. **Increase the span of healthy life for Americans.**
II. **Reduce health disparities among Americans.**
III. **Achieve access to preventive services for all Americans.**

These goals mark a fascinating evolution in thinking about health and health promotion in the U.S. Whereas the original *Healthy People* stressed the role of individual behaviors and the potential for changing behaviors to extend life, the above statements imply that quality and equality define health more than direct physical indices of well-being, and that we, as a country, can only be healthy when all of us have access to preventive services. In spite of conservative political trends, health leadership in the U.S. evidences a shift toward a more activist stance, one more in line with positions held by international organizations.

In the original *Healthy People*[4] the Surgeon General of the United States reported the results of an investigation into major health problems for American infants, children, adolescents, adults, and the elderly. As shown in Figure 2–1, age-adjusted mortality rates have declined in the U.S., indicating apparent improved health among the four younger age groups. Whereas infectious diseases such as pneumonia and influenza were the leading causes of death at the turn of the century, heart disease and cancer now claim that position among Americans.

Deaths from the three major chronic diseases (heart disease, cancer, and stroke) have declined somewhat since the first half of the century, or at least seem to be stabilizing. However, most motor vehicle and other accidents, liver diseases, and suicides/homicides do not seem to be changing substantially from decade to decade.

Infant mortality rates have declined dramatically in the past twenty-five years, as has the racial inequality in these rates. One could choose to be gratified by these statistical improvements or shocked by continued discrepancies, as white non-Hispanic infants are only half as likely to die before the age of one as are African-American infants. Figure 2–2 presents the leading causes of infant deaths for 1950, 1979, and 1985. Although the infant mortality rate in the U.S. has dropped from 100 deaths per 1,000 births in 1900 to only 10 in 1985, the first year of life is the most hazardous until reaching the age of 65 due to the various causes listed in Figure 2–3. African-American infants in 1984 were 3.4 times more likely to die from disorders related to short gestation and unspecified low birth weight than were white infants.[5] Moreover, even for infants who survive the first year, a far larger percentage of African-Americans and other minorities are likely to suffer from low birth weight than are whites. Inadequate prenatal care and teenage maternity both contribute to this discrepancy.

From 1950 to 1985, the death rate for American children (age 1 to 14 years) fell from 87.7 to 34.8 deaths per 100,000. This reduction is largely attributable to the control of pneumonia and influenza, which are no longer among the top five killers of children in industrialized societies. Conversely, homicide rates for this age group have jumped dramatically since 1950. Although deaths due to accidents have dropped substantially since 1950, a large number of children still die from automobile accidents, drownings, burns, falls, and poisoning (Figure 2–3).

The development and widespread use of vaccines for various infectious diseases has led to far lower incidence rates for these diseases among children. However, aggressive efforts for total immunizations at the national level must be sustained in order to prevent these disabling and at times fatal diseases from reappearing in developed countries.

Accidents constitute the major causes of adolescent and young adult deaths, just as they do for children (see Figure 2–4). Almost three-fourths of these are motor vehicle crashes. Other significant killers of people in this age group are suicide and

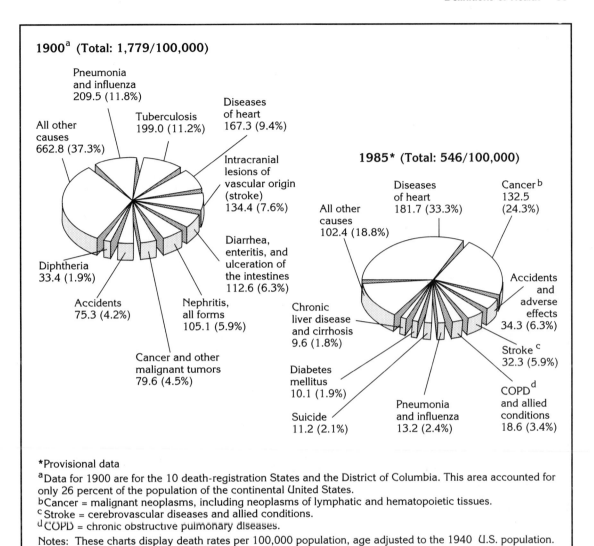

1900[a] (Total: 1,779/100,000)

Pneumonia
and influenza
209.5 (11.8%)

Tuberculosis
199.0 (11.2%)

Diseases
of heart
167.3 (9.4%)

All other
causes
662.8 (37.3%)

Intracranial
lesions of
vascular origin
(stroke)
134.4 (7.6%)

Diarrhea,
enteritis, and
ulceration of
the intestines
112.6 (6.3%)

Diphtheria
33.4 (1.9%)

Accidents
75.3 (4.2%)

Nephritis,
all forms
105.1 (5.9%)

Cancer and other
malignant tumors
79.6 (4.5%)

1985* (Total: 546/100,000)

Diseases
of heart
181.7 (33.3%)

Cancer[b]
132.5
(24.3%)

All other
causes
102.4 (18.8%)

Accidents
and
adverse
effects
34.3 (6.3%)

Chronic
liver disease
and cirrhosis
9.6 (1.8%)

Stroke[c]
32.3 (5.9%)

Diabetes
mellitus
10.1 (1.9%)

COPD[d]
and allied
conditions
18.6 (3.4%)

Suicide
11.2 (2.1%)

Pneumonia
and influenza
13.2 (2.4%)

*Provisional data

[a]Data for 1900 are for the 10 death-registration States and the District of Columbia. This area accounted for only 26 percent of the population of the continental United States.

[b]Cancer = malignant neoplasms, including neoplasms of lymphatic and hematopoietic tissues.

[c]Stroke = cerebrovascular diseases and allied conditions.

[d]COPD = chronic obstructive pulmonary diseases.

Notes: These charts display death rates per 100,000 population, age adjusted to the 1940 U.S. population. Numbers in parentheses indicate percentages of total age-adjusted death rate. The sum of data for the 10 causes may not equal the total because of rounding.

Source: National Center for Health Statistics.

FIGURE 2–1.   Age-adjusted rates for major causes of death in the United States in 1900 and for leading causes of death in 1985. Reprinted by permission of Macro International Inc.

homicide. Male adolescents in all of these three categories have higher mortality rates than do females, while the major killer of African-American youths is homicide rather than motor vehicle accidents. Homicide rates in the U.S. are approxi-mately ten times those of other major Western countries. Underlying these trends are high rates of alcohol and drug use, legally- or illegally-obtained handguns and assault weapons, and ex-traordinarily high rates of unemployment in inner

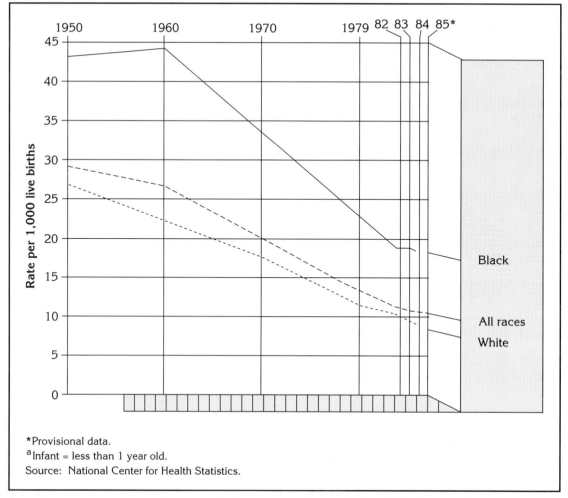

FIGURE 2–2. Infant[a] mortality rates, by Race: selected years 1950–1985. Reprinted by permission of Macro International Inc.

cities (see Fig 2–6). The decline of adolescent smoking rates has leveled off dramatically since 1980. This is especially due to the contribution of girls taking up the habit.

Figure 2–5 shows the leading causes of adult deaths in the U.S. for the years 1950, 1979, and 1985. This category accounts for nearly half of the American population. As can be seen, heart disease, followed by cancer, accidents, stroke, and liver diseases, account for the majority of deaths in this population. Since 1950, there has been a 47 percent reduction in heart disease and a 69 percent reduction in stroke mortality.

Whereas Figures 2–7 and 2–8 show that heart disease and stroke have declined for all races and both genders, African-American populations are still threatened by these chronic diseases more than whites.

Since 1950, a variety of advances have been made in determining specific causes for cancer and heart disease. Dietary fat and cholesterol have been linked to serum cholesterol and subsequently to heart disease risk, while dietary fat seems to be implicated in various forms of cancers, as well. In the past ten years, careful attention has been paid to the amount of animal

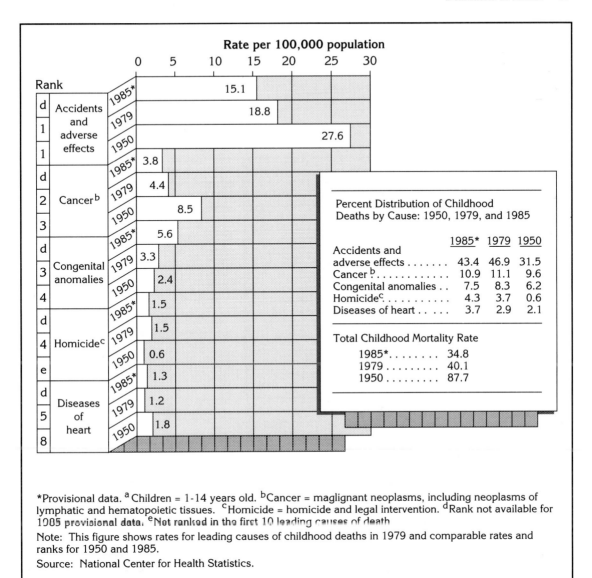

FIGURE 2–3. Leading causes of childhood deaths: 1950, 1979, and 1985. Reprinted by permission of Macro International Inc.

fat and cholesterol that adults consume in American and other Western populations. Both males and females have substantially reduced their intake of beef, whole milk, and eggs, while they have increased their consumption of fish and low-fat or skim milk.

Heart disease and cancer hold in common cigarette smoking as their major causal factor. Since the early 1950s, irrefutable evidence has linked cigarette smoking with lung cancer, heart disease, and a variety of other respiratory and chronic diseases. Since the 1964 Surgeon General's Report was released linking cigarette smoking with lung cancer, the percentage of adult smokers has declined substantially, largely due to the reduction in smoking prevalence among males. The data for

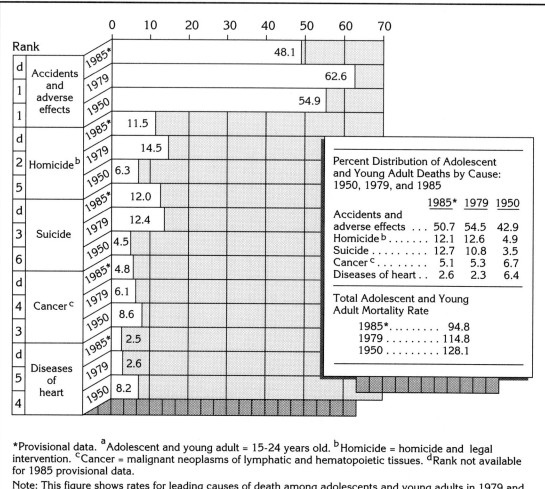

FIGURE 2–4. Leading causes of adolescent and young adult[a] deaths: 1950, 1979, and 1985. Reprinted by permission of Macro International Inc.

five selected years between 1965 and 1985 are presented in Figure 2–9.

Figures 2–10 and 2–11 show age adjusted cancer death rates for males and females by the site of the cancer and the race of the population. Lung cancer continues to increase, perhaps representing the fact that the disease may form latently from cigarette smoking even though a person has not been smoking for some years. Again, it is

noteworthy that African-American males are more likely to die from various cancers than are their white counterparts. As a function of the relative increase in cigarette smoking among women, lung cancer has surpassed breast cancer as a killer of women.

In general, the people of the U.S. and other industrialized countries are less likely to die prematurely than they were twenty to thirty years

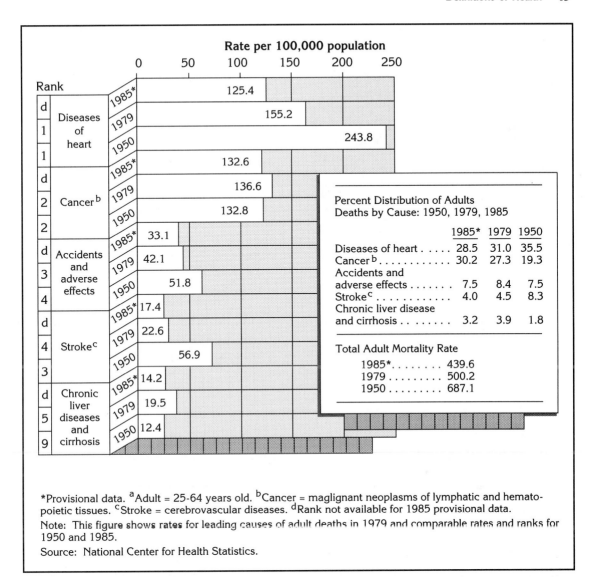

FIGURE 2–5. Leading causes of adult[a] deaths: 1950, 1979, and 1985. Reprinted by permission of Macro International Inc.

ago. However, further progress is possible, especially given that the majority of risk factors for these diseases are so-called "life style" factors. In other words, the way a person lives will dictate whether he or she will fall victim to one of these illnesses or disabilities.

Promotion, Prevention, and Protection

Healthy People and *Healthy People 2000* classify activities for health enhancement in three general categories: promotion, prevention, and protection. Health **promotion** targets individuals

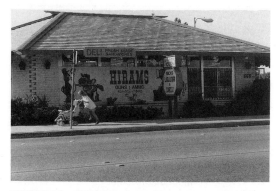

FIGURE 2-6. One-Stop Shopping: Fire-arm related homicides and drunk driving are major killers of adolescents and other Americans. *Photo courtesy of John Elder.*

who are already healthy and maintaining or even enhancing their state of well-being through community and individual approaches for healthy life style development. Health promotion targets include smoking cessation, reduction of alcohol and drug abuse, improved nutrition for diet and cancer prevention (especially reduction of excessive calorie, saturated fat, cholesterol, salt, and sugar consumption with relative increases in complex carbohydrate and fish, poultry, and legume consumption), exercise, and stress control. The implication of this section of the Surgeon General's Report is that health promotion *per se* requires active involvement of the individual and the community in health enhancement.

Prevention (now labeled preventive services) is more a matter for the health services sector,

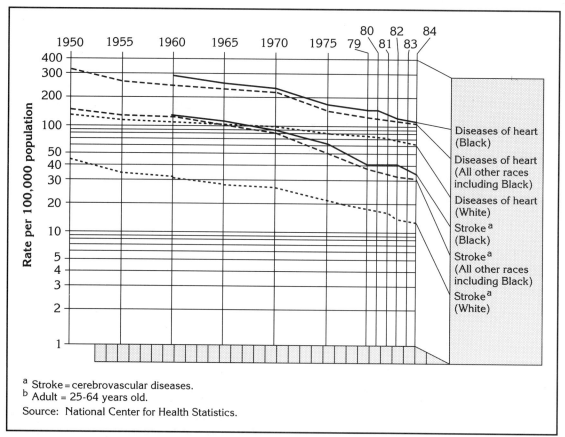

a Stroke = cerebrovascular diseases.
b Adult = 25-64 years old.
Source: National Center for Health Statistics.

FIGURE 2-7. Trends in death rates for diseases of heart and stroke[a] among adult[b] females, by race: selected years, 1950–1984. Reprinted by permission of Macro International Inc.

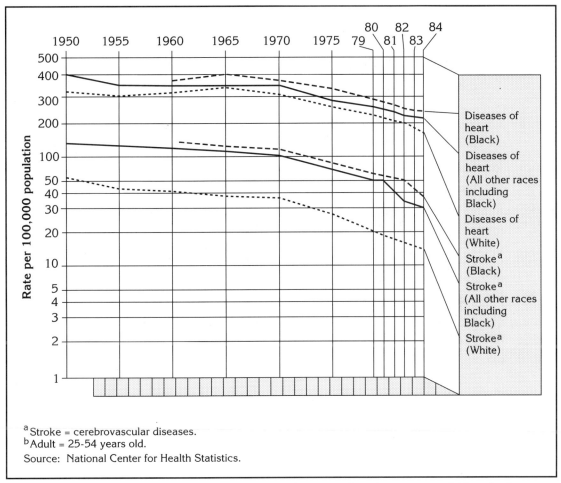

FIGURE 2–8. Trends in death rates for diseases of heart and stroke[a] among adult[b] males by race: selected years, 1950–1984. Reprinted by permission of Macro International Inc.

and thus connotes a relatively passive consumer. Five priority preventive services include maternal and infant care, HIV infection control, heart disease and stroke, cancer, and diabetes and other chronic disabling conditions. **The *Healthy People* approach to prevention, that of developing and tailoring pertinent screening, detection, diagnostic and treatment services to specific risk for specific individuals at various ages, emphasizes health services more than individual behavior change.**

Finally, **health protection emphasizes decreasing or eliminating health hazards in our physical environment. Toxic agent control, occupational safety and health, injury control, fluoridation of water supplies, and infectious agent control are advocated with the implication that additional government and organizational regulations would help to make our environment safer.** Again, minimal emphasis is placed on the consumer's participation in working toward this end (see chapter 22). Therefore, one could place the

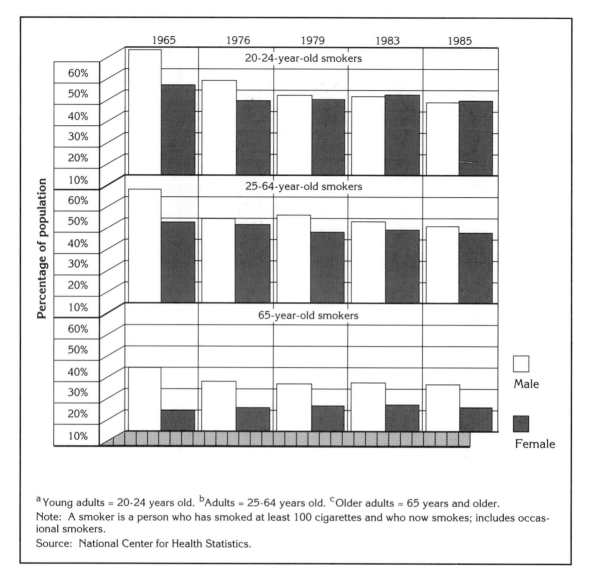

^aYoung adults = 20-24 years old. ^bAdults = 25-64 years old. ^cOlder adults = 65 years and older.

Note: A smoker is a person who has smoked at least 100 cigarettes and who now smokes; includes occasional smokers.

Source: National Center for Health Statistics.

FIGURE 2–9. Cigarette smoking among young adults,[a] adults,[b] and older adults,[c] by sex: 1965, 1976, 1979, 1983, and 1985. Reprinted by permission of Macro International Inc.

activities related to promotion, prevention, and protection on a continuum ranging from active consumer involvement to service provision to passive clients.

Table 2–2 presents the current priority areas within the three major categories of *Healthy People 2000*, as well as the fourth category related to data systems needed to monitor progress in these areas. In turn, these areas are categorized according to four "age related" targets: children,

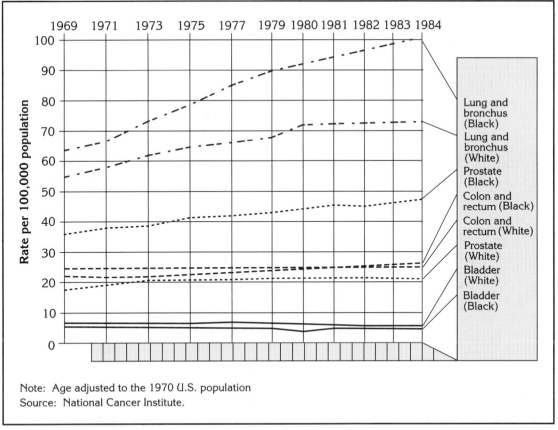

FIGURE 2-10. Age-adjusted cancer death rates for males, by site and race: selected years, 1969–1984. Reprinted by permission of Macro International Inc.

adolescents and young adults, adults, and older adults.

How appropriate is this classification system? Our position is that health behavior is relevant to *all* areas of health enhancement (promotion, prevention, and protection), although different types of health behaviors are appropriate for different domains. Generally, smoking cessation and exercise are health promotive behaviors which may be deemed "under the control" of specific consumers and communities.[6] However, just because preventive health services are provided by clinics and health agencies, individuals may still not practice appropriate family planning or "safer sex," nor is the simple provision of immunization services sufficient to ensure that everyone is immunized. Additional regulations may help strengthen health protection efforts, yet unsafe driving and work habits or a lack of enforcement of safety policies are still human behaviors needing modification in order to realize the potential of health protection measures. Moreover, we still lack regulations for banning tobacco advertising and even sales of certain tobacco products to minors. Citizen participation in passing bills to enact such laws or enforce existing statutes may be engendered through appropriate uses of incentive and community organizational strategies. Therefore, it is our position that while the type of health behavior change may vary from category

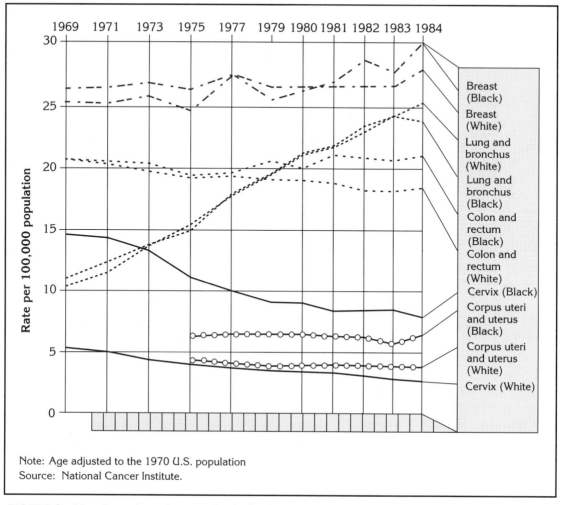

FIGURE 2–11.   Age-adjusted cancer deaths for females, by site and race: selected years, 1969–1984. Reprinted by permission of Macro International Inc.

to category, behavior change is the unifying theme which links all health enhancement activities together.

Criteria for Healthy People 2000's Objectives

Healthy People 2000 establishes specific goals for each of the twenty-two priority areas listed in Table 2–2. Objectives fall into one of three categories: those which aim at improving health status through the reduction of death, disease, and disability; those which aim for specific behavioral and other risk reduction and for increasing behaviors which improve health; and those which aim to increase the comprehensiveness, quality, and accessibility of preventive services and interventions. Among the specific criteria listed by *Healthy People 2000* for the development of these objectives are the following:

1. **Credibility:** Objectives should be both scientific and realistic.

TABLE 2-2
Priority Areas from *Healthy People 2000*

I. Health	II. Health Protection	III. Preventive Services	IV. Surveillance and Data Systems
1. Physical activity and fitness 2. Nutrition 3. Tobacco 4. Alcohol and other drugs 5. Family planning 6. Mental health and mental disorders 7. Violent and abusive behavior 8. Educational and community based programs	9. Unintentional injuries 10. Occupational safety and health 11. Environmental health 12. Food and drug safety 13. Oral health	14. Maternal and child health 15. Heart disease and stroke 16. Cancer 17. Diabetes and chronic disabling condition 18. HIV infection 19. Sexually transmitted diseases 20. Immunization 21. Clinical preventive services	22. Surveillance and data systems

2. **Public comprehension:** Objectives should be understandable and relevant to a broad audience, including individual citizens, planners, managers, and insurers.
3. **Balance:** Objectives should include both outcome and process measures, recommendations for achieving change, and standards for evaluating change.
4. **Measurability:** Objectives should be quantified.
5. **Continuity and compatibility:** Measures are linked to previously established objectives and those established by other agencies.

In the context of these criteria, *Healthy People 2000*[7] presents highly detailed objectives for health promotion and disease prevention, subcategorized by specific risk behaviors and disease conditions, age and ethnicity of target groups, and other dimensions. Let's review the representative objectives for the health promotion category, presented in Table 2-3.

In summary, health promotion objectives entail risk reduction, policy changes, and the provision of services and programs. Such services must meet the "5 As" criteria: they must be affordable, appropriate, acceptable, accessible, and adequate to meet the needs of the target population (see chapter 11). The overriding emphasis of this set of goals, however, is on specific behaviors of the population in terms of what actions should be increased and which decreased. Also, among these objectives are various preventive actions, which entail getting people to continue doing what they are doing, such as *not* taking drugs ("maintenance targets"). Finally, knowledge change to set the stage for this behavior change also receives attention among these health promotion objectives.

TABLE 2–3
Representative *Healthy People 2000* Health Promotion Objectives

Category	*Priority Area*	*Objectives for the Year 2000*
HEALTH PROMOTION	Physical Activity	"Increase moderate physical activity to at least 30% of people (a 36% increase)."
		"Reduce sedentary life styles to no more than 15% of people (a 38% decrease)."
		Among the other objectives: combining dietary and activity changes for overweight people; increasing physical activity and facilities in schools, worksites and communities; more emphasis by service providers on physical activity.
	Nutrition	"Reduce overweight to a prevalence of no more than 20% of people (a 23% decrease)."
		"Reduce dietary fat intake to an average of 30% of calories (a 17% decrease)."
		Among the other objectives: increase vegetable, fruit and grain consumption; increase calcium intake, breast feeding, and the availability of low fat foods; reduce sodium intake and iron deficiency; increase availability, identification, and promotion of healthy foods in schools, worksites, health services and restaurants.
	Tobacco	"Reduce cigarette smoking prevalence to no more than 15% of adults (a 48% decrease)."
		"Reduce initiation of smoking to no more than 15% by age 20 (a 50% decrease)."
		Among the other objectives: reduce deaths from lung cancer and chronic obstructive lung disease; smoking during pregnancy and smokeless tobacco use; increase policy implementation and enforcement in schools, worksites, and public places; enforce prohibition of sales to minors and restrict advertising targeting youth; promote cessation by primary care providers.
	Alcohol and Other Drugs	"Reduce alcohol-related motor vehicle crash deaths to no more than

Category	Priority Area	Objectives for the Year 2000
		8.5/100,000 people (age adjusted; a 12% decrease)." "Reduce alcohol use by school children age 12–17 to less than 13%; marijuana use by youth age 18–25 to less than 8%; and cocaine use by youth age 18–25 to less than 3%. (50% decreases)." Among the other objectives: increase average age of first use of addictive substances; reduce heavy drinking by young people and per capita alcohol consumption; increase awareness of effects of addictive substances; increase access to treatment programs; increase quality and enforcement of D.U.I. laws; increase access of workers to assistance for substance use problems and involvement of primary care providers in dealing with these problems; increase policies for reducing minors access to alcohol.
	Family Planning	"Reduce teenage pregnancies to no more than 50/100,000 girls age 17 and younger (a 30% decrease)." "Reduce unintended pregnancies to no more than 30% of pregnancies (a 46% decrease)." Among the other objectives: reduce sexual intercourse among teenagers and non-use of contraception among unmarried; increase effectiveness with which contraceptives are used and improve communication between adolescents and parents; increase availability of appropriate preconception counseling; increase referral rates to such counseling and other appropriate services; increase the availability of information on adoption for unmarried pregnant patients and reduce rates of infertility.
	Mental Health and Mental Disorders	"Reduce suicides to no more than 10.5/100,000 (a 10% decrease)." "Reduce adverse effects of stress to less than 35% of people (an 18% decrease)." Among the other objectives: Reduction of the prevalence of mental disorders; increase treatment and use of

Continued

TABLE 2-3—*Continued*

Category	*Priority Area*	*Objectives for the Year 2000*
		community support programs; increase attention to such problems by primary care providers, employers, and others.
	Violent and Abusive Behavior	"Reduce homicides to no more than 7.2/100,000 people (a 15% decrease)."
		"Reduce assault to no more than 10/100,000 people (a 10% decrease)."
		Among the other objectives: reducing weapon-injury related deaths; reducing child and spouse abuse; reducing rape; reducing weapon-carrying by adolescents; reducing inappropriate storage of weapons; improving emergency treatment, housing, and services for battered women, children, and older people; improving school programs for conflict resolution; and strengthening state-based efforts in violence prevention.
	Educational and Community-based programs	"Provide quality K–12 school health education in at least 75% of schools."
		"Provide employee health promotion activities in at least 85% of workplaces with 50 or more employees (a 31% increase)."
		Among the other objectives: increase reading levels and high school graduation rates; increase preschool programs for disadvantaged children; strengthen the public health system; increase accessibility of health promotion programs for older people; develop state-based strategies for health promotion; and have a stronger focus on the health promotion needs of minorities.

Table 2–4 presents the specific health protection objectives. The health protection objectives place some emphasis on target population behavior, but primarily focus on policy and technology developments for eventually improving the health status of the nation. Where health-related behavior is addressed directly, it is in the context of promoting the appropriate consumer use of technology. For example, installing smoke detectors, wearing motorcycle helmets or construction "hard hats," or using appropriate waste management all require an increase in specific human behaviors. Thus, educational, skills training, motivational, and marketing procedures apply to

TABLE 2–4
Representative *Healthy People 2000*
Health Protection Objectives

Category	Priority Area	Objectives for the Year 2000
HEALTH PROTECTION	Unintentional Injuries	"Reduce unintentional injury deaths to no more than 29.3/100,000 (a 15% decrease)."
		"Increase automobile safety restraint use to at least 85% of occupants (a 102% increase)."
		Among the other objectives: reduce deaths from motor vehicle crashes, falls, drownings, and residential fires; reduce hip fractures, poisonings, head and spinal cord injuries; increase the use of protective helmets; extend safety belt and motorcycle helmets laws; expand installation of fire detection and control systems; improve roadway design; involve schools and primary care providers in education.
	Occupational Safety and Health	"Reduce work-related injury deaths to 4/100,000 workers (a 33% decrease)."
		"Reduce work-related injuries to no more than 6/100 workers (a 22% decrease)."
		Among the other objectives: reduce cumulative trauma disorders, occupational skin disorders, and hepatitis-B infection among workers; increase use of occupant protection systems; reduce exposure to lead; implement state laws for identification and control of major work-related illnesses and injuries, and standards to prevent disease; increase the number of work sites with formal plans for worker health and safety; etc.
	Environmental Health	"Eliminate blood lead levels below 25UG/dL in children under age 5."
		"Increase protection from air pollutants so that at least 85% of people live in counties that meet EPA standards (a 71% increase)."

Continued

TABLE 2–4—*Continued*

Category	Priority Area	Objectives of the Year 2000
		"Increase protection from radon so that at least 40% of people live in homes which are tested by homeowners and found to be, or made, safe (a 700% increase)."
		Among the other objectives: reduce contamination of drinking water and surface water; reduce exposure to air, water, and soil-borne toxic agents; reduce solid waste contamination; eliminate risk from hazardous waste sites; improve household management of recyclable materials and toxic waste materials; and track environmental exposure and diseases through state-based systems.
	Food and Drug Safety	"Reduce salmonella infection outbreaks to fewer than 25 yearly (a 68% decrease)."
		Among the other objectives: reduce incidence of food-borne diseases; improve food handling techniques; improve pharmacy-based systems to alert customers to potential adverse drug effects; and increase reviews by primary care providers of patients' medications.
	Oral Health	"Reduce the prevalence of dental caries to no more than 35% of children by age 8 (a 34% decrease)."
		"Reduce edentulism to no more than 20% in people age 65 and older (a 44% decrease)."
		Among the other objectives: expand treatment of dental caries; reduce periodontal disease and tooth loss; increase use of protective sealants on permanent teeth in children; improve parental practices for prevention of tooth decay related to baby bottle feeding; and increase and improve oral health screenings.

health "protection" just as they do to "promotion." But without political mobilization and community organization, voter, legislator, and governmental actions would probably be inadequate.

Preventive services (Table 2–5) target the procedures and the service structure of primary health care services. Specific health issues addressed in this category include maternal and child health, HIV infection, and the control of cardiovascular disease. Note again, however, the specific behavior change targets: the actions of the mother which protect (or harm) her unborn fetus or infant, the sexually mature individual or intravenous drug user who fails to take precautions against HIV infection, and the providers and consumers of screening and medical regimens for high blood pressure control. With these em-

phases, both preventive services and protection overlap with promotion. And both entail carefully planned, implemented, and evaluated behavior change strategies, such as those outlined in the **ONPRIME** model.

Healthy People 2000 goes on to discuss the "shared responsibilities" we all have in achieving these very ambitious and multitudinous objectives. This comprises a mix of personal and family responsibility, the involvement of health professional, media and government programs at all levels, and community efforts (including those undertaken by local health officials; voluntary organizations; business, community, and labor leaders; and schools and churches). These objectives are applicable to the bulk of the populations of the developed world (e.g., Japan, United States, Can-

TABLE 2–5
Representative *Healthy People 2000*
Preventive Services Objectives

Category	*Priority Area*	*Objectives for the Year 2000*
PREVENTIVE SERVICES	Maternal and Infant Health	"Reduce infant mortality to no more than 7 deaths to 1000 births (a 31% decrease)." "Reduce low birth weight to no more than 5% of live births (a 28% decrease)." "Increase the first trimester of prenatal care to at least 90% of live births (an 18% increase)." Among the other objectives: reduce rates of fetal death, maternal mortality, and fetal alcohol syndrome; increase abstinence from tobacco and other drugs during pregnancy; increase the proportion of mothers who gain an adequate amount of weight during pregnancy; increase the number who breast feed their babies; reduce severe complications of pregnancy and cesarean delivery rates; increase the availability of pre-conception care and counseling as well as genetic services and counseling; improve the management of high-risk cases and increase the proportion of babies who receive recommended primary care services.

Continued

TABLE 2-5—*Continued*

Category	Priority Area	Objective for Year 2000
	Heart Disease and Stroke	"Reduce coronary heart disease deaths to no more than 100/100,000 people (a 26% decrease)."
		"Reduce stroke deaths to no more than 20/100,000 people (a 34% decrease)."
		"Increase control of high blood pressure to at least 50% of people with high blood pressure (a 100% increase)."
		"Reduce blood cholesterol to an average of no more than 200mg/dcl (a 6% decrease)."
		Among the other objectives: appropriate management of people with high blood cholesterol and high blood pressure; reduce dietary fat intake and overweight and increase physical activity; reduce tobacco use; increase number of adults who have been screened for high blood pressure and high cholesterol; use worksites for detection and follow-up programs; and improve adherence to recommended protocols for primary care providers and laboratories involved in cholesterol testing and management.
	Cancer	"Reverse the rise in cancer deaths to no more than 130/100,000 people."
		"Increase clinical breast exams and mammography to at least 60% of women age 50 and older (a 140% increase)."
		"Increase PAP tests every 1–3 years to at least 85% of women age 18 and older (a 13% increase)."
		"Increase fecal occult blood testing every 1–2 years to at least 50% of people age 50 and older (an 85% increase)."
		Among the other objectives: reduce dietary fat intake; increase consumption of vegetables, fruits, and grain products; reduce tobacco use; decrease sun exposure; increase counseling by primary care providers on these risk factors and offer screening procedures; and improve the quality of PAP test and mammograms.
	Diabetes and Chronic Disabling Conditions	"Reduce disability from chronic conditions to no more than 8% of people (a 15% decrease)."
		"Reduce diabetes-related deaths to no more than 34/100,000 (an 11% decrease)."
		Among the other objectives: reduce complications of diabetes and disability

Category	Priority Area	Objectives for the Year 2000
		from asthma, chronic back conditions, osteoporosis, hearing and vision impairment and mental retardation; increase physical activity; reduce overweight; improve early diagnosis and referral for disabling conditions; improve community and self help resources from chronic and disabling conditions; and improve employee policies related to people with disability needs.
	HIV Infection	"Confine HIV infection to no more than 800/100,000 people."
		Among the other objectives: reduce sexual intercourse among adolescents; increase use of condoms among unmarried people; increase access to treatment programs for I.V. drug abusers; expand testing and counseling for people at risk for HIV infection; increase school and college education about HIV infection; and extend regulations to protect workers at risk for occupational transmission of HIV.
	Sexually Transmitted Diseases	"Reduce gonorrhea infections to no more than 225/100,000 (a 25% decrease)."
		"Reduce syphilis infections to no more than 10/100,000 people (a 45% decrease)."
		Among the other objectives: reduce chlamydia trachomatous, genital herpes and warts, and hepatitis-B; reduce incidence of pelvic inflammatory disease; increase use of condoms among sexually active unmarried people; increase availability of STD related services and education, including middle and secondary school education.
	Immunization and Infectious Diseases	"Eliminate measles."
		"Reduce epidemic-related pneumonia and influenza deaths to no more than 7.3/100,000 people age 65 and older (a 20% decrease)."
		"Increase childhood immunization levels to at least 90% of two year olds (a 20% increase)."
		Among the other objectives: eliminate diphtheria, tetanus, polio, and rubella; reduce viral hepatitis, tuberculosis, bacterial meningitis, diarrhea among children at licensed care centers, and middle ear infections; increase

Continued

TABLE 2–5—*Continued*

Category	*Priority Area*	*Objectives for the Year 2000*
		immunization levels of pneumococcal pneumonia and hepatitis-B; expand immunization laws for schools, preschools, and child care settings; eliminate financial barriers to immunizations; fully involve primary care providers in meeting immunizations needs of the patients; expand laboratory capabilities for rapid diagnosis of influenza.
	Clinical Preventive Services	"Eliminate financial barriers to clinical preventive services." Among the other objectives: increase proportion of people with specific source of ongoing care; increase primary care providers' delivery of recommended preventive services; increase number of people receiving clinical preventive services; increase delivery of preventive services among public funded providers; increase representation of minorities among primary care providers.
SURVEILLANCE AND DATA SYSTEMS	(Surveillance and data systems)	"Develop and implement common health status indicators for use by federal/state/local health agencies." Among other objectives: create data sources to track progress on previously described objectives; expand state-based activity to track progress of population; improve data for African-Americans, Hispanics, Indians and Alaska Natives, Asian-Americans, and people with disabilities; improve information transfer capabilities among various agencies; and increase speed of processing of survey and surveillance data.

ada, Western Europe). Many of the recommendations (especially for infants and children) overlap with those established for underdeveloped countries, as well.

THE PICTURE IN UNDERDEVELOPED COUNTRIES

Shifting our focus from the U.S. and other Western nations to the underdeveloped nations in Africa, Asia, and Latin America, we observe a much different pattern of health, illness, and mortality. Overall, half of all deaths in Africa are among children under the age of five. Children born in many countries of Africa and Southern Asia are twenty times more likely to die before their fifth birthday than are children born in the U.S. Infectious disease, parasitic diseases, malnutrition, and wasteful fertility, in the context of poverty and inequitable resource distribution, guarantee a continuance of these patterns in the foreseeable future in spite of ambitious goals set by the World Health Organization and governments of the underdeveloped countries (see Figure 2–12).

Because of these high infant and child mortality figures, poverty, and low levels of education, the fertility of women in developing countries is al-

most twice that of women in developed countries (see Figure 2–13). Relatedly, the percentage of total populations represented by children under five is twice or more greater in certain African and Asian countries as it is in various developed countries (see Figure 2–14).

Nearly 16,000,000 infants and young children will die in underdeveloped countries in the coming

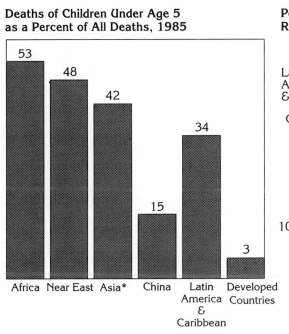

Deaths of Children Under Age 5 as a Percent of All Deaths, 1985

- Africa: 53
- Near East: 48
- Asia*: 42
- China: 15
- Latin America & Caribbean: 34
- Developed Countries: 3

The 11.9 percent of world's population under age 5 contributed almost one-third of all deaths.

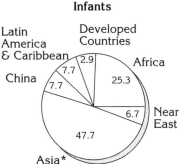

Percent Deaths Occurring In Each Region, 1985

Infants

- Developed Countries: 2.9
- Africa: 25.3
- Near East: 6.7
- Asia*: 47.7
- China: 7.7
- Latin America & Caribbean: 7.7

10 million infants died during 1985

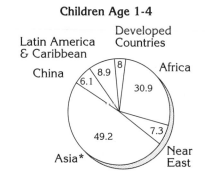

Children Age 1-4

- Developed Countries: 8
- Africa: 30.9
- Near East: 7.3
- Asia*: 49.2
- China: 6.1
- Latin America & Caribbean: 8.9

5 million children age 1-4 died during 1985

Mortality during the first year of life exceeds mortality during ages 1-4. Globally, there are approximately 2 infant deaths for each death of a 1-4-year-old. Higher levels of overall mortality are associated with proportionately higher **levels of child mortality. In Africa, the** ratio of infant to child deaths is 1.6 to 1; in developed countries the ratio is 6.6 to 1.

FIGURE 2–12.   Child mortality and numbers of deaths by region. Reprinted by permission of Macro International Inc.

Percent of World Births Occurring in Each Region

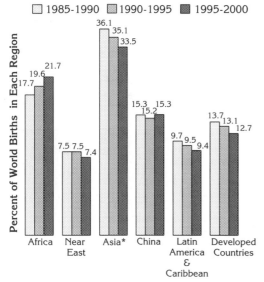

Legend: ☐ 1985-1990 ▨ 1990-1995 ■ 1995-2000

Y-axis: Percent of World Births in Each Region

- Africa: 17.7, 19.6, 21.7
- Near East: 7.5, 7.5, 7.4
- Asia*: 36.1, 35.1, 33.5
- China: 15.3, 15.2, 15.3
- Latin America & Caribbean: 9.7, 9.5, 9.4
- Developed Countries: 13.7, 13.1, 12.7

Including China, more than 50 percent of the world's children are projected to be born in Asia between 1985 and 2000. Due to an increasing number of women of childbearing age and high birth rates, the percentage of the world's children born in Africa is expected to increase rapidly.

Average Number of Children Women Bear

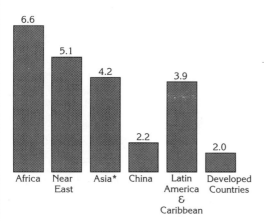

- Africa: 6.6
- Near East: 5.1
- Asia*: 4.2
- China: 2.2
- Latin America & Caribbean: 3.9
- Developed Countries: 2.0

Fertility of women in developing countries is almost twice that of women in developing countries. In some African countries women bear enough children to replace their generation fourfold, while in some European countries and the United States, fertility is below replacement level.

*Excluding China

Source: United Nations

(Data are included in Table 6 of Appendix 1)

Number of Births During 1985-2000
(in thousands)

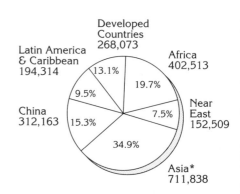

- Developed Countries 268,073 — 13.1%
- Latin America & Caribbean 194,314 — 9.5%
- China 312,163 — 15.3%
- Africa 402,513 — 19.7%
- Near East 152,509 — 7.5%
- Asia* 711,838 — 34.9%

More than 2 billion children are projected to be born in the world between 1985 and 2000. Some 87 percent, or 1.8 billion, will be born in developing countries.

Number of Women of Reproductive Age: 1985-2000 (in millions)

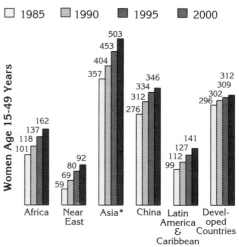

Legend: ☐ 1985 ▨ 1990 ■ 1995 ■ 2000

Y-axis: Women Age 15-49 Years

- Africa: 101, 118, 137, 162
- Near East: 59, 69, 80, 92
- Asia*: 357, 404, 453, 503
- China: 276, 312, 334, 346
- Latin America & Caribbean: 99, 112, 127, 141
- Developed Countries: 296, 302, 309, 312

The number of women of reproductive age will increase through the end of the century, reflecting momentum from higher birth rates in the past. As a result, the total number of births occurring each year is projected to grow, despite overall declines in fertility taking place in all regions of the world.

Demographic Data for Development Project

FIGURE 2–13.   Births by region. Reprinted by permission of Macro International Inc.

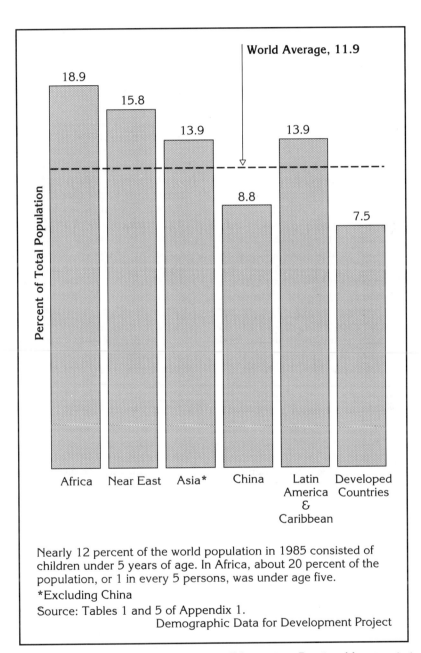

Nearly 12 percent of the world population in 1985 consisted of children under 5 years of age. In Africa, about 20 percent of the population, or 1 in every 5 persons, was under age five.
*Excluding China
Source: Tables 1 and 5 of Appendix 1.
Demographic Data for Development Project

FIGURE 2–14.   Percent of total population under age 5 by region. Reprinted by permission of Macro International Inc.

year. In the next sixty seconds, nearly thirty tragic deaths will occur in this age group. This has almost nothing to do with the genetic inheritance or behavior of the children. However, the great majority of these deaths are preventable through the control of diarrhea, acute respiratory infections, and malaria as well as the widespread use of appropriate vaccines and the prevention of malnutrition and excess fertility. As will be discussed later, however, all of these preventable causes of illness and death are imbedded in deeper structural factors, such as poverty and the low status of women (see chapter 21).

Diarrheal Disease

Diarrhea is a symptom of a large number of intestinal diseases, including infections by virus, bacteria, a parasite, or a combination of these. Although nearly all children get diarrhea, the frequency and duration of diarrhea episodes vary dramatically from region to region (see Figure 2–15). **Diarrheal disease is the leading cause of infant and child death in the world, as five million children die from diarrhea-related problems every year.** Dehydration is generally the direct cause of diarrhea-related mortality. The risk of mortality, however, increases during weaning, as the child is less protected from contaminated food and water and has less of an immunological response than during the breast feeding period. Diarrhea and malnutrition are generally very closely interrelated, as diarrhea causes malnutrition due to the lack of ability to absorb food and a loss of appetite, while malnutrition, prior to diarrhea, lowers the child's overall resistance.

Specific health promotion measures for promoting child survival strategies in the underdeveloped world are described in chapter 21. Oral rehydration therapy (providing a solution of sugar, salt, and water with regular feeding during the diarrheal episode) is advocated by the World Health Organization and other international health agencies as being the best single approach to reducing mortality caused by dehydration and malnutrition following a diarrheal episode. Cleaning the water and food supply, handwashing, breast feeding, and immunizing will also promote health through the primary prevention of diarrhea.

Vaccine-Preventable Diseases

The World Health Organization's Expanded Program on Immunization (EPI) seeks to establish universal protection against diphtheria, pertussis, tetanus (DPT), polio, and tuberculosis. This effort is based on two facts: these are among the most common and deadly diseases killing infants and young children, and the vaccines against these diseases are inexpensive and relatively easy to use. However, less than 20 percent of total possible deaths potentially prevented by these vaccines are, in fact, prevented.

The tremendous implication of these diseases for child survival stems from four principal factors: levels of immunization are very low, these diseases attack especially young children, they are especially deadly during cases of malnutrition, and there is little health care available to combat the effects of these diseases. In spite of these contributing factors, vaccination alone can be extremely effective in preventing diseases among young populations. However, overall coverage remains low, especially in Africa, the Near East, and Asia (see Figure 2–17). The Expanded Program on Immunization (EPI) effort faces other significant challenges. First, the target diseases strike primarily in infancy; therefore, immunization must occur before the child is one year old. However, vaccinations cannot be given too early as the infant is not strong enough to neutralize the vaccine immediately after birth. Therefore, the window of opportunity for vaccination is open a relatively short period of time. Additionally, the "cold chain" for most vaccines must be maintained if the vaccines are to retain their effectiveness. Therefore, house-to-house coverage is made difficult or impossible as refrigeration is generally not very mobile. Finally, the DPT and polio vaccines must be given at three different times. Uneducated parents often fail to return for the second and third vaccinations and thereby are leaving their children unprotected.

Acute Respiratory Infections (ARI)

Acute respiratory infections as a group are the second leading threat (behind diarrhea) to child survival in the world. They are caused by a wide

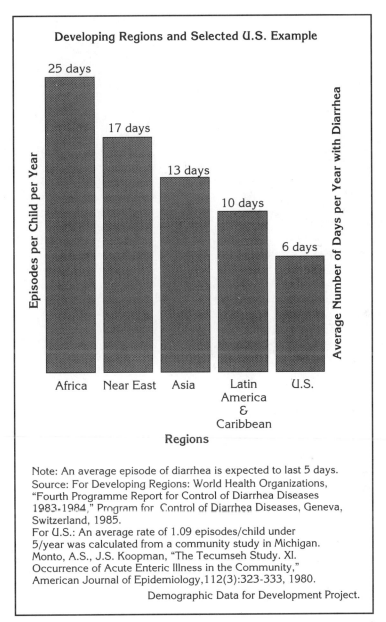

FIGURE 2–15. Estimated annual episodes of childhood diarrhea and average number of days of diarrheal illness. Reprinted by permission of Macro International Inc.

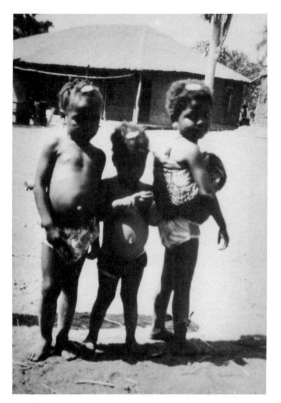
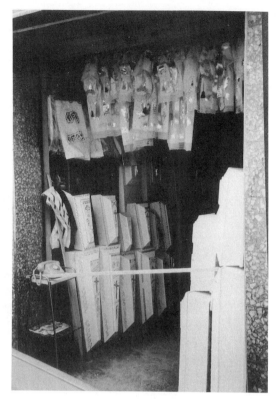

FIGURE 2–16.   Children such as these in Sierra Leone are naturally healthy and full of vitality, given appropriate nutrition and protection. But the preponderance of child-sized coffins and shrouds in this store in Bolivia grimly attest to the high rate of infant mortality in under-developed countries. *Photos courtesy of Karen Keay and John Elder.*

variety of disease agents, including various bacterial and viral sources. These infections are generally classified as infections of either the upper or lower respiratory tract and are typically spread through the air. Like diarrhea and vaccine preventable diseases, ARI mortality is closely related to nutritional status. Vitamin A deficiency and crowded living conditions also contribute greatly to the spread of ARI.

ARI-related health promotion efforts generally focus on getting mothers to recognize ARI as it develops and to respond with ensuring that the child is warm and continues to get plenty of fluids and regular feeding during the ARI episode. Second, the mother is encouraged to react quickly to

more severe forms of ARI and seek medical care from the closest available clinic, as the child will likely need immediate attention.

Malaria

Malaria threatens the health of populations in tropical areas of the world, such as equatorial South America, Africa, Southern Asia, and the Southwest Pacific. It is spread through the interaction of the human and the mosquito, with infants and young children at greatest risk of severe infection. Although healthy adults can develop immunity to malaria, it is likely to cause loss of

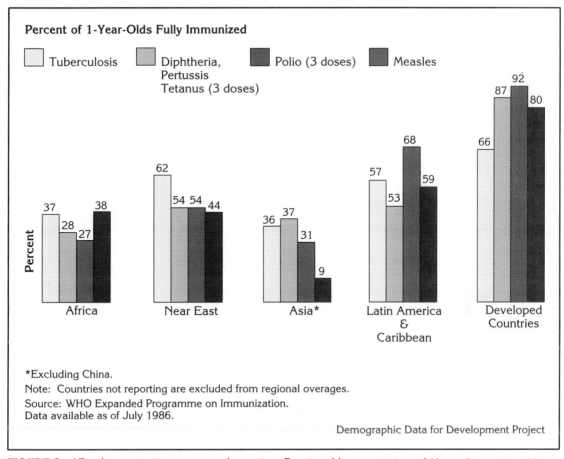

Percent of 1-Year-Olds Fully Immunized

☐ Tuberculosis ▨ Diphtheria, Pertussis Tetanus (3 doses) ■ Polio (3 doses) ◼ Measles

*Excluding China.
Note: Countries not reporting are excluded from regional overages.
Source: WHO Expanded Programme on Immunization.
Data available as of July 1986.

Demographic Data for Development Project

FIGURE 2 – 17.   Immunization coverage by region. Reprinted by permission of Macro International Inc.

healthy days and thereby diminish one's ability to work or lead a productive life. In areas where it is endemic, it presents a significant threat to child survival.

Malaria control activities consist of "vector control" (i.e., eliminating mosquitos, such as by draining areas with stagnant water and spraying mosquito-infested areas with insecticides), and other efforts. A variety of antimalarial drugs are available for treatment and prevention programs. Despite these advances, it is doubtful malaria will be eradicated in the foreseeable future. Indeed, the number of cases reported in Latin America and the Caribbean have increased substantially in the past fifteen years, whereas data from Africa show malaria to be at least as big a threat as it was over a decade ago.

Malnutrition

Malnutrition represents a common link for most of the problems threatening child survival in developing countries. An absence of adequate proteins, calories, or other nutrients increase the likelihood of children dying following sickness. While Western populations are threatened by consuming too much fat, calories, sodium, or other substances, the opposite is true in underdeveloped countries.

A lack of proteins, calories, or micro-nutrients can contribute to malnutrition. Malnutrition in children occurs when the weight of the child is below 80 percent of the median weight for that child's age group. Whereas Vitamin A, iron, and iodine deficiencies may not contribute directly to mortality as quickly as do a lack of proteins and calories, severe problems and eventual life-threatening illnesses can result from these types of malnutrition, as well.

The vicious cycle of malnutrition begins before the child is even born. Inadequate or improper nutrition on the part of the pregnant mother can result in low birth weight, which in turn makes malnutrition and subsequent illnesses much more likely. Inappropriate or inadequate breast feeding and supplementation as the child gets older can also contribute to malnutrition, as does abrupt or inappropriately supplemented weaning.

Improved health and nutrition during pregnancy, breast feeding with appropriate weaning, feeding the child during the previously described

illnesses, and growth monitoring with nutritional supplementation and corrective action as necessary may all contribute to alleviating the malnutrition cycle. While malnutrition is most prevalent in Asia and Africa (see Figure 2–18), it is only partly related to the availability of appropriate foodstuffs.

In the West, we tend to think of malnutrition as equivalent to starvation and may respond sporadically to appeals, such as U.S. for Africa's attempt to supply food to drought-stricken Ethiopia and more recent U.N. attempts to assist Somalia. However, simply increasing the availability of nutritional substances is not sufficient to counteract malnutrition. Malnutrition may occur in areas where foodstuffs are ample or potentially available

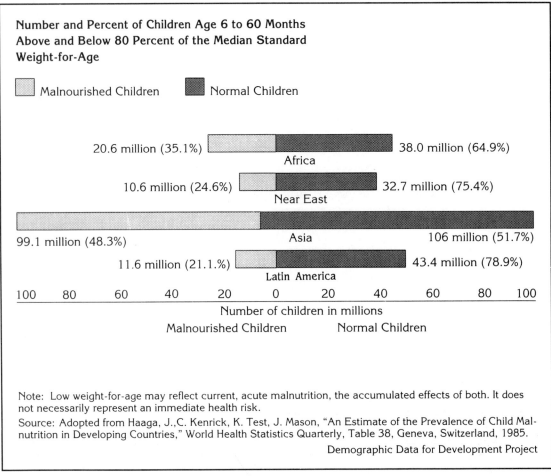

Number and Percent of Children Age 6 to 60 Months Above and Below 80 Percent of the Median Standard Weight-for-Age

☐ Malnourished Children   ■ Normal Children

20.6 million (35.1%) — Africa — 38.0 million (64.9%)

10.6 million (24.6%) — Near East — 32.7 million (75.4%)

99.1 million (48.3%) — Asia — 106 million (51.7%)

11.6 million (21.1.%) — Latin America — 43.4 million (78.9%)

100   80   60   40   20   0   20   40   60   80   100
Number of children in millions
Malnourished Children   Normal Children

Note: Low weight-for-age may reflect current, acute malnutrition, the accumulated effects of both. It does not necessarily represent an immediate health risk.

Source: Adopted from Haaga, J.,C. Kenrick, K. Test, J. Mason, "An Estimate of the Prevalence of Child Malnutrition in Developing Countries," World Health Statistics Quarterly, Table 38, Geneva, Switzerland, 1985.

Demographic Data for Development Project

FIGURE 2–18.   Estimates of childhood malnutrition in developing regions, 1980. Reprinted by permission of Macro International Inc.

due to inadequate distribution of income or endemic diseases which inhibit nutritional uptake.

Excessive Fertility

Excessive fertility can be defined as excesses in pregnancy and birth rates, which in turn contribute to malnutrition, high rates of miscarriages and abortions, maternal illness, death, and infant and child morbidity and mortality. Children who are born at least two years apart from their nearest sibling are much less likely to die before the age of five than are children who follow closely the birth of a sibling or who are followed by the birth of another child shortly thereafter. Teenagers and older women are also much more likely to give birth to unhealthy children than are women aged twenty through thirty-nine.

Family planning and child spacing can save as many as 2,000,000 lives per year. However, fertility behavior is deeply imbedded in the cultural patterns of a society, and major changes in women's work status and education and attitudes of men must occur before widespread use of contraceptives can take place. Moreover, women who expect a significant number of their children to die are negatively reinforced for having a large number of children. This vicious cycle is very difficult to break without first making child survival a reality (and thereby temporarily *increasing* the overall fertility of a population). However, as will be seen in chapter 21, significant changes in wasteful fertility are possible and have been realized in various regions of the world.

General Factors

It is impossible to adequately address the major threats to child survival and maternal health without improving the overall education and literacy levels; and ensuring that health services are available and accessible, that per capita income and income distribution are adequate and equitable; and that food, clean water, and appropriate sanitation facilities are available to all segments of the population. Additionally, individuals who do manage to survive these incredible threats to their health and live to middle age face all of the same chronic disease risks discussed earlier. For instance, the environments of developing and underdeveloped countries are quickly having their resources depleted while being polluted by more and more toxic fertilizers, pesticides, and other

materials. The worldwide use of cigarettes is being promoted very effectively by American, British, and other tobacco companies who perhaps see "the writing on the wall" for their markets in Western countries. Occupational hazards for workers in underdeveloped countries are even greater than those in developed countries, where at least some levels of protection exist. In summary, the outlook in underdeveloped countries is, perhaps, much more complicated than the term "child survival" may imply. But maternal and child health has been chosen as the place to start.

THE ALMA ATA CONFERENCE

In 1978, the World Health Organization and the United Nations Children's Fund sponsored the International Conference on Primary Health Care in Alma Ata, the capital of Kazakhstan. Experts from both developed and underdeveloped countries throughout the world participated in the drafting of a declaration addressed to the world community for the purposes of protecting and promoting the health of the world's population. This ten-part declaration, which in describing "health care" also defines health, is summarized below:

I. Health is a state of complete physical, mental, and social well-being and not merely the absence of disease or infirmity. Health is a fundamental human right and constitutes a worldwide goal of the utmost importance. A wide variety of social and economic sectors as well as the health sector must contribute to the attainment of health.

II. The existing gross inequality in the health status of people, both between populations of developed and developing countries as well as within countries, is politically, socially, and economically unacceptable.

III. Economic and social development is of basic importance to the full attainment of health for all.

IV. People have the right and duty to participate individually and collectively in planning and implementing their health care.

V. Governments have responsibility for the health of their people.

VI. Primary health care, based on practical sound and acceptable methods, should be universally accessible to individuals and families.

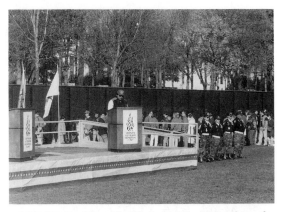

FIGURE 2–19. Health is much more than the absence of disease or infirmity. Standing before the Vietnam War Memorial in Washington, D.C., this ex-Marine reads the names of a few of the more than 58,000 Americans killed in Vietnam. *Photo courtesy of John Elder.*

VII. Primary health care (a) reflects and evolves from the economic conditions and social-cultural and political characteristics of the country; (b) addresses main health problems in the community and provides promotive, preventive, curative, and rehabilitative services; (c) includes education, promotion of proper nutrition, safe water and sanitation, maternal and child health care, immunizations, control of diseases and appropriate treatment of disease and injury; (d) involves all related sectors of national community development; (e) requires and promotes maximum community and individual self-reliance; (f) should be sustained by mutually supportive referral systems; and (g) relies on all levels of health workers working as a team.

VIII. All governments should formulate national policies, strategies, and plans of action to launch and sustain primary health care.

IX. All countries should cooperate in the spirit of partnership to insure primary health care for all people.

X. Health for all by the year 2000 can be attained through a fuller and better use of the world's resources, including those which are now devoted largely to military arms and conflicts.

In the fifteen years following this declaration, the world changed dramatically. The Iron Curtain fell. Alma Ata is now the capital of an independent nation, not just a city in the Soviet Union. Nevertheless, the elements of the Alma Ata declaration continue to ring true. The authors of this book support the Alma Ata declaration and the manner in which health is defined therein. Health, indeed, is not simply the absence of disease, but a more general physical and mental condition of well-being in which individuals and their social groups actively work to improve their condition. Economic and political inequality can contribute greatly to health problems and may be considered health problems in and of themselves. Health promotion involves far more than changing the behavior of a few primary care personnel or other change agents. Indeed, health promotion efforts are incomplete and may well be ineffective without full involvement of mayors and city council members, employers and union representatives, teachers and church officials, food retailers and policemen, and all other key and representative individuals in a community who can contribute to the planning, implementation, and maintenance of health promotion programs. Specific techniques for organizing such efforts are described in more detail in chapter 4. At this point, let it suffice to say that a comprehensive definition of health should include elements of social equality and involvement. This assertion is applicable to the health of peoples from all parts of the world.

Community Health Workers

If health is as we have defined above, how do we define our roles in its promotion? Whether we are educators, physicians, nutritionists, social workers, psychologists, or nurses, our roots are closely associated with community health work, defined in the Alma Ata framework as follows:

> Community health workers come from the community and are trained to work in it, in close relationship with the health care system. . . . Their functions have been shaped by the . . . eight essential components of primary health care. . . . Community health workers are in a unique position because they have a role both in the community and within the health care system. They make a bridge between one and the other. In the community they help to identify problems, and people at risk or in need. They involve the community in planning how to deal

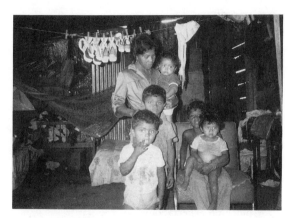

FIGURE 2–20. Severe poverty and wretched living conditions are major risk factors for disease and early death regardless of individual health behavior and preventive actions. *Photo courtesy of John Elder.*

with its own problems, and they help the community to be in touch with the health services.[8]

We now proceed to examine how we as community health workers view health-related behavior.

SUMMARY

Deaths from heart disease, stroke, and injuries continue to decline in the U.S., while progress on other fronts has been realized, as well. Nevertheless, the U.S. is slipping in health status compared to other industrialized nations. *Healthy People 2000* establishes health promotion, prevention, and protection goals for the current decade which are designed to increase America's life span, reduce health disparities among socioeconomic groups, and increase access to preventive services.

In underdeveloped countries, infants, children, and women suffer from illnesses and premature death. The major killers there are malnutrition, vaccine-preventable diseases, and excessive fertility. The Alma Ata Declaration holds health to be a fundamental right for all of the Earth's citizens.

Indices of health in the developed and underdeveloped world alike are directly related to two factors: the disadvantaged segments of the population suffer more than the advantaged, and all

aspects of health and health care have critical behavioral components. The next chapter establishes the definitions and critical dimensions of behavior, the other cornerstone of health promotion.

ADDITIONAL READINGS

R. Kaplan, J. Sallis, Jr., & T. Patterson. (1993). *Health and Human Behavior.* New York: McGraw-Hill, Inc.

U.S. Department of Health and Human Services. (1991). *Healthy People 2000.* Washington, D.C.: U.S. Government Printing Office.

EXERCISE

Self-Change Project. Select a personal health-related problem or behavior which you would like to change, and think about how you would measure it.

ENDNOTES

1. U.S. Department of Health, Education and Welfare, Public Health Service. (1979). *Healthy people: The Surgeon General's Report on Health Promotion and Disease Prevention.* Washington, D.C.: U.S. Government Printing Office, Foreword.

2. National Center for Health Statistics. (1989). *Health, United States, 1989 and Prevention Profile.* Atlanta, GA: Centers for Disease Control, National Center for Health Statistics.

3. U.S. Department of Health and Human Services. (1991). *Healthy People 2000.* Washington, D.C.: U.S. Government Printing Office, p. 5.

4. World Health Organization. (1988). *Education for Health.* Geneva: WHO, p. 5.

5. Demographic Data for Development Project. (1987). *Child Survival: Risks and the Road to Health.* Columbia, MD: Institute for Resource Development/Westinghouse.

6. Even these behavioral factors are strongly influenced by the environment, however. When the tobacco industry bombards inner cities with ads and streets are too unsafe to jog on for example, health behavior is less likely.

7. *Healthy People 2000*, pp. 70–79.

8. World Health Organization, p. 195.

Chapter 3

Dimensions of Behavior

OBJECTIVES

By the end of this chapter, the reader should be able to:

1. Define the following terms:
   - ABC recording
   - behavior
   - behavioral asset
   - binary recording
   - checklist
   - duration recording
   - frequency recording
   - operational definition
   - outcome expectations
   - permanent product recording
   - rate of behavior
   - reliability
   - self-monitoring
   - self-efficacy
2. Given a list of health-related terms, operationalize these terms with behavioral precision.
3. Construct a graph and graph behavioral data.
4. Describe and give examples of the uses of five types of direct observation.
5. Given a health-related problem, design observational instruments for assessment of this problem and its related behaviors.
6. Describe the similarities and differences among the main theories of health behavior.

THEORIES OF HEALTH BEHAVIOR AND HEALTH PROMOTION

In placing the technology of behavior modification and the theory of "behaviorism" among the various other behavioral and social sciences, it is apparent that there are many similarities between our approach and other theoretical systems such as the Health Belief Model,[1] the Theory of Reasoned Action,[2] Communications/Persuasion Model,[3] Social Learning Theory,[4] and Field Theory.[5]

Health Belief Model

The Health Belief Model was perhaps the first behaviorally-oriented conceptual system in health education. **It holds that health behavior is a function of both knowledge and motivation. Specifically, the Health Belief Model emphasizes the** role of perceptions of vulnerability to an illness and the potential effectiveness of treatment in decisions regarding whether to seek medical attention.[6]

Developers of the Health Belief Model, such as Becker[7] and Rosenstock[8] assert that health-related behavior is determined by whether individuals: (a) perceive themselves to be susceptible to a particular health problem; (b) see this problem as a serious one; (c) are convinced that treatment or prevention activities are effective yet not overly costly in terms of money or effort; and (d) receive a prompt or cue to take health action.[9] For example, a woman living in a rural area of a developing country may choose to take her child to a health center for Diphtheria-Pertussis-Tetanus (DPT) vaccinations if she (a) has seen neighbors' children die from one of these problems (increasing the perceived susceptibility her child has to these illnesses and her sense of their seriousness); (b) has seen other children remain healthy after receiving the vaccinations (perceived effectiveness); (c) does not have to walk too far for or pay too much for the services (personal and material costs); and (d) has heard over the radio that a vaccination campaign is underway (cue for action). These processes are summarized in the decision-tree in Figure 3–1.

The Health Belief Model was one of the first successful attempts to orient health professionals and researchers to the roles of cognitions and motivation in health-related behavior. It has served as the basis for many successful health promotion campaigns and anticipated many of the elements of the currently popular Communications/Persuasion Model and Social Learning Theory, two of the most important health behavior models today.

(2.) Theory of Reasoned Action

Fishbein and Ajzen[10] developed the **Theory of Reasoned Action, which emphasizes the role of personal volition in determining whether a behavior will occur.** In turn, this "behavioral intention" can best be predicted by the person's expectancies regarding the outcome of a behavior, other attitudes toward the behavior, and "normative" beliefs the person may have with respect to what "influentials" (e.g., peers) would do in this situation.

(3.) Communications-Persuasion Model

The **Communications/Persuasion Model, developed by William McGuire[11] and others, considers how mass media and other forms of public communication can be used to change attitudes and behaviors.** The effectiveness of a given communication effort will depend on various inputs and their characteristics, as well as the types of outputs one is interested in. Output factors reflect the specific sequence of changes the receiver of the communication is expected to go through, from the initial exposure to the communication to the long-term behavior change. Implicit in this sequence is the assumption that knowledge change is a prerequisite for attitude change, which in turn is a necessary precondition for decision-making and behavior change.

McGuire's input variables include the *source* of a message, the *message* itself, the *channel* by which it is sent, *receiver* characteristics, and *destination.* Source variables focus on characteristics of the individual perceived as sending the message. Sources vary in terms of the numbers of people sending the message, their credibility, their physical attractiveness, and characteristics they have in common with the receiver. *Messages* themselves vary in their specific appeal (e.g., negative vs. positive appeal), the information they present, what is included and what is omitted in the message, how the messages are organized, and how frequently they are repeated. *Channel* factors were initially thought to vary primarily between print (e.g., newspaper, pamphlets) and electronic (radio and television) media. Today, however, many social marketers would include face-to-face communication as one of the channel factors (chapter 10).

Receiver factors in some sense present a mirror image of source factors. Again, these include the demographic characteristics of the people at whom the messages are aimed, as well as their capacity to understand and assimilate the information, their "personality," and their life style. Finally, *destination* factors refer specifically to the target behaviors on which the communication is expected to impact. Tables 3–1 and 3–2 summarize McGuire's critical input and output variables.

The Communications/Persuasion Model has been one of the most influential models to date in public health promotion efforts in both developed

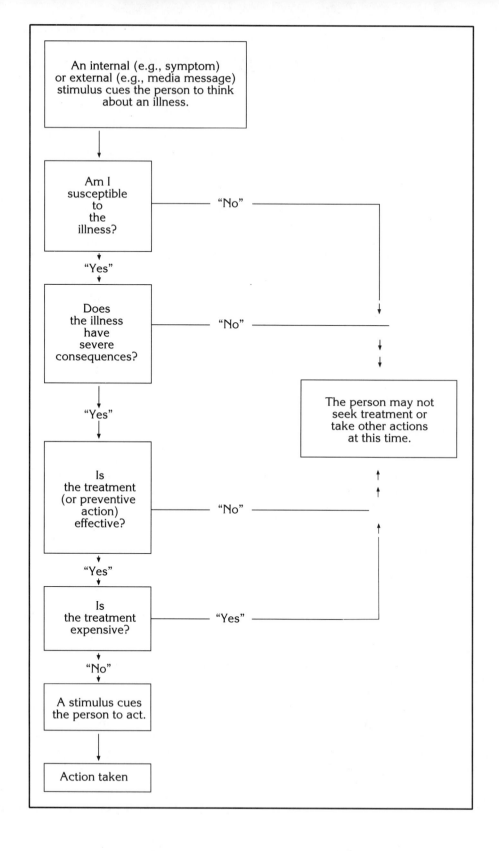

TABLE 3–1
Input Variables from the Communication/Persuasion Model
(adapted from McGuire, 1989)

Source	Message	Channel	Receiver	Target Behavior ("destination")
	1. Appeal	1. Modality (audio, visual, etc.)	1. Demographics	1. Short-/long-term
1. Number	2. Information	2. Direct vs. indirect/ interpersonal	2. Knowledge	2. Promotion vs. prevention policy
2. Unanimity	3. What's included/excluded	3. Context	3. Skills	
3. Demographics	4. Organization		4. Motivation	
4. Appeal	5. Repetition		5. Lifestyle	
5. Credibility				

and developing countries (e.g., the HEALTHCOM Project). Combined with Social Learning Theory, this model and its social marketing applications (detailed in chapter 10) has served as the foundation for such pioneering efforts in community health promotion as the Stanford Heart Disease Prevention Program. The Communications/Persuasion inputs are summarized in simplified form in Figure 3–2.

4 Social Learning Theory

Social Learning Theory stresses the interrelationships between people, their behavior, and their environment through a process labeled "reciprocal determinism." In other words, while the environment largely determines or causes behavior, the person in turn can act in ways to change the environment (see Figure 3–3). Social Learning Theory also holds that behavior depends on a person's "self-efficacy", their self-confidence, and outcome expectations (see Figure

TABLE 3–2
Output Variables from the Communication/ Persuasion Model
(Adapted from McGuire, 1989)

1. Exposure to the Communication
2. Attention
3. Developing interest and attraction
4. Understanding/Learning from the Communication
5. Skill Acquisition
6. Attitude change: "Yielding"
7. Remembering the message and Attitude toward it
8. Retrieval of information
9. Deciding what to do
10. Acting in accord with decision
11. Being reinforced for behavior
12. Behavioral "consolidation"

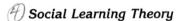

FIGURE 3–1.   Health belief model processes

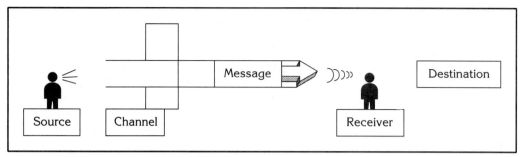

FIGURE 3-2.   Communications/Persuasion input variables

3-4). For example, a sixty-year-old man who does not have much confidence in his ability to master his own destiny (low self-efficacy), who has smoked for thirty years, thereby leading him to expect he would suffer severe withdrawal (negative outcome expectations) and would not live much longer (no positive outcome expectations) if he quit smoking, would be unlikely to try to quit. Conversely, a thirty-two-year-old woman who, after having been trained to do so, became very confident in her ability (self-efficacy) to detect a lump in her breast through regular breast self-examination (BSE) and was convinced of the potential afforded by BSE for preventing mortality from breast cancer (positive outcome expectation) would be likely to perform regular BSE.

Field Theory

Kurt Lewin and other social psychologists working in the first half of this century developed the conceptual system referred to as Field Theory, which anticipated much of social learning (cognitive) theory and behaviorism. **Field Theory explains behavior in terms of the present situations in which people find themselves as well as the needs they bring to those situations.**[12] Behavior can only be understood in terms of the "field" which surrounds it. In this field are various forces which will include direction (either to accelerate or decelerate a behavior), strength (e.g., salience of a reinforcer which is related to a person's needs), and "point of application"[13] (which can be defined

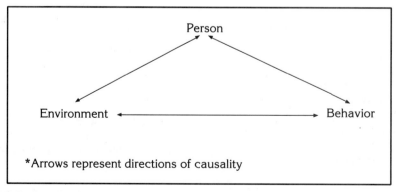

FIGURE 3-3.   Reciprocal determinism processes from social learning theory*

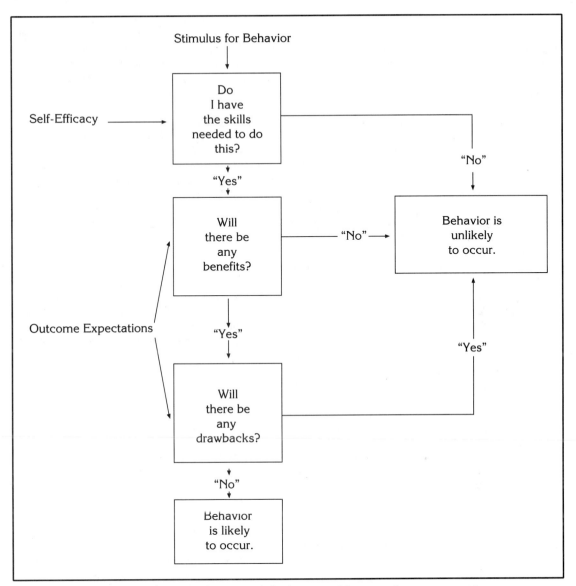

Stimulus for Behavior

Self-Efficacy ⟶ Do I have the skills needed to do this?

"No"

"Yes"

Will there be any benefits?

Outcome Expectations

"No" ⟶ Behavior is unlikely to occur.

"Yes"

Will there be any drawbacks?

"Yes"

"No"

Behavior is likely to occur.

FIGURE 3–4. Cognitive-behavioral processes from a social learning theory perspective

as the contingency between a consequence and a behavior). Although Lewin argued that a person's needs were more important than stimulus-response associations,[14] Skinner and Bandura subsequently showed how these concepts overlap. Lewin's many contributions to understanding social behavior have especially been felt in studies of group dynamics, social networks, and health.

Although the Health Belief Model, Communications/Persuasion Model, Social Learning Theory, and Field Theory share important features with behaviorism, there are important distinctions to be drawn, as well. Unlike these and other theoretical approaches, behaviorism de-emphasizes unobservable processes such as "emotions," "attitudes," and "knowledge," as such variables are very subjective and therefore difficult to measure scientifically. Instead, behaviorists focus on specific behaviors or their products which can be objectively observed or otherwise measured. The purpose of this focus is twofold: first, behaviorism emphasizes the scientific approach, which perhaps is best accomplished in the behavioral sciences by applying methods of measurement and intervention that can be reliably and validly described and evaluated. For example, it is much easier to measure attendance at a health clinic than attitudes people have about the clinic. Second, to be effective in the public health arena, behavior change technology must be developed in such a way as to be accessible to the largest number of people. Therefore, highly sophisticated concepts and techniques which may be appropriate only for a select few (such as those who can afford private, small group therapy for obesity) and require sophisticated advanced professional training to be useful may not prove effective in accomplishing the broader goals of public health behavior change.

Behavior modification is an **appropriate technology** for public health behavior change. For such a designation it meets two related criteria. First, behavior modification can have an impact on large numbers of people (i.e., the "public") in various ways related to improving health. Second, fundamental principles and techniques of behavior modification can be learned in a relatively brief time by professionals trained primarily in other disciplines or, for that matter, by the public at large. Although years of study can be devoted to a mastery of motivational technology, it is the purpose of this text to equip practitioners and other consumers with fundamental abilities in behavior modification which can be applied with supervision in a variety of community settings or personal situations. This technology is presented in detail in chapter 8.

BEHAVIOR IS OBSERVABLE

"Our patients have bad attitudes about our services."
"My kids don't eat the right foods."
"We need our clinic staff to perform at peak efficiency."
"I live a very healthy life."

What do the above statements have in common? They all pertain to health, they all generally imply or refer to behavior, but are all inadequately precise for effective health promotion. The present chapter now turns to the concept of behavior, how it may differ from other more general definitions, and why and how to be specific in describing health behavior.

What exactly is behavior? Our simple definition is as follows: **Behaviors are the observable actions of people. In other words, we can see, hear, or otherwise sense what people do or do not do, i.e., their actions or inactions.** Within this definition smoking, talking, performing job-related tasks, riding a bicycle, or purchasing fresh vegetables are behaviors. Sleeping or not working may be classified as the absence of behavior, and are also observable and have relevance to health promotion. Thinking, feeling, and being in a bad mood are not observable, are not behaviors, and therefore have secondary importance. Although these latter processes can be relevant to certain health promotion efforts, they have limited public health utility.

OPERATIONAL DEFINITIONS OF BEHAVIOR

For two decades chronic disease epidemiologists have debated the importance of various risk factors for heart disease. Many of these risk factors are fairly straightforward and objectively measured, such as smoking, high blood pressure, and elevated serum cholesterol. Other purported risk factors, such as a lack of exercise and excessive consumption of dietary sodium and fats, are perhaps less easily measured given a need to rely on an individual's recall of recent actions. Yet behaviors in these categories are still fundamentally objective in nature. In other words, researchers are able to agree that "exercise" includes the frequency, duration, and intensity of physical activity, whereas the recall of what substances we ingested can be objectively related to the weight or volume of these substances.

An additional category of purported heart disease risk factors have been lumped into a category labeled the "coronary prone behavior pattern," or more commonly, "Type A Personality."

Although the evidence is still subject to debate, some researchers have maintained that the "Type A Personality" may be responsible for as many heart disease-related illnesses and deaths as the physically-related risk factors described above.

But what is meant by the Type A personality? Those of us not intimately familiar with this line of research may think of a variety of labels such as "stressed," "aggressive," "impatient," "pressured," and "hard-working" or "overworked." Indeed, researchers have tried to look into all of these factors at various times to determine their relationship to this overall constellation called "Type A."

From a behavioral perspective, the problems with designations such as Type A personalities are more fundamental than the argument as to whether such personalities or behavior patterns increase heart disease risks. The basic issue is whether we can objectively define and measure something as obscure as "personality" or "behavior pattern." In this case, not only is the definition of the personality a little fuzzy, but its supposed components, such as "aggressiveness" and "drive," are equally vague and difficult to measure.

Behavior analysis is a subdiscipline within psychology closely associated with the work of B. F. Skinner and others, which emphasizes the direct observation of behavior-environment relationships. Before behavior analysts would consider a concept such as the Type A personality, an operational definition of this concept would have to be provided. **An operational definition is the "product of breaking down a broad concept . . . into observable and measurable component behaviors."**[15] Operational definitions identify the procedures involved in observing the behavior, thereby allowing two or more observers to come up with the same results. Operational definitions usually quantify a variable or characteristic rather than referring to it in general or subjective terms (e.g., "slept 9½ hours" rather than "slept a lot"; "has a body weight of 20 percent greater than normal" rather than "is fat"; "finishes a 12 oz. beer in less than three minutes" rather than "is a heavy drinker"). The two related characteristics of operational definitions, therefore, are observability and objectivity.

Returning to our Type A example, how could we operationally define the various components of this so-called personality type or behavior pattern? Perhaps we could look at stress as consisting of less than normal amounts of sleep, excessive muscle tension, and excessive consumption of alcohol, cigarettes, or coffee. Aggressiveness could be broken down into the use of loud and rapid speech when interacting with peers or subordinates or frequently using a horn when driving an automobile in rush-hour traffic. Somewhat easier to operationally define would be "heavy work." The operational definition for heavy work would involve accepting work assignments far in excess of that which could be done in forty hours per week, which might in turn include simply staying longer than quitting time three or more nights per week, or working in the evenings and weekends. In all these cases, we can begin to develop objective measurement procedures (i.e., measures that observers could use to ascertain objectively the frequency or duration of the above behaviors) to assess the various components of the coronary prone behavior pattern. Subsequently, we would be able to determine objectively whether these phenomena are indeed related to heart disease morbidity and mortality. In fairness to the founders of this line of research, some work has been done to operationally define the coronary prone behavior pattern, such as through the Jenkins Activity Schedule. But rather than specifically saying that "this behavior" and "that behavior" may be related to heart disease, researchers try to integrate these various behaviors back into the "coronary prone behavior pattern" context, as though these behaviors were naturally related to one another.

As health professionals working in health promotion, we are often confronted with the problem of dealing with a physical outcome (i.e., a disease, injury, or death) which may be the result of several contributing behaviors and environmental factors rather than one or two easily understood causal agents. However, it is essential that we are able to operationally define behavioral factors which contribute to disease or to health in order to optimize prevention and enhance promotion efforts.

BEHAVIORAL ASSESSMENT

We have discussed why it is important to be specific about our target behaviors in health promotion. But how do we go about being specific? How can we represent complex behaviors such as patient care, healthy diets, and infectious disease control with "numbers"? We now turn to the topic of **behavioral assessment, which is the process of identifying, specifying, and quantifying health behaviors relevant to our health promotion efforts.**

Why Assess?

Assessment serves two categories of individuals: health professionals (or other change agents) and consumers. The latter group can consist of almost anyone—clients, parents, advisory boards, funding agencies, and the public in general. Through thorough assessment, the consumer can be assured of the most appropriate treatment or program planning. Whereas an initial assessment starts programs off in the right direction, a continual "time-series" assessment points to areas where intervention plans should be modified. Consumers and communities can be shown objective evidence of their progress and will be able to generate ongoing input for planning continuous improvement in an intervention plan.

Ongoing program assessment serves a critical self-correcting vehicle for the health professional and the responsible institution or agency. Incorporating continual behavioral assessment as an integral component of planning and evaluation can keep health professionals on target or allow them to change the focus of programming when appropriate (e.g., when little progress is being made using one approach rather than another). More importantly, monitoring improvements via objective assessment can be a very rewarding experience for health workers who, like everyone else, must usually rely on themselves for a pat on the back.

Objective Assessment

Objective assessment is to subjective assessment as "has improved" is to "seems to have improved." The clinical or field interview may be the most convenient method of gathering assessment information relevant to individual behavior

change-programs. However, self-report is highly susceptible to various biases. For example, clients may attempt to "look good" in soliciting favorable comments from professionals or to "look bad" when attempting to emphasize the severity of their problems. Moreover, health workers may be prone to detect improvements when the opposite is true. While objective assessment is not foolproof, it can serve to hold in check many of the problems mentioned above.

Sources of Objective Assessment

There are two basic dimensions of sources for assessment data: setting and informant. **Setting refers to the place where the data have been collected.** This dimension can be divided into two mutually exclusive categories, "office" (i.e., the health professional's base, such as a research clinic or office) and "natural" (i.e., the consumer's) setting. Collecting data from the natural as well as clinical environments help us determine the generality, or "external validity," of an intervention program.

Informant is the person(s) who actually makes the observations or fills out the self-report forms. This dimension may be divided into three mutually exclusive categories: health professional (or other external change agent), consumer, and others (e.g., spouse, neighbor, parent). Using more than one informant in an assessment strategy may increase the reliability (accuracy) of the data. Table 3–3 shows six possible sources of assessment data, given two types of settings and three informants.

A. *Health professional—office.* This refers to any assessment of the consumer performed by the health professional in the clinic or other setting not a part of the consumer's "natural" (i.e., day-to-day) environment. This category refers primarily to direct observations of the consumer's verbal and non-verbal behavior. It does not include subjective summations of unstructured clinical interviews.

B. *Consumer—office* or more appropriately, self-report. This category refers primarily to the completion of interviews, questionnaires, etc., by the consumer. Much of this self-

TABLE 3-3
Sources of Assessment

SETTING	INFORMANT		
	Health worker/ Professional	Consumer	Other
Health Agency, Clinic or Laboratory or Other "Office"	A	B	C
Natural Environment	D	E	F

assessment must still be interpreted by the health professional, as it relies on the consumer's recall or interpretation of past behaviors.

C. *Others—office.* Inter-rater reliability means two people observing the same phenomenon in the same way. Before we can be really comfortable with our assessment, we may want to determine how reliable or accurate it is. Such reliability assessment is especially useful when the behavioral observations are difficult or complex.

One easy way to determine the reliability of our client's self-report is to have significant others, neighbors, or community volunteers provide information on various aspects of the client's health behavior and functioning. Various circumstances may demonstrate a need for such reliability checks.

First, the client may indicate a perceived need for assistance in data collection, or agree that with the professional's suggestion, a second data source would help ensure the best possible information. If the client does so agree, he or she selects the person in the best position to provide confirmatory information.

Depending on the nature of the assessment

(and the commitment of the reliability checker), this third person conducts regular observations or retrospective summaries of the target behavior.

The "other's" data can then be compared to the client's. Should discrepancies exist, further inquiries into the true nature of the behavior or problem should be made. On the other hand, should a client's data closely correspond with his or her significant other's, the need for future checks would be relatively minimal.

D. *Health professional—natural setting.* This category is identical to "A" (in the clinic), with one exception. Obviously, these structured observations are conducted in "natural" settings such as the home, school, worksite, or village.

Since the collection of these data requires a field or home visit, it would be done most frequently by outreach or village health workers. However, all health professionals are encouraged to make such naturalistic observations whenever possible. If developing the consumer's ability to change in the natural setting is the ultimate goal of an intervention, objective data from this setting are essential.

E. *Consumer—natural setting,* or more simply,

self-monitoring. This technique not only provides the professional with extremely useful information, it may actually contribute directly to attainment of the behavior-change goal. **Self-monitoring involves teaching the consumer to observe and record the frequency, duration, or "permanent products" of his/her behavior.**

F. *Others — natural setting.* The use of "significant others" or volunteers, neighbors, or health workers to furnish assessment data collected in the natural setting serves the same purposes as the "others/office" category. Reliability estimates can be made to increase confidence in the validity of the results.

Which of the above categories should we use? This will depend on a variety of factors, including the scope of the program, available resources, the reliability of the consumer's self-report, and other factors. Large-scale programs with few resources apply self-report to a greater extent than do smaller or resource-rich ones, since objective observations and supervised self-monitoring require substantial resources. Actually, mature and motivated consumers are likely to provide reliable data, circumventing the need for external confirmation by others. For instance, if the program primarily emphasizes one-to-one clinical work with adults, the selection of a recording system

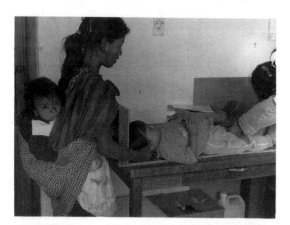

FIGURE 3–5. A Guatemalan mother assists in the measurement of her toddler at a regular growth monitoring check-up. Active involvement of clients in the monitoring of their own data will enhance their involvement in a behavior change effort. *Photo Courtesy of John Elder*

would be much easier than when working with several classes of sixth graders. Additionally, the direct observation of seven-year-old children by a teacher or health professional may be advisable, whereas adults enrolled in a smoking cessation class should be capable of recording their own behavior. A nurse in an understaffed primary health care clinic in a developing country may only be able to observe how well a mother can administer oral rehydration solutions to her child while she is in the clinic. However, a clinic with itinerant health workers may arrange for one of them to actually visit the mother in her home to conduct a more valid observation of the mother's treatment in this natural setting.

Graphing

Graphing gives us a "picture" of what is happening with the consumer over time. It also makes it easy to spot trends or patterns (e.g., "more behavior on weekdays, less on weekends"). Generally, any behavioral information that can be (a) expressed as a frequency or score, and (b) obtained several times should be represented on a graph. Examples include scores on tests, self-monitoring data, observational data, and permanent product data.

How to Graph

1. On graph or ruled paper, draw in the "axes" which are the horizontal and vertical lines, and which are the graph's boundaries (Figure 3–6).
2. Label the vertical axis to show what target behavior or dependent variable is being graphed. Be sure to leave enough space to allow for the scores to go as high or as low as they can go. Generally, the bottom of the graph should represent zero (see Figure 3–7).

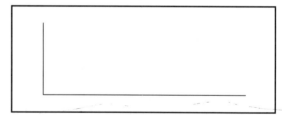

FIGURE 3–6. Drawing the lines

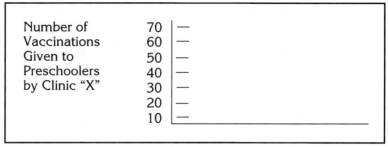

FIGURE 3–7.   Labeling the dependent variable

3. Label the horizontal axis to show when the data were collected, either enumeration, hours, days, weeks, etc., or specifying times or dates. Leave some space between each unit (Figure 3–8).
4. Chart the data corresponding to the date (week, month) which they represent and connect the dots (Figure 3–9).

Example.   Joe Tirante is a 34-year-old blue collar worker who suffers from chronic muscle soreness and back pain. His physician has put him on an exercise schedule where he is expected eventually to perform one hour a day of stretching and other exercises. The doctor cautioned Joe not to jump into this regimen too quickly as he would run the risk of injuring himself if he put too much

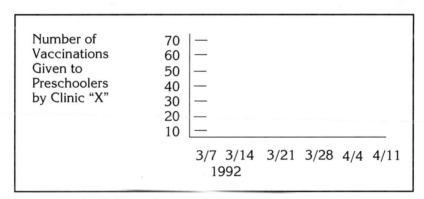

FIGURE 3–8.   Labeling the time dimension

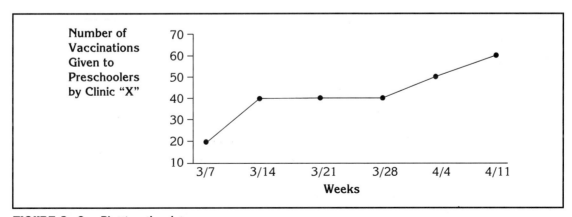

FIGURE 3–9.   Plotting the data

pressure on his already sore muscles. The doctor also gave Joe a graph on which to chart his progress. As instructed, Joe graphed the amount of stretching time he put in every week and brought the graph back to the doctor at the end of every six-week period. Feeling exceptionally well at the end of twelve weeks, Joe decided to add extensive running into his new exercise pattern. However, he overdid it and strained his achilles tendon, which limited his ability to stay with the program for that week. The next week, however, he was back on track. Figure 3–10 shows how Joe charted his data. It is sometimes handy to make a notation directly on the graph to identify notable or unusual events.

Categories of Behavioral Assessment

Overview.   The direct observation of behavior (by the professional or consumer or other person) has several advantages over assessment via self-report. With observational assessment, we need not infer from surveys and other self-reported data how the client behaves in his/her natural setting. Rather, we have direct evidence of this behavior. We can pinpoint more directly the problems by observing the consumers' responses and the antecedent and consequent situations under which the responses occur. At times, of course, the direct observation of health behavior may be impossible. When this is the case, it is necessary to rely on consumers or other appropriate persons to recall what they did or saw to the best of their ability.

Direct assessment of the target person's behavior encompasses four of the six assessment categories (Table 3–3), namely, all three of the natural setting categories and "professional/office." Therefore, it is critical that health promotion specialists be familiar with observational techniques and variations.

Use of Observational Assessment.   Behavioral excesses, deficits, or assets of the consumer are all potential targets for behavioral observation. Excesses, deficits, and assets are defined as follows:

A. *Behavioral excess.* **A class of related behaviors described as problematic by the consumer or an informant because of excess are (1) frequency, (2) intensity, (3) duration, or (4) occurrence in inappropriate situations.** Examples of behavioral excesses along one or more of these dimensions include consuming alcoholic beverages, smoking, exercising at an excessively high-pulse rate, drinking polluted water, driving beyond the speed limit, or having unprotected sex.

B. *Behavioral deficit.* **A class of responses are considered problematic by someone because of failure to occur (1) with sufficient frequency, (2) with adequate intensity, (3) in appropriate form, or (4) situations.** Behaviors related to reduced social responsiveness, fatigue, and other restrictions in function can all be categorized as "deficient." Examples of behavioral deficits include insufficient breast feeding, exercise which results in a pulse rate

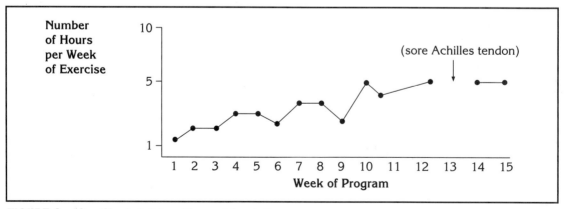

FIGURE 3–10.   Charted data with special notations

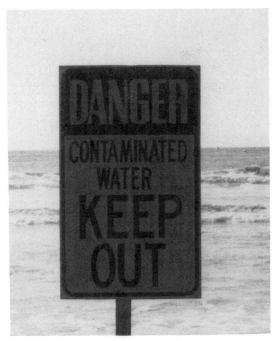

FIGURE 3–11. Excesses in some human behaviors, such as those which lead to the contamination of our oceans, can prevent healthy behaviors (such as exercise and relaxation) from occurring. *Photo courtesy of Betsy Clapp.*

below the targeted range, poor clinic attendance, or non-action in response to a life-threatening illness. Deficits often become the acceleration targets, to be increased via a health promotion effort.

C. *Behavioral asset.* **Behavioral assets are health-promotive or other adaptive consumer behaviors.** What does the consumer do well for personal or group health? What are his/her effective social behaviors? What other resources does the person have? Any segment of a person's activities can be used as an arena for building up new behaviors. In fact, work and other day-to-day community activities provide a better starting point for behavior change than does a clinical setting. For example, an ill person who lives alone but resides in a neighborhood and has frequent, supportive interactions with several friends can be linked with them to insure appropriate compliance to a treatment regimen.[16] In other behavior

change plans, we often include behavioral assets as maintenance targets, to be sustained or strengthened in health promotion programs.

Types of Observational Assessment

For health promotion purposes, we recommend five types of observational assessment and two schedules of assessment. The types of assessment are (1) narrative recording (a.k.a. "ABC" recording); (2) binary recording (usually done with "checklists"), (3) frequency recording; (4) duration recording; and (5) permanent product recording. While observations can be conducted continuously, a time schedule which may make recording easier is called "interval recording."[17]

Definitions and examples of these recording procedures are listed below. Remember, the procedures can be used by health professionals, supervisors, group leaders, the clients themselves, or anyone directly concerned with the behavior change program.

1. *Narrative recording.* **For narrative recording, the observer writes a narrative or a "story" describing in sequence all behaviors observed. These observations can be organized into a three-column chart (an "ABC" chart) consisting of the events occurring prior to the behavior (Antecedents), the subject's responses (Behaviors) following these antecedents, and the events following the behavior (Consequences).** Narrative recording allows further specification of conditions in which the behavior occurs, including discriminative stimuli and the possible reinforcers that maintain behavior, and it provides general information for choosing efficient recording methods (e.g., frequency, duration, and/or intensity). It is used (1) prior to formal assessment and modification, when unfamiliar with the subject, or (2) when the behaviors still need to be more precisely defined (e.g., when two observers cannot agree on what is an instance of the behavior).

2. *Checklist (binary recording).* **In many cases, observers are simply interested in whether a specific behavior occurred.** For instance, in driver education courses, we want to make sure a student fastens her safety belt appropriately, checks the rearview mirror, adjusts the seat according to her height and comfort, and

uses turn signals before pulling out into traffic. Indeed, during tests to obtain a driver's license, the testing officers observe whether these safe driving behaviors. **They often use a binary (i.e., "yes/no") recording format, to simply indicate whether a certain behavior occurred** at a particular location of the driving route. Checklists are fairly easy to use and therefore very popular among professionals and lay people alike, whether observing behavior directly or auditing environmental conditions. For instance, in a tobacco control campaign, we might want to see whether tobacco ads reached particular blocks of an inner city. A checklist would be constructed specifying the community locations to check and whether a tobacco advertisement was present in the area (e.g., on a billboard or elsewhere).

This binary format is not only appropriate for a general statement of behavioral occurrence (e.g., overall frequency), but can also be used in interval recording to determine whether behaviors occurred in smaller subsets of larger blocks of time. Interval recording and a binary format, allows one to estimate overall frequency or duration (see below).

3. *Frequency recording.* **The observer simply counts each occurrence of the target behavior during a predefined time period,** often extended over long durations if the behavior is of low frequency. **Such frequency recording gives an accurate record of response occurrence within designated time periods, thus allowing for an estimate of the rate at which the behavior occurs.**

Frequency recording is used (1) when behavior is of moderate to low frequency and occurrences are similar in duration and intensity; and/or (2) when an observer needs to observe more than one behavior or more than one person at a time. For example, one can record different people engaging in the same easily-observed behavior (such as patients entering the clinic), or one can record more than one behavior for one individual (such as the number of drinks consumed and cigarettes smoked by one patron in a bar).

Examples of frequency recording include counting numbers of apples eaten, push-ups performed, vaccinations given, or questions a physi-

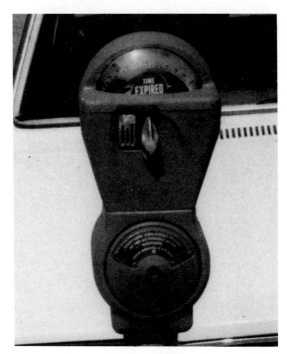

FIGURE 3–12.   Duration recording can be done with a watch or a special timing mechanism. *Photo courtesy of Betsy Clapp.*

cian asks her patient during an examination. The rate of behavior can then be computed by dividing this frequency by the duration of the observation period.

4. *Duration recording.* **The observer measures the total length of time the behavior occurs during a predefined observational period.** The purpose of duration recording is to provide a record of behavioral duration within a given time period. Duration recording is used primarily when (a) a behavior or behavioral process has an easily determined beginning and end, (b) the behavior is variable (e.g., length of interactions between workers and clients in clinics), and (c) the behavior is an excess of long duration and moderate to low frequency (e.g., alcohol-drinking "binges"). Examples of duration recording include an individual's total talk time in a conversation as observed by the clinician in a role-play, the number of hours of sleep per night, the duration of a single breast

feeding episode, the length of exposure to ill cohabitants in a small house, and the length of wait in clinic's waiting room.

5. *Permanent product recording.* **Permanent product recording is a simple observation (or notation) of the physical product, outcome or permanent record of a behavior (e.g., the weight of a person, the test scores of a health worker trainee, or the number of clinic visits recorded on clinic records), usually measured at the end of a predetermined time period.** Its purpose is to provide a retrospective measure of the effect of a behavior in lieu of concurrent observation. Permanent product recording is often used when direct observation can interfere with the target behavior or when the target behavior is too difficult or too time-consuming to observe directly. Also, the measurement approach can readily be used in conjunction with another method. Permanent product data provide excellent means of validating other types of recording, or in some cases actually represent the principal form of measurement (e.g., weight loss programs). Given these applications and advantages, permanent product recording can be very useful in public health promotion. Examples of permanent product recording include counting the cigarette butts in an ashtray, measuring a child's height and

weight at a growth monitoring station, counting the number of discarded beer bottles in a parking lot, tabulating the volume of sales of lard and vegetable oil from a supermarket's sales records, and measuring the remainder of milk left in a baby's bottle. Measuring these and other "behavioral traces" has the distinct advantage of unobtrusiveness: the person being observed may no longer be on the scene when permanent product recording takes place.

Schedules of measures include continuous or interval recording. Continuous recording is just as the word implies: the observer notes all data pertaining to a target behavior throughout an entire observational period. Interval recording is where the observers divide the observation period (e.g., one-half hour) into a number of equal time intervals, usually ranging from five seconds to one or two minutes. Then it is noted whether or not the target behavior(s) occurs in each interval, usually with a binary code format. Interval durations should be selected so time is available for one occurrence of the target behavior. Interval recording gives a rough estimate of the frequency of the responses and the latency between responses, in terms of the number or percentage of intervals scored. It can be used when multiple behaviors are recorded, or for multiple individuals (e.g., recording one to five behaviors for a different person for

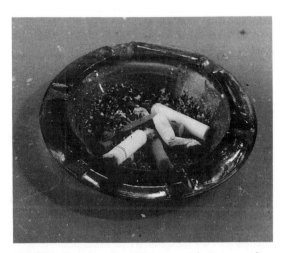

FIGURE 3–13. Permanent product recording can be conducted when the person performing the behavior is not actually present. *Photo courtesy of Betsy Clapp.*

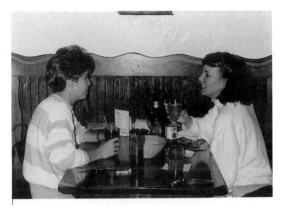

FIGURE 3–14. Frequency, duration, or permanent product recording may be used to record drinking behavior. *Photo courtesy of Betsy Clapp.*

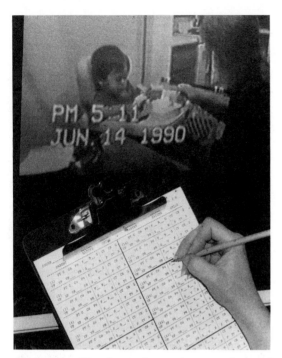 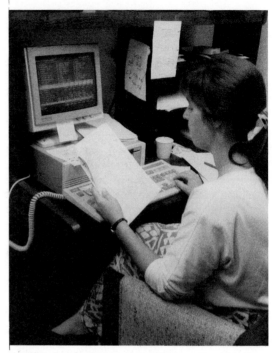

FIGURE 3–15. Interval recording may be used to estimate the duration, frequency, or other dimensions of behavior. Above, a researcher records the occurrence or non-occurrence of several behaviors from a video tape showing a mother and toddler interacting during lunch, and later enters these data into her computer. *Photo courtesy of Betsy Clapp.*

each interval), for behaviors with highly variable frequencies, when the behavior does not have an easily determined beginning and end, or for when frequency and duration recording do not work (and when, of course, a watch or alternative "time-piece" is accessible).

An example of interval recording is provided through research conducted by Dr. Philip Nader and his colleagues.[18] These researchers were interested in how much physical activity various preschool children emitted. Observers watched the children for thirty seconds. Then, using a binary format, they recorded whether each child was inactive or active during that interval. Later, by totalling the percentage of intervals scored as "active" during a twenty-minute period (with forty intervals), the investigators estimated total amount of activity per child and for the entire group.

Summary: Choosing a Recording Technique

In choosing a procedure for recording behavior, there are three important decisions the person designing the observational approach must make: (1) Who is going to do the recording? (2) When and how often are records going to be taken? and (3) What kind(s) of data will be recorded?

To make these decisions, we must take into account the nature of the target behavior, how frequently it occurs, who is around to record its occurrence(s), and whether the duration of the behavior varies from time to time. The following guidelines can facilitate these decisions.

1. *Who will record?* If the consumer is the only one around when the behavior or problem occurs, and he or she is capable of reliable

recording, you can implement a self-monitoring procedure.

If others (e.g., friends or relatives) are around to observe the behavior and the consumer agrees this would be helpful, others can be enlisted to assist.

It may be useful to use both self-monitoring and observations by others to get a more complete picture. Health workers, for example, may have time available to do some behavioral observation. Remember, though, health workers are often "actors" in a system we want to assess in general. Therefore, their behavior may also be a target for behavioral observation.

2. *When and how often to record?* If the target behavior or problem occurs fairly infrequently (less than several times a day), record each instance (e.g., nausea/vomiting, exercising, water boiling) using frequency or binary recording. If the target or problem occurs frequently (many times each day), take a time sample (e.g., one hour). An example of such a target would be medical charting by nurses in the nurses' station of a hospital ward.

3. *What to record?* If the target or behavior is continuous but varies in duration, record its duration (e.g., sleep, coughing spells). If the target varies in outcome or results (e.g., light snacking vs. heavy eating) or is difficult to observe (e.g., pill-taking), get a permanent product measure.

Table 3–4 summarizes these behavioral observation measures and their advantages and disadvantages.

Examples of Behavioral Observation

The Thin Thighs Professional Fitness Corporation relies extensively on behavioral observation and behavior modification for promoting weight loss in its clientele. Emil Rollizo, an executive in a local bank, is one of their first clients in the new year. Emil is approximately seventy-five pounds overweight, a problem which has hounded him in the ten years since he left high school.

On his first visit to the Thin Thighs office, Emil was given a narrative recording form to get a better idea of the specific nature of his obesity-related behaviors and possible environmental causal factors related to these behaviors. Emil was instructed to fill out this narrative recording and

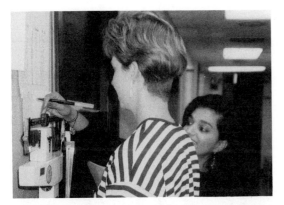
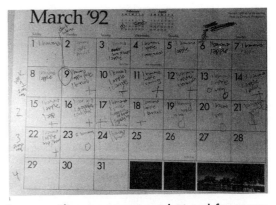

FIGURE 3–16. Nutritional health promotion projects may utilize permanent product and frequency recording. A client's weight is checked on a regular basis in weight loss programs, while individuals may self-monitor their consumption of various healthy target foods. *Photos courtesy of Betsy Clapp.*

TABLE 3-4
Summary of Behavioral Observation Methods

Recording Method	Description	Examples	Advantages	Disadvantages
Narrative or "ABC"	Verbal description of behavior and events which precede and follow it	Observing what is happening when students are paying attention and what seems to lead to inattention	1. Helps define behavior and gives clues to intervention 2. Easy to do	1. No quantification 2. Subject to observer bias
Binary "yes/no" or "Checklist"	One time check in predefined period of time as to whether a behavior occurred	Checking whether each of 20 different vegetables is available in supermarket	1. Easy to use 2. Good if one occurrence of behavior/event suffices 3. Lends itself to interval recording	1. Does not quantify beyond present/"absent" classification
Frequency or "Event" (converts to "Rate")	One time check in predefined period of time as to number of behaviors that occurred	Number of critical statements coach makes to grammar school soccer team members	1. Useful when behavior is well-defined 2. Self-recording alone may decrease behavior in desired direction	1. Not useful for extremely high rates of behavior
Duration	Amount of time over which the behavior occurs	Time it takes for parent to go from house to clinic taking child for vaccination	1. Useful when duration of behavior is most important variable	
Permanent Product (Outcome) Recording	Provides a measure of the product, effect or "residue" of a behavior	# pieces of litter on 1 mile stretch of highway; serum cholesterol measure	1. Unobtrusive; may be taken after behavior occurs 2. In some cases, most valid representation of health goal	1. May not directly reflect target behavior of person(s)

given brief training on the meaning of antecedents, behaviors, and consequences. The Thin Thighs counselors were interested in episodes of Emil's binge eating, since in the intake interview this seemed to be a root cause of Emil's obesity.

Emil took the Thin Thighs ABC diary home with him and filled it out for the first week of his program. Since he was interested in showing not only what was wrong with his life, but also what he occasionally did well with respect to his dieting and exercise behavior, he also recorded incidents of the latter. His first week's diary is shown in Table 3–5.

Given these new data, the Thin Thighs staff was ready to help Emil with a customized intervention and additional assessment exercises. First, however, they wanted to see for themselves what Emil's typical meal consumption pattern looked like. They loaned Emil a videotape camera to record a typical dinner at the Rollizo residence. Thin Thighs is especially keen on getting people to slow their rate of eating and use non- or low-caloric substances (e.g., water, fresh vegetables) to develop a feeling of "full." Therefore, they were especially interested in recording how much time Emil and his family spent talking during dinner and how frequently Emil took a drink of water with his dinner, both of which could be future acceleration targets for a differential reinforcement procedure. They also wanted to look at direct indices of how much and how fast Emil ate, so their interval recording procedure included the amount of time a fork or other eating utensil was in Emil's hand and how frequently he took a bite of food.

The Thin Thighs Dinner Observation Form is presented in Table 3–6.

The trained interviewers observed this videotape and checked every ten seconds whether they had observed Emil talking or taking a sip of water, and whether he had touched an eating utensil or taken a bite of food in that interval, as well. From these data, the staff were able to compute an estimate of the total amount of talk time and relate water drinking to food consumption rates.

After bringing in the videotape, Emil was given another specific diary as part of his initial weight loss program (Figure 3–17). This diary included

TABLE 3–5
Thin Thighs Diet Diary Form #1

Instructions: Describe what happens before, during, and after each occurrence of excessive calorie consumption in the coming week. Add extra pages as needed.

Antecedents (and time/day)	Behaviors	Consequences
Fought with wife; felt upset (10 a.m. Saturday)	Went to cookie jar; ate 10 Oreos.	Calmed down a bit.
Had a rough day at work; went to "happy hour" with buddies (6 p.m. Tuesday)	Had 4 martinis. Stopped by McDonalds for two orders of large fries on way home.	Ate dinner and went to sleep.
Had a hangover (all day Wednesday)	Had an extra large lunch to calm my stomach.	Felt more relaxed but a little disgusted; "What the heck" and had a big dinner.
Wife encouraged me to get exercise workout in before work (7 a.m. Thursday)	Went for 40 minute power walk.	Felt good; wife gave me a hug.

TABLE 3–6
Thin Thighs Dinner Observation Form

Minute #1

0–10″	11″–20″	21″–30″	31″–40″	41″–50″	51″–60″
Talk	Talk	Talk	Talk	Talk	Talk
H_2O	H_2O	H_2O	H_2O	H_2O	H_2O
Fork	Fork	Fork	Fork	Fork	Fork
Food	Food	Food	Food	Food	Food

Minute #2

0–10″	11″–20″	21″–30″	31″–40″	41″–50″	51″–60″
Talk	Talk	Talk	Talk	Talk	Talk
H_2O	H_2O	H_2O	H_2O	H_2O	H_2O
Fork	Fork	Fork	Fork	Fork	Fork
Food	Food	Food	Food	Food	Food

Minute #3

0–10″	11″–20″	21″–30″	31″–40″	41″–50″	51″–60″
Talk	Talk	Talk	Talk	Talk	Talk
H_2O	H_2O	H_2O	H_2O	H_2O	H_2O
Fork	Fork	Fork	Fork	Fork	Fork
Food	Food	Food	Food	Food	Food

Minute #4

0–10″	11″–20″	21″–30″	31″–40″	41″–50″	51″–60″
Talk	Talk	Talk	Talk	Talk	Talk
H_2O	H_2O	H_2O	H_2O	H_2O	H_2O
Fork	Fork	Fork	Fork	Fork	Fork
Food	Food	Food	Food	Food	Food

Minute #5

0–10″	11″–20″	21″–30″	31″–40″	41″–50″	51″–60″
Talk	Talk	Talk	Talk	Talk	Talk
H_2O	H_2O	H_2O	H_2O	H_2O	H_2O
Fork	Fork	Fork	Fork	Fork	Fork
Food	Food	Food	Food	Food	Food

Instructions to observer: Cross out each behavior that occurs during the ten second interval.

Codes: Talk = if the person said anything to table companion

H_2O = if a sip or drink of water was consumed

Fork = whether the fork, knife, or spoon were held at any time in the interval

Food = whether any food was ingested during the interval

DATE:

Breakfast

Food #1: _____ Portion _____ Total
Size (gms)   Calories _____

Food #2: _____ Portion _____ Total
Calories _____
                                                   Total
Food #3: _____ Portion _____ Calories _____

Total Breakfast Calories _____

Time Started: _____ Time Ended: _____

Total Breakfast Time: _____

Lunch

Food #1: _____ Portion _____ Total
Size (gms)   Calories _____

Food #2: _____ Portion _____ Total
Calories _____
                                                   Total
Food #3: _____ Portion _____ Calories _____

Total Lunch Calories _____

Time Started: _____ Time Ended: _____

Total Lunch Time: _____

Snack

Food #1: _____ Portion _____ Total
Size (gms)   Calories _____

Dinner

Food #1: _____ Portion _____ Total
Size (gms)   Calories _____

Food #2: _____ Portion _____ Total
Calories _____
                                                   Total
Food #3: _____ Portion _____ Calories _____

Total Dinner Calories _____

Time Started: _____ Time Ended: _____

Total Dinner Time: _____

_____ _____ _____

Alcoholic Beverages:
Use stroke tally:
(\\\\) marks   Total # alcohol calories   Total calories for day

FIGURE 3–17. Thin Thighs diet diary form #2

63

both permanent product, frequency, and duration recording.

Emil was instructed to weigh each serving of food and compute calories based on one of the books he received as part of the program. He was also instructed to time the beginning and the end of each meal, since the Thin Thighs staff were trying to get him to slow down his eating. Finally, a frequency count of the number of alcoholic beverages he consumed (standardized for 12 oz. beer or equivalent in other beverages) was also tallied. From all of these data, Emil was able to calculate total calories consumed per day.

Hoping both to confirm directly the reliability of Emil's data and enlist his wife Debbie's support in his weight-loss effort, the Thin Thigh staff also trained Emil's wife to use a checklist which noted four specific eating and exercise events. Debbie's checklist is presented in Figure 3–18. Thus, all forms of direct observation described above were used in Emil's weight loss program.

BEHAVIORAL ASSESSMENT AND PUBLIC HEALTH PROMOTION

Techniques of behavioral assessment come from the field of behavior therapy and individual behavior modification. Therefore, many of the techniques described here are more appropriate for one-to-one, clinic-based health promotion efforts than perhaps for larger scale programs designed to have a public health impact. In the community settings, we are more likely to be interested in the use of interviews, questionnaires, telephone surveys, and measures of the "behaviors" of large numbers of people. In fact, we have little choice but to use these types of techniques for which behavioral observation has only an indirect relevance. However, with a behavioral assessment foundation, the design of various questionnaires or larger scale measurement devices which include frequency, duration, and permanent product measures may be invaluable to planning a comprehensive evaluation of large-scale programs.

An example of the use of principles of behavioral assessment in designing a questionnaire is presented in the following "intake assessment," (i.e., the initial interview) which a clinic for the treatment of problem drinking uses to assess the behaviors of their potential clients. Because it is impossible for the staff of this clinic to conduct direct behavioral observations of their clients' drinking behaviors (although self-monitoring may be tried), they use the following types of questions in gaining behavioral information:

1. "In what types of situations do you usually take a drink? What times of day? Who else is around? In what types of situations are you unlikely to drink?" (This is the assessment of antecedents to drinking in "ABC recording.")
2. "How do you feel if you go a long time without drinking? How do you feel after you've taken one drink? How about after you've had five? How do you feel the next morning after drinking heavily? What are other people's reaction to your drinking? How about to your periods of abstinence?" (Parallel to "ABC recording," this emphasized the consequences of drinking.)
3. "How many bottles of beer, glasses of wine, or shots of hard liquor do you usually have on a typical weekday morning? Weekday afternoon? Weekday evening? Weekend morning, afternoon, and evening?" (This results in

---

Date: _____: On this day, did your spouse eat seconds at

dinner?	_____ Yes	_____ No
Have alcoholic beverage?	_____ Yes	_____ No
(If yes, #:_____)		
Snack before bedtime?	_____ Yes	_____ No
Exercise 20 minutes or more?	_____ Yes	_____ No
Fill out diet diaries end of day?	_____ Yes	_____ No

Initials

FIGURE 3–18. Thin Thighs spouse confirmation list

estimates of frequencies and rates of behavior.)

4. "How long does it take you to finish a drink? From the time you have your first drink, how long do you usually go before you quit drinking?" (This parallels duration recording.)

5. (Questions asked of spouse or other significant other)

"Does this information match your perception of your spouse's drinking? Do you ever look at the number of bottles in the wastebasket or garbage can? How about the amount of alcohol gone from the bottles of liquor in the liquor cabinet?" If so, what do you observe?" (Here we obtain examples of permanent product recording.)

Specific behavioral assessment procedures will vary greatly depending on the problem behavior and the number of people targeted. Generally, the broader the scale of a program (see Section III) the more reliance the health professional has to put on permanent product- and self-report. (See also chapter 6 regarding the use of behavioral assessment as applied to the field of behavioral epidemiology.)

GOAL SETTING

Once operational definitions are established for various behaviors and a baseline rate for the frequency, duration, or permanent product of these behaviors has been graphed, we need to develop goals for our behavior change programs. This section discusses the processes involved in establishing practical and ethical goals for health promotion, whether conducted for individuals, organizations, or entire communities.

A "goal" or "general goal" is typically a health criterion (or the converse of a health problem) toward which progress can hopefully be made. Once a general goal has been selected, a "subgoal" or "behavioral objective" should be established which more clearly specifies levels of behavior change to be achieved. For example, our general goal could be "decrease the number of smokers in Davenport, Iowa," with objectives such as "increase smoking cessation rates in Davenport clinics from an average of 33 percent to an average of 50 percent," "increase 'spontaneous cessation rates' in the general population from 10 percent to 15 percent via contests and other procedures," and "decrease the incidence of new

smokers among adolescent age groups from 20 percent to 10 percent." These are examples of community-wide goal setting. Goal setting for organizations, groups, and individuals should be progressively more specific with respect to well-defined desired outcomes, the situations in which the responses are to occur, and the criteria for determining when the objective has been accomplished (see chapter 7).

The specific nature of the desired response or outcome is a product of developing a good operational definition of this outcome or response. Again, individual or small group goals can be stated in terms of the frequency, duration, or product of the response. Health promotion with groups or organizations may also involve these behavioral dimensions, but are more likely to focus on the products of behavior, institutional records, or institutional changes (e.g., participation in worksite blood pressure screenings stated in terms of the percentage of the total work force). Behavioral objectives designed for entire communities will by necessity involve larger-scale analysis and reliance on archival records for determining whether various goals and objectives have been met.

Specific **criteria** should also be developed for determining whether or not a goal or objective has been reached. For example, instead of stating "the incidence of teenage pregnancies in three public high schools should be reduced," we should propose something like "the incidence of teenage pregnancies should be reduced from 18 percent to 5 percent of the high school age females during three years of high school age." By specifying specific criteria and conditions for accomplishment, we force ourselves to be realistic and practical rather than idealistic. Clearly, criteria can be adjusted upward (or downward) if we have been fortunate and met the criteria fairly rapidly. On the other hand, criteria should be set sufficiently stringent in order to be of some social and public health significance. This level of such significance can be established by various participants in the goal setting process (see chapter 4).

Next, we need to specify the **situation** with which goal attainment can be expected. We may need to provide certain materials, financial support, and educational programs as a part of our health promotion effort. For example, we may wish to improve attendance at a vaccination clinic. Clearly, however, we cannot expect this attendance to improve unless we meet certain specifications, such as opening the clinic during announced times, having vaccines available, and having a certain number of trained staff present to administer the vaccinations. Without the specification of such situational requisites, we may find our health improvement efforts to fail, and may unfairly blame a specific change approach (e.g., in this case, we could have used a residential prompt and/or a lottery system to increase clinic attendance).

Ethical considerations also need to be observed in developing goals and objectives. Dimensions on which to consider ethical issues include whether constructive or suppressive approaches are used, whether direct versus indirect interventions are emphasized, and what are the benefits to clients, staff, and/or society.

A **constructive approach** should be given priority over a suppressive approach.[19] Constructive approaches generally involve the maintaining or building of an adaptive health behavior (or "asset") rather than the inhibiting of a maladaptive (or "excessive") one. Emphasizing acceleration and maintenance targets leads us away from continually "telling people what's bad for them" and instead allows us to help people find things they can do more of in order to improve their health.

An emphasis on suppressive approaches, on the other hand, is generally perceived as more manipulative or negative and get us into the bind of trying to get people to do less of something they are being reinforced for. Programs to combat smoking, drinking, excessive calorie, fat and sodium consumption, high speed driving, and drug use make us appear puritanical in our approach to building a healthier life style. However, as discussed later, pleasant consequences can be used to reduce inappropriate behavior through targeting other behaviors which "compete" with unhealthy behaviors. Health promotion efforts to restrict or eliminate certain behaviors can thereby be developed in such a way as to reduce the likelihood of backlash, sabotage, or unpopularity of the behavioral program being developed. These issues are discussed in chapter 8.

Another consideration in goal selecting is who ultimately benefits from goal attainment. We often operate under the illusion that consumers are truly benefiting from our health promotion program, when in fact we are simply trying to meet the requirements of a state contract or federal grant. In other cases, we find ourselves trying to please the staff of an agency rather than promoting the health of the target populations in a way which they would find acceptable. Consumers or their representatives therefore should be directly involved in goal selection, serving as co-equals with professional staff. Such participation not only can serve to enhance ethical and legal safeguards to our health promotion efforts, but also can optimize program effectiveness by engendering a sense of "community ownership" of the program.

Finally, ethical considerations must include minimization of "coercion." Coercion may include "making people an offer they can't refuse" because the consequences of not accepting our program are too fearsome to risk, or the reward is too great to forego in spite of misgivings or concerns the consumers may have. We typically think of coercion as getting someone to engage in behavior through the use of a very powerful aversive stimulus such as the threat of imprisonment or a heavy fine. However, coercion can also consist of disproportionately large incentives: "offers that we can't refuse." For example, a community advocacy agency in a very poor neighborhood might not be able to refuse a large offer of financial aid from the tobacco industry and, therefore, will allow exploitation of that and similar populations. In our system this is defined as coercion, given the disproportionate incentive of a large program of much needed financial aid. (Figure 8–3 provides more detail on how to select minimally intrusive intervention strategies.)

SUMMARY

The Health Belief Model, the Communications/Persuasion Model, the Theory of Reasoned Action, Field Theory, Social Learning Theory, and Behavior Modification have all played important roles in the development of the fields of health education and health promotion. While these theories have more in common than not, behavior modification stresses the importance of observable behavior and how directly to change it. Behavioral assessment emphasizes the direct observation of behavior by the consumer or others in "artificial" or natural settings. Behavioral observations may emphasize the frequency, duration or permanent product of behaviors, collected continuously or in selected intervals. Narrative recording provides the opportunity to develop a better understanding of the why's and wherefore's of a potential target behavior. While many consumers of health behavior change interventions may have certain behavioral excesses and deficits, they all most certainly have assets as well, which should not be ignored.

The next section's presentation of the **ON-PRIME** planning, implementation, and evaluation sequence builds on the information presented in the Health and Behavior chapters.

ADDITIONAL READINGS

For those with greater outcome expectations for health behavior theory information, reach for the following sources:

1. B. Sulzer-Azaroff, & G. Mayer. (1977). *Applying behavior analysis procedures with children and youth.* New York: Holt, Rinehart & Winston.
2. A. Bandura. (1977). *Social learning theory.* Englewood Cliffs, NJ: Prentice-Hall.
3. M. Fishbein, & I. Ajzen. (1975). *Beliefs, attitudes, intention, and behavior: An introduction to theory and research.* Reading, MA: Addison-Wesley.

EXERCISE

Self-Change Project. Select a personal health-related target behavior for change. Choose a behavior change goal, an observational/measurement system, and sources of data if other than yourself. Remember to define the behavior specifically. Construct a graph and graph your data on a regular basis. After reading Chapter 8, you will be ready for your intervention!

ENDNOTES

1. Becker, M. (1979). Psychosocial aspects of health-related behavior. In H. Freeman et al. (Eds.), *Handbook of medical sociology.* Englewood Cliffs, NJ: Prentice-Hall.
2. Fishbein, M., & Ajzen, I. (1975). *Beliefs, attitudes, intention, and behavior: An introduction to theory and research.* Reading, MA: Addison-Wesley.; and Fishbein, M., & Ajzen, I. (1980). *Understanding attitudes and predicting social behavior.* Englewood Cliffs, NJ: Prentice-Hall.

3. McGuire, W. J. (1964). Inducing resistance to persuasion: Some contemporary approaches. In L. Berkowitz (Ed.), *Advances in experimental social psychology* (Vol. 1). New York: Academic Press.
4. Bandura, A. (1977). *Social learning theory.* Englewood Cliffs, NJ: Prentice-Hall.
5. Lewin, K. (1951). Behavior and development as a function of the total situation. In D. Cartwright (Ed.), *Field Theory in Social Science.* New York: Harper & Row.
6. Rosenstock, I. M. (1977). What research in motivation suggests for public health. *American Journal of Public Health, 50,* 295–302.
7. Becker, M. H. (Ed.). (1974). The Health Belief Model and personal health behavior. *Health Education Monographs, 2,* 324–473; and Janz, N. K., & Becker, M. H. (1984) The Health Belief Model: A decade later. *Health Education Quarterly, 11,* 1–47.
8. Rosenstock, I. M. (1966). Why people use health services. *Milbank Memorial Fund Quarterly, 44,* 94–124; and Rosenstock, I. M. (1974). Historical origins of the Health Belief Model. *Health Education Monographs, 2,* 328–335.
9. Becker, Psychosocial aspects of health-related behavior.
10. Fishbein & Ajzen, *Understanding attitudes and predicting social behavior.*
11. McGuire, Inducing resistance to persuasion.
12. De Rivera, J. (1976). *Field theory as human-science.* New York: McGraw-Hill.
13. Lewin, K. (1935). *A dynamic theory of personality.* New York: McGraw-Hill; and De Rivera, p. 16.
14. De Rivera, p. 22.
15. Sulzer-Azaroff, B., & Mayer, G. (1977). *Applying behavior analysis procedures with children and youth.* New York: Holt, Rinehart & Winston.
16. Kanfer, F. H., & Saslow, G. (1969). Behavioral diagnosis. In C. M. Franks (Ed.), *Behavior therapy: Appraisal and status* (pp. 431–432). New York: McGraw-Hill.
17. Not included in this text is "intensity recording," presented by some as an additional observational category. Audio volume and measures of strength are examples of intensity recording.
18. McKenzie, T., Sallis, J., Nader, P., Patterson, J., Elder, J., Berry, C., Rupp, J., Atkins, C., Buono, M., & Morris, J. (1991). BEACHES: An observation system for assessing children's eating and physical activity behaviors and associated events. *Journal of Applied Behavior Analysis, 24,* 141–151.
19. Sulzer-Azaroff & Mayer, *Applying behavior analysis procedures with children and youth.*

Section II:

Step-By-Step Through ONPRIME

Chapter 4

Organizing for Health Promotion

OBJECTIVES

By the end of this chapter, the reader should be able to:

1. Define the following terms:
   - community organization
   - locality development
   - social action
   - social planning
2. Select an appropriate organizing strategy for a particular social or health issue and its circumstances.
3. Assess the gap between "real" and "ideal" community health or social conditions.
4. Indicate how legislation can influence or support health behavior and health promotion.

INTRODUCTION

Having completed an overview of the fundamental topics in health promotion, we are now ready to proceed with our "how to" sections: a step-by-step journey through the **ONPRIME** model. The departure point is our organizational structure and the direction it gives us in terms of what we should be doing—or more fundamentally—how we should go about determining what we should do.

Organization—the "**O**" of **ONPRIME**—is one of the most frequently used yet least understood terms in health promotion. *Motivating Health Behavior* proposes the following definition for **"organization" (used synonymously with "community organizing"):**

The development of new or mobilization and integration of existing organizations to deal with health or social issues through strategies which raise the public's or establishment's awareness of the issue, increase a local capacity for problem-solving, or protect a vulnerable segment of society.

This definition includes three components: a structure (new or existing organizations), a purpose (dealing with health/social issues), and a mechanism for change (increasing awareness, problem-solving, or protection). By its nature, public health promotion differs from "pure" community organization, which always starts with the community's agenda. In public health promotion, health is almost always the agenda.

Some organizations, committees, or councils are established especially to deal with a health problem on a time-limited basis. Often, it is the case that the health professional will be called on to organize a community (or, in most cases, its representatives) even before defining the community's health issues. In other situations, the health promoter is working for a corporation, agency, or public health office which is already firmly established as an organizational entity, affording the opportunity to proceed more rapidly toward the intervention phase of the ONPRIME sequence.

Well-staffed health promotion teams may include health educators, marketers, nutritionists, medical personnel, psychologists, and others. Such an abundance in professional resources is the exception, however; health promoters are far more likely to find themselves working alone or with only one or two other professionals. The degree of specificity of professional roles will influence the way health promotion programs are structured as well as the pacing through the ON-PRIME process.

Clearly, getting in on the ground floor of the development of an organization is the more complex of the two general possibilities. It is also potentially the more rewarding. We begin with some information on community organization for health promotion, followed by a discussion of strategies used by various organizations to set the health promotion process in motion.

Background.   As we have discussed in chapter 2, promoting health in entire populations requires far more than getting a lot of people to exercise,

eat healthier foods, quit smoking, or in other ways take charge of their personal health habits. Indeed, many typical health promotion activities are in the mode of the "medical model" (chapter 1). The medical model of treatment or health services connotes the interaction between a highly trained and sophisticated health professional and a relatively passive "patient," who waits for the health professional to perform some service to improve health or alleviate illness or pain. This model of health delivery is appropriate for a person who is very ill or has a disorder that is very unusual or difficult to understand without a high level of expertise. However, this top-down, authoritarian approach is less appropriate when the patient actually needs to develop skills for continuing treatment at home (e.g., a cardiac rehab patient learning how and when to exercise) and when the clinician needs to assess the level of the patient's understanding and ability to carry out a treatment regimen. Therefore, the medical model has been relegated to the emergency and surgery rooms, whereas more egalitarian — and effective — approaches to a patient-physician communication are being advocated for most other settings.

Health promotion efforts often suffer from the same basic flaw as the medical model. When we "tell" people they need to exercise more and eat less fat, we are assuming they understand what we are talking about, and they will be duly impressed with (and motivated by) our expertise in health promotion and motivated to take the prescribed action. Community organization models, in contrast, **generally hold that individuals and entire populations need to take charge of their own lives in order to deal with not only the problem(s) at hand — such as the high rate of heart disease in a community — but also with the root causes related to this problem and future problems** as they may arise. Through community-based behavior change techniques (described in chapters 7 through 10) combined with political and citizen support, community organization efforts can serve to empower a community to design its own best health promotion process. Without a relatively strong emphasis on community organization activities in a health promotion effort, it is unlikely that the majority of the Alma Ata principles (chapter 2) stressing local capacity building can be realized.

The processes and structures of community organization may include anything from traditional or even paternalistic approaches to community change to radically progressive and non-traditional strategies. They can be applied to the decision-making or planning of the project, the implementation of the project, or the evaluation of the project. The term "community participation" has often been used interchangeably with community organization and often will be interchangeable in *Motivating Health Behavior*, as well. However, community participation refers more specifically to the involvement of community residents in health promotion activities and less to the specific structure of the organization developed to promote health.[1] Before detailing different approaches to organizing communities for health promotion, let's describe some fundamental questions which generally should precede planning for community organization efforts.

REAL AND IDEAL SITUATIONS

Some ten years ago, one of the authors (JE) was running a smoking cessation group for some factory workers in northeastern United States. At the end of the second session, a fifty-year-old male participant was already beginning to disparage his prospects for quitting. At the end of the session, he dismissed our arguments with an, "Oh well, you have to die of something." I interpreted this as meaning he could not quit this time but perhaps would try later.

Although my opposition to tobacco has not wavered in the ensuing years, this man's words have often haunted me. Perhaps his real message was, "My wife wants me here, my foreman wants me here, but this is not *my* health goal," or even, "Look, buddy—you try thirty years of back-breaking work in the kind of job I have and then see how important your health promotion is to you!" Regardless of our idealism, health promoters should never lose sight of this popular axiom: "Everyone has to die of something." This is presented not to jaundice or discourage the reader, but so that important questions will be asked, real problems addressed, and the citizens' perspective kept in the forefront.

How do we know our health promotion interest coincides with those which the community really needs? Are we really thinking about something that will make a difference in the lives of the citizens of our community or target population? Is

our program going to benefit the same old privileged few and never really have an effect on the "person in the street"? Before developing a community organization and health promotion strategy, we need to examine the real situation, the "vision," and the analysis of the gap between the real and ideal.[2] Addressing the following questions should help us arrive at an appropriate strategy for a particular community.

First, consider the situation as it currently exists. Are the population's needs generally being met, especially with regard to education, meaningful and rewarding work, easy access to health services and transportation, appropriate and healthy nutrition, and adequate housing? Most importantly, to what extent do the citizens of the community feel they control necessary resources, and how much influence do they actually have in the community's decision-making? By not considering these issues, health promoters run the risk of extending the *quantity* of years of a group of people without improving *quality* of life.

Next, consider what the ideal community would look like. What would be the ideal decision-making process in this community? How should common community resources be allocated? What kind of access do people have to their local, regional, and national government? What kind of economic equality exists in the community and ideally, what should it be like? In terms of the physical environment, how safe, clean, and green is the community?

Third, consider and analyze the gap between the real and the ideal. Do the health and related problems correlate with political power and decision-making processes and structures? Are they associated with economic problems and power? Are there problems related to cumbersome and large bureaucracies which simply do not change? Who is benefiting from the current situation and how? Who is being hurt by the current situation and how?

Considering these data then leads us to our analysis of potential strategies for community organization. Questions we now want to ask ourselves include: How can community organizers and community citizens go about overcoming obstacles to improve health and the quality of life? What actions can we use to confront the problems and obstacles discussed earlier? What kinds of organizational, social, and political structures can be applied (e.g., private vs. public sector; labor, religious, economic and social organizations; political parties)? Who should be involved in the specific activity, and who can be counted upon for support? Who is unlikely to have an interest in the program, or might even seek to impede progress? What sorts of goals can be established, and how will we know when progress is being achieved?

Finally, cutting across all of these content areas is the mode of asking the questions. Are we as health professionals actually listening, or are we simply collecting a little bit of data to confirm our largely preset conclusions? Getting the community talking and maintaining this flow of input and information is a critical skill for health promoters.

As we can now see, community organization generally assumes a much different orientation than does problem- or disease-specific health promotion. On the other hand, it is likely the slower and more gradual improvements in health through active and aggressive community organization for health promotion will in the long term result in greater maintenance and generalization of health change than a more traditional approach.

MODELS OF COMMUNITY ORGANIZATION

One of the most influential writings in the area of community organization was published twenty-five years ago by Jack Rothman.[3] Rothman pointed out that community organization approaches have taken many forms in social work and related professional activities in that there is no "pure" approach to community organization. Community organization can include anything from politically conservative to relatively progressive activities, or a mixture of the two in one single effort. Rothman categorized the three general approaches to community organization as locality development, social action, and social planning, reflecting different activities along a conservative-activist dimension. (The acronym LAP will assist the reader's memory, with "L" for "locality" and "action" and "planning" represented by "AP.")

Social planning approaches look at specific problems and attempt to determine appropriate solutions to them. Social planners are likely to be advocates of specific policies or legislation which will protect or facilitate the population's health. **Social action** advocates, in direct contrast, assume that whatever problems exist are largely a function of inequality in a given system and therefore seek changes in the system.

Locality development[4] is a process-oriented approach to community organization involving self-help and grass-roots efforts in solving problems.

Differences in strategies among these categories parallel the differences in their orientation toward goals. Social action proponents tend to favor confrontation approaches which, in turn, lead to clarification of the positions and hopefully a recruitment of converts to the "cause." For example, anti-abortion and pro-choice protestors

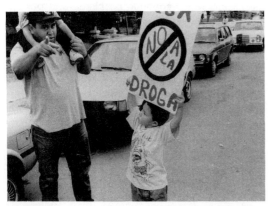
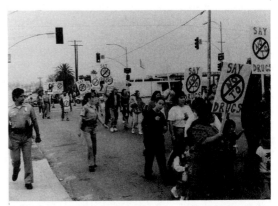

FIGURE 4–1. Locality development approaches emphasize a need for communities to assume responsibility for combating their own health problems. *Photo courtesy of Betsy Clapp.*

EXHIBIT 4-1

Multi-racial Community Coalition Building

Community organizers emphasizing environmental issues or other topics may find themselves at odds with economically disadvantaged, racially diverse groups in target areas. African Americans, Latinos, and Native Americans may have other priorities far more important to them than the white activists' agenda. Freudenberg* discussed methods to find a common ground. First, individuals from all groups need to educate one another about what they perceive to be pressing issues. Second, coalition building and priority setting must always address issues such as jobs and education. Finally, white environmentalists and other activists must oppose measures which place an undue burden on other ethnic neighborhoods; for example, by opposing a waste dump only because it is to be located in a white neighborhood.

*N. Freudenberg. (1984) *Not in our backyards! Community action for health and the environment.* New York: Monthly Review Press, pp. 212–215.

frequently confront police (and each other) purposefully and get arrested in order to get the abortion issue in the media.

Similarly, anti-apartheid demonstrators in the 1980s frequently crossed Washington, D.C. police lines in front of the South African Embassy in order to highlight their opposition to apartheid and hopefully gain support from the public in general. Social planners, in contrast, collect facts on the negative economic and social effects of, for instance, inadequate family values, sex education, or discriminatory policies, and present these data to people in powerful positions in our government and abroad. More in keeping with a "pure" community organization approach, locality development proponents would focus more on mobilizing a large cross-section of the population to discuss an issue and express itself at the polls rather than proposing a specific solution or arousing the public's emotions.

Another contrast in these three approaches is how they define the population being served by the community organization activities. Rothman sees social action constituents as victims seeking to redress previous ills, whereas social planning constituents are relatively passive consumers. In contrast, locality development clients are perceived as citizens engaging in a democratic, problem-solving process to address present or future community problems. In this sense, the social planning model is conceptually closer to a "medi-

cal" model of public health, often emphasizing the development and implementation of specific, expert-derived policies. In contrast, the locality development model tends to parallel more closely the social learning theory model of individual self-control. Social action proponents, in contrast, are often fighting against a specific policy (frequently, a governmental policy). Therefore, examples of social action approaches are perhaps less common in the health promotion literature.[5] Indeed, the bulk of health promotion research is funded by federal and state governments, while much of health promotion practice is sponsored by public or semi-public institutions (e.g., hospitals) which rely in part on governmental money for support. The implications of this funding, of course, are that such approaches would tend not to confront governmental policies.

Perhaps the writings of Saul Alinsky (based on his many experiences in social action in the turbulent 1960s) best reflect the political nature of the social action approach. For example, the following guidelines (partly tongue-in-cheek) are among the "rules" for community organization developed by Alinsky and give us some ideas of how he would go about organizing for change:[6]

Rule 1. Power is not only what you have but what the enemy thinks you have.

Rule 2. Never go outside the experience of your people.

Rule 3. Whenever possible go outside the experience of the enemy.

Rule 4. Make the enemy live up to their book of rules.

Rule 5. Ridicule is your best and most potent weapon.

Rule 6. A good tactic is one that your people enjoy. If your people are not having a ball doing it, there is something very wrong with the tactic.

Rule 7. A tactic that drags on too long becomes a drag. People can sustain militant interest in any issue for only a limited time.

Rule 8. Keep the pressure on with different tactics and actions and utilize all events of the period for your purpose.

Rule 9. The threat is usually more terrifying than the thing itself.

Rule 10. The major premise for tactics is the development of operations that will maintain a constant pressure upon the opposition . . . constant pressure sustains action.

The use of aggressive social action strategies, such as those proposed by Alinsky, have perhaps waned somewhat since the end of the Vietnam War era. However, individuals with active interest in specific health promotion issues—such as the tobacco problem—have used many of Alinsky's ideas to highlight specific health problems that for a variety of reasons have not been successfully dealt with by governmental or community problem-solving approaches. Although it can be argued that much progress has been realized in this country in the war against tobacco, there is no doubt we have a very long way to go. Indeed, it may be questioned whether the health promotion profession is leading the way or being led in the fight against tobacco use. The tobacco industry actually had a hand in many of the "victories" of the anti-tobacco conflict, following a highly organized and minimally expensive retreat from the social fabric of the American and other Western cultures. However, the industry is not without enemies. Doctors Ought to Care (DOC) is a good example of a social action-oriented organization

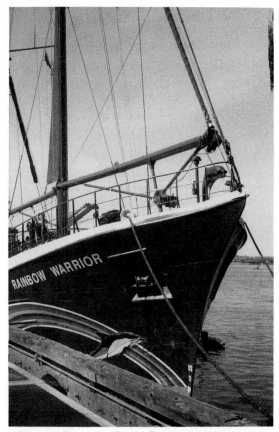

FIGURE 4–2. With their ship, the *Rainbow Warrior*, the social activist Green Peace organization has attracted headlines in their fight against pollution, the killing of endangered species, and the proliferation of nuclear weapons. *Photo courtesy of Betsy Clapp.*

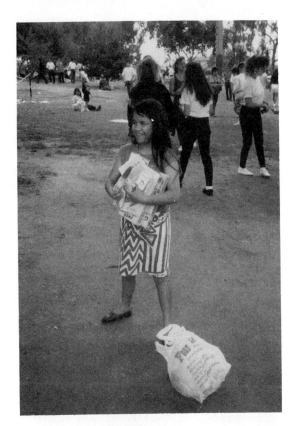
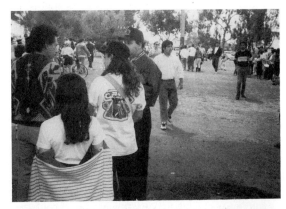
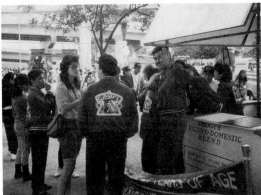
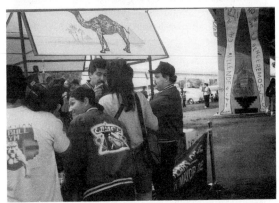

FIGURE 4–3.   Social activism disrupts a tobacco promotion. Many tobacco companies promote their products by showing up at special community events and giving away free samples and other tobacco related paraphenalia. While the promotions are not necessarily aimed at children, cigarettes often end up in their hands. At a recent promotion at Chicano Park in San Diego, anti-tobacco activists followed "roamers" who were strolling around the park at the festival and giving out free samples of tobacco. The young girl in the center above is handing a "stop smoking" flier to a man as he is receiving a free pack of cigarettes. Later, these "roamers" felt harried and gave up, returning to their central booth. At that booth, another activist took pictures of the Camel employees as they gave out packs of cigarettes to individuals standing in line. Eventually, the exchange between the activist and the employees became heated and the camera was shoved in her face. Realizing that they had perhaps overstepped their bounds, the Camel group closed up their booth and left. *Photo courtesy of John Elder.*

which frequently attacks the tobacco industry with a variety of strategies, including ridicule and constant and varied pressure (see chapter 16). Social action against the tobacco industry is necessitated by the fact that the government is largely (albeit quietly) supportive of the industry's viability and "rights." At times, the principles of health promotion advocated in the Alma Ata declaration simply cannot be realized through social planning or locality development strategies, even though the current text generally supports the capacity-building philosophy of these approaches. In such cases, social action and other more political strategies require consideration by responsible health professionals.

Political Strategies

General "Rules of Thumb."   A toxic dump has been found near the city, and the county government has yet to take any action. Activists from across the state embark upon an initiative to increase taxes on cigarettes, and we would like to see our community get involved. A neighborhood within the city where very few primary health care services are available is underrepresented in the electorate, and we would like to see an increase in the number of voters in this group. Where do we start?

With appropriate political skills, health promoters and other professionals, or any citizen for that matter, can be influential in health-related public affairs. Although specific political strategies vary according to the situation, they often follow the basic logic[7] of: (a) starting at the beginning, (b) sustaining and focusing the action, (c) understanding governmental actions, (d) providing public information, (e) forming alliances, and (f) promoting membership *esprit de corps.*

Understanding the political process allows us to get our citizens' group involved at the beginning of that process. During drafting of legislation or citizen-based initiatives, citizen input can be very helpful in ensuring that initiatives and bills will have substantial popular support as well as assistance from the "powers-that-be." Sustained action refers to planning a political activity to have continued "presence" in the public eye. Resistance can easily overcome action which is short-lived and perhaps does not even last until election day. "Focused action" refers to the need to select a limited number of clearly defined targets and maintain efforts toward achieving goals related to these targets. Clear-cut goals increase the likelihood of accomplishment.

Understanding the process of government is a prerequisite to political change. We need to know when and where to intervene on the drafting of legislative bills, committee hearings, voter registration drives, and other potential points of impact for changing city hall. Public information can be an important method of ensuring community participation and interest in the topic. At times, dramatic Alinsky-esque events may be needed to ensure media interest in our program or initiative. Environmental activities in the Greenpeace organization have demonstrated the effectiveness of this strategy on numerous occasions.

In order to ensure we have adequate power and resources to accomplish our political-change goals, we need to determine what other agencies or entities in the community are involved in the issue at hand. Sometimes this alliance formation leads to "strange bedfellows"; indeed, we may be unable politically to afford the formation of certain alliances. However, we must be able to contact other people doing work in our area of interest, since at a minimum we will want to make sure we do not unnecessarily anger others by invading their "turf." Finally, we may manage to ensure the participation of a few very active volunteers or other participants in our community organization process. There will be a need to make these people feel they are a "cadre" and have a certain status, based on their participation in our program. In order to develop this esprit de corps, it is sometimes necessary to remind people of the substantial contributions they can make to the well-being of a community. This often requires a very skillful and energetic leader who is quick to reinforce participants for their contributions to the health promotion/political organization effort.

Getting Out the Vote.   The two fundamental approaches to political action are: (a) influencing legislation or policy, and (b) going directly to the voters to influence them to vote a certain way. One approach to ensuring the community has true "ownership" of a given political process is to focus on an underrepresented population in the electorate and increase their voting numbers. Whether we are interested in simply increasing the overall representation of our target population in the electorate or specifically motivating them to vote for a certain issue, we can benefit greatly from efforts to "get out the vote."

Three rules of thumb apply to effective voter mobilization efforts. First, door-to-door canvasing with face-to-face contact works much better than either mail or phone work. Of course, the resources required for appropriate door-to-door canvasing can be extensive. Second, multiple contacts are more effective than one or a few contacts. Campaign workers, candidates, and others should make a concerted effort to get back to target voters as many times as possible. Finally, focused efforts work better than diffuse efforts. Through a marketing analysis (chapter 10), we can determine where our supporters are likely to reside, and we can avoid working areas where a large percentage of opposition voters live.[8]

Obviously, some individuals may not be eligible to vote simply because they have not registered. Again, we might wish to target them for voter registration drives in order to ensure our side of the story is being represented in the election outcome. In voter registration drives, we may wish to enlist the support of the League of Women Voters, churches, various civic or business groups, public interest groups, unions, or even political parties to ensure we are maximizing the potential gain from our resources.

The following questions should precede the implementation of a voter registration activity:

1. What are the goals of the voter registration drive (e.g., to elect a specific candidate, to get rid of an official who has been in the way of needed reforms, to pass or defeat a referendum or initiative, to raise people's consciousness about a specific issue, to put pressure on the government by making officials take notice)?
2. Whom do we want to reach?
3. Where do we want the voter registration drive to take place?
4. What should we do to conduct a voter registration drive?
5. When is the best time for the voter registration drive?
6. Who are the existing leaders of our target groups, and how will they feel about our voter registration activities?[9]

Influencing the Legislative Process. The law is a potentially powerful tool for supporting or even leading the way in health promotion efforts. In tobacco control, for instance, legislation can:

1. establish policy on production, promotion, and use of tobacco;
2. encourage smokers to stop and youth not to start;
3. provide protection against environmental smoke;
4. monitor and control the content of tobacco products;
5. contribute to the development of an anti-tobacco social climate;
6. provide tobacco control resources;
7. provide a legal basis for the enforcement of tobacco control policy; and
8. put government on the side of health.[10]

In order to influence the legislative process, we need to know something about politicians and other decision makers in our community. First, we need to know our national as well as state senators and representatives, what form of government our community has and its chief officials, the members of the school board, and representatives of other political offices or entities in the community. We also need to know what the critical issues affecting our population have been in the past few years and what stance local politicians have taken with respect to these issues. Next, we should know who in the community are the major formal and informal religious, social service, business and labor, legal, health, and other civic leaders. Why are they considered leaders, and what issues have they focused on in the past? Who are their constituents and to what powers do they respond?

Next, we need to know the economic decision makers in the community and in what issues they have been involved. Leaders of banks, major property owners or heads of real estate companies can give us a clue as to who the real powers are in a community. We also want to see what their involvement with major social issues in the community has been, and for what reason.

Once we have constructed a "who's who" of the community's formal and informal leadership, we want to know how these influential people perceive the community's problems and their potential solutions. Are there differences in the way these various people approach this problem solu-

TABLE 4–1
Strategies for Different Actions

Legislative Step	Action Required of Us	Key People to Contact	How to Contact
1. Research the best way to get a bill sponsored	Make decisions: What should the bill say? Who (legislator) should sponsor the bill? When should the bill be introduced?	Legislative aide/committee staff for committee reports, general information on committee; newspaper for information on committee issue; legislative directories;	Phone/Meeting Visit Library Research
	How should strategy be developed? Which committee should it go to? Who will look the most favorable on it? What is the committee like? Who are supporters? Opposers? How do we activate supporters/		
	Do a head count of the committee. Ask each one if he will vote for or against.	All members	Phone/meeting

78

2. Getting a bill written	Impress legislators with the need for the bill.	Individual legislator and/or the legislative or committee aide	Meeting
	Compile evidence on the need for the bill in legislative packet	Meet with other possible supporters and those who can provide evidence of need for bill.	Meeting
3. Getting the bill through subcommittee	Get the leadership to endorse the bill or at least not oppose it.	Leadership through your legislator	Attend hearings, provide written information (legislative packet)
4. Getting bill through committee	Work with subcommittee designee to develop strategy.	Leadership through your legislator and committee staff	Meeting
	Work to get the leadership to endorse.	People to testify (updated)	More legislative packets
	Be ready to accommodate amendments.		
5. Mark-up on the bill	Meet with aides to get bill written in your favor.	Right aides	Meeting/phone
6. Getting bill through full legislative body	Hold a strategy meeting.	Aide, leadership of bill	Meeting/phone
7. Executive passage	Gather public support.	Supporters, media	Cards, letters, calls
	Be ready to accommodate amendments.	Executive aides	Meeting/phone
	Contact Executive office.		

SOURCE: In G. Speeter. (1978). *Playing their game our way*. Amherst, MA: Citizens Involvement Training Project, p. 70.

tion? This could prove very helpful in determining whom we should contact in a policy change effort and from whom we should expect resistance.

After we compile our "who's who," it is time to get the legislative process rolling. Table 4–1 presents the strategies for different actions that community organizers can take with respect to legislative actions, which may be applied to city councils, regional planning boards, state or even federal legislatures. These steps range from pre-draft to executive passage of the bill.

Few health promoters pay much attention to political action. Such activities are often beyond the scope of or even prescribed by our various jobs. Second, we may see this as less relevant or less professionally reinforcing than "patient contact" or other more typical duties to which health promoters are assigned. Although there is no doubt health promotion politics can be very trying and frustrating compared to more tangible results from working with individuals or small groups, we want to emphasize that perhaps no other activity can be more important than political actions which influence entire communities or even larger population segments. Always remember: *someone* makes political decisions which influence our health, whether or not we participate.

LOGISTICAL CONSIDERATIONS IN COMMUNITY ORGANIZATION

"Community Organization for Primary Health Care" (PRICOR)[11] has detailed a variety of logistical problems, decisions, and constraints to be considered when developing a community organization strategy. They have divided these variables into categories of initiating contacts, setting objectives, determining strategies and functions, determining the community organization's structure, and implementing community organization activities.

In our initial work with the community, we need to consider a variety of issues, such as how to initiate contacts with political, civic, business, and voluntary organization leaders, the amount of time and resources we will need for this, an analysis of the "power networks," a needs assessment of the community's health and related problems, and how to secure commitment from various decision makers and representatives.

A very important phase following the above is the establishment of organizational objectives. Decision makers will set resource and operational objectives (e.g., staffing, budgetary) and establish health objectives (e.g., determining key health problems, choosing among health promotion, protection or prevention activities, and selecting subpopulations for special focus). Implicitly at least, this group will also set "equity objectives." In other words, this group will determine the program's donors and beneficiaries. PRICOR cautions that generally the community's privileged class benefits most from primary health care programs, different constituents will have different priorities, and objectives will change over time. Strategies must be chosen in this context.

Once objectives are set, problem-solving approaches or other decision-making methods can be used to brainstorm these strategies, while the various participants in the decision-making group may have differing roles at this time (e.g., "experts" in a given health problem may come to the forefront, whereas political leaders who know less about health per se may not actually participate in a specific brainstorming of strategies). Consistent with social action strategies, PRICOR advises us to start with activities that can yield quick success in order to keep our initial participants interested. More difficult and time-consuming efforts should be tackled later.

Subsequently, we should develop a structure for our community organization. Will this structure be formal or informal, will it be established for a one-time only health promotion effort, or will it be ongoing? Should we work within an existing agency or program or should we create a new one? Who will be our constituency and how will they be represented in decision making? How large an area or population should we work with? How will our leadership be chosen, what duties should they have, and how and when will they be replaced? Next, how will we determine what decision-making processes we should use? PRICOR notes that building on existing structures and working with multi-purpose rather than single-purpose organizations tend to result in more successful and efficient efforts.

Finally, we need to consider day-to-day operational issues, including personnel and their schedules, the location of our physical facility, methods we will use to stay in touch with the community, and what training our personnel should have and when.

SUMMARY

In our years of work in physical and mental health promotion, we have often heard clinicians describe their work as "half science, half art." In other words, patient contact involves far more than rote memorization of a diagnosis-treatment algorithm, especially when patients need to be involved in their own treatment. The human interactive process and its corresponding subtleties may determine whether we will be successful.

The complexities involved in understanding the processes and power relationships attending community organization efforts are perhaps a hundredfold greater than those related to examining clinician-patient interactions. Neither social planners, social activists nor grassroots "developers" can prescribe a step-by-step approach to community change, as each community is different, each changes at different rates and in different ways, and each community organizer has a unique style and impact on other people.

After reading this text, you will have been introduced to community organization, behavior modification, social marketing techniques, and other community health promotion tools. These approaches can be applied to entire communities as well as their constituent organizations, support networks/groups, and individuals simultaneously or sequentially.

By its very nature, community organization for health promotion is a complicated and value-oriented topic, much more so than the other core health promotion techniques. It is difficult to present a step-by-step solution for analyzing and resolving community problems. The **ONPRIME** process is sufficiently flexible to allow the community to participate in determining its own problems. Although community participants may not have the expertise to actually conduct or analyze needs assessments or develop specific communication or behavior change strategies, they can realize an ownership of the program by participating in planning, goal setting, research, and implementation of intervention activities. In fact, they can (and should) participate in needs and resource assessment and other data gathering activities, presented next.

ADDITIONAL READINGS

When you join the protest march, keep these in your pocket:

1. Jack Rothman. (1968). Three models of social work practice. In *Social work practice: Proceedings, National Conference on Social Welfare.* New York: Columbia University Press.
2. Paulo Freire. (1970). *Pedagogy of the oppressed.* New York: Herter.
3. Nicholas Freudenberg. (1984). *Not in our backyards! Community action for health and the environment.* New York: Monthly Review Press.

EXERCISE

Divide your class or a subset of it into three groups: locality developers, planners and activists. Select a health issue, and as you proceed through chapters 4 through 11, sketch out your approach to a health promotion effort for each of the **ONPRIME** steps.

ENDNOTES

1. PRICOR. (1986). *Community organization for primary health care.* Arlington, VA: PRICOR.
2. Speeter, G. (1978). Power: *A repossession manual.* Amherst, MA: Citizens Involvement Training Project (UMASS).
3. Rothman, J. (1968). Three models of social work practice. In *Social work practice: Proceedings.* National Conference on Social Welfare. New York: Columbia University Press.
4. "Locality" as used in this context does not refer to a specific geographic location, but instead implies "grassroots" or "local" capacity.
5. An interesting observation of the development of the field of health promotion: as with other disciplines, our research conventions, published literature, and health agencies tend to be dominated by people with doctoral degrees or who are in other ways "experts." In turn, health promotion leader-

ship and the development of the field takes on a social planning flavor, with the activists in the streets having less access to established lines of communication and mechanisms of power. On the other hand, social activist groups are often guilty of assuming expertise in a given conflict, and implicitly, assuming the public would support them if only the facts were known. While looking and behaving differently, they may at times emulate social planners.

6. Alinsky, S. (1971). *Reveille for radicals.* New York: Vintage Press.

7. Speeter, G. (1978). *Playing their game our way.* Amherst, MA: Citizens Involvement Training Project [UMASS].

8. As the reader will note in Chapter 10, these rules apply to social marketing interventions as well.

9. Speeter, *Playing their game our way.*

10. U.S. Department of Health and Human Services. (1992). *Smoking and Health in the Americas.* Atlanta: USDHHS/CDC (92-8419).

11. PRICOR, *Community organization for primary health care.*

Chapter 5

Assessing Needs and Resources and Setting Priorities

OBJECTIVES

By the end of this chapter, the reader should be able to:

1. Define, describe, and give examples of:
   a. needs/resources assessment
   b. key informant interview
   c. community forum
   d. rates-under-treatment
   e. archival research
   f. surveys
2. Describe the steps for setting needs/resources assessment objectives.
3. Describe similarities and differences between needs/resources assessment and research.
4. Given a description of a community and its health problem, develop a needs/resources assessment (N/RA) strategy and appropriate N/RA instruments. Then add additional questions or variables based on the organizational strategy used.

BACKGROUND

We now turn our attention to the intertwined processes of determining the specific needs of a community or group, setting health promotion priorities, and assessing the resources available for meeting a community's health needs. This critical step in health promotion is frequently overlooked or given insufficient emphasis. Health professionals are often more highly skilled in intervention design or research, or are funded for these activities from external agencies. Nevertheless, the success of a program may hinge on knowing what the target population needs and wants, how to set priorities, and what steps can be taken to optimize the attainment of program goals.

Needs and resources assessment (N/RA) for health promotion is research and planning activities used to determine (a) a community's health behavior patterns, (b) the extent and kind of health needs and priorities in the community, and (c) approaches and resources to deal with these needs.

Thus, needs and resources assessment comprises a category of research — specifically, that used for setting priorities and program planning. Therefore, the techniques described in this chapter will overlap with those in chapters 7 and 11 and with formative research approaches described in chapter 6. Needs and Resources Assessment, however, is research with a "small r": it is less structured, requires less technical training to conduct, and varies substantially from program to program and community to community. Nevertheless, it is a priority activity in the ONPRIME sequence and takes (at least temporal) precedence over research with regard to understanding a given community's priorities and potential. Once organizational and program governance considerations have been addressed, understanding a community's priorities and potential is the next step in the planning-intervention-evaluation process.

The ONPRIME model includes the term "resources" in what is typically called needs assessment. This affirmative version of the more common phrase symbolizes the fact that all communities have strengths, capabilities, and a track record of successful approaches to deal with health-related challenges. Thus, we should avoid invoking the medical model approach of trying to do things to the community, rather than working as a partner with the community and its representatives. This partnership process begins early, with establishing the objectives for the needs and resources assessment.

SETTING OBJECTIVES FOR THE NEEDS/RESOURCES ASSESSMENT ACTIVITY

While health professionals may have the necessary skills to coordinate and carry out the needs/resources assessment, the steering committee, advisory committee, or board of directors should provide the direction for defining, conceptualizing, and operationalizing the objectives for the N/RA. Together with the professional staff, they should begin by addressing questions like the following:

1. What do we want and need to know?
2. Why do we want to know this particular information?
3. How will this information be used?
4. Where and how can we obtain this information?
5. What useful data sources (state, federal, local) already exist? Who in the community could

serve as "key informants"? Who among us should contact these individuals?
6. What other community agencies or entities have an interest in this issue? Should they be involved? Why or why not?
7. Do we need technical assistance? Where can we get it?
8. How much will the N/RA cost?[1] How much time and what resources exist to put into this program's effort?

The process of setting N/RA objectives may occur in a variety of ways, depending on who constitutes the governing body (or management team), what roles they have in the project, and what background and health expertise they have. A pre-existing and sophisticated health agency board may add a number of other questions to those listed above and increase the level of complexity, with minimal guidance from the professional staff. An ad hoc advisory committee, consisting of individuals with less education and little or no experience in establishing community health goals, may initially lack the assertiveness to express themselves fully in conversations leading to goal setting. A personnel manager in a large worksite may simply hand the health staff a list of expectations relating to the N/RA (or may suggest skipping this important step altogether!). The health professional is saddled with the delicate task of ensuring that (a) a valid assessment of practices, problems, and resources takes place; (b) the individuals or group helping set the N/RA objectives represent the ultimate target population; and (c) if external funding has been obtained, the requirements attached to this funding are met. At times, health promoters are faced with an inability to meet each of these three criteria totally. However, we should ensure that at a minimum we do not leave any criterion unaddressed altogether.

TYPES OF NEEDS/ RESOURCES ASSESSMENT

Needs/Resources Assessment techniques generally consist of variations of key informant interviews, archival research, rates-under-treatment assessment and surveys (represented by the acronym KARS). Community forums and participant or non-participant observations may also be used to gather important information at the N/RA stage of a program. However, due to logistical and political considerations, the forum is used less frequently than the previous four categories. (Observational procedures are detailed in chapter 3.)

Key Informant Interviews

Key informant interviews (KII) are conducted with people "in the know"—individuals who are very familiar with a community and its people, its health behavior patterns, health needs, and intervention techniques appropriate or inappropriate for the community. The program's governance should be able to provide invaluable input regarding who should be contacted, whereas the health professional staff can provide guidance as to what types of individuals are generally contacted in KII. Religious and political leaders, business and labor representatives, public health staff and physicians, and heads of service agencies and social organizations are among those typically able to provide insight into a community's health. Yet more important and at the same time more difficult to identify are the community's informal leaders, those who may not have a specific title but are very important "opinion leaders." The roster of key informants will vary substantially from one community to another.

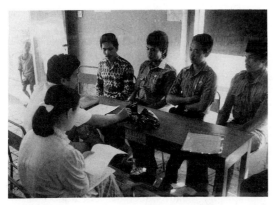

FIGURE 5–1. Key informant interviews, such as those being conducted with four village chiefs in Indonesia, can provide valuable short cuts for determining a community's health needs or designing interventions. *Photo courtesy of John Elder.*

The specific steps involved in the KII are as follows:

1. Discuss the implications of the N/RA objectives for the KII effort.
2. Construct a questionnaire consisting largely of open-ended "discussion" questions, with direct objective items added as needed. The wording of the questions should strike a balance between getting at the information needed and not appearing confrontative or "nosey." Also, care should be taken to minimize the time required of these typically busy individuals.
3. Draw up a list of potential interviewees with direction from the program governance. This list should contain the types of individuals described in the preceding paragraph. However, this list need not be exhaustive, only representative and inclusive of important political considerations.
4. Determine which staff and directors are going to contact the interviewees, and then conduct the interviews.
5. Decide whether KIIs will be face-to-face, conducted by phone, or processed through the mail. Face-to-face interviews are preferable, and phone interviews are superior to mail surveys. The former two provide a more personal touch and generally elicit more expansive responses, while allowing the key informant to get to know something about the program and its staff. However, some interviewees will prefer to respond to the questions by mail. (Some N/RAs may use two or all three of these modes of KII administration.)
6. Conduct the interviews and summarize the data, emphasizing the consistencies and inconsistencies among the respondents' answers.

Archival Research

Archival research (also known as "secondary research") takes advantage of work already accomplished. By locating existing sources of data (or "archives"), extracting relevant information and presenting these data to the program governance, we save invaluable time and resources. Indeed, many forms of archival data (such as state health department morbidity and mortality

TABLE 5–1
Advantages and Disadvantages of Major Needs and Resources Assessment (N/RA) Techniques

Method	Advantages	Disadvantages
Key Informant Interview	1. Straightforward 2. Inexpensive 3. Encourages broad discussion of issues 4. Lines of communication established 5. Unifies staff and orients them to more focused and well-defined issues	1. Selection or response bias may limit validity of data
Archival Research	1. Relatively more reliable data 2. Reference to such data enhances program credibility	1. Data may not be relevant to specific purposes of progam 2. May be difficult or time consuming to access, especially confidential data 3. Certain inherent biases, depending on nature and purpose of the data
Rates Under Treatment	1. Relatively available and inexpensive data 2. Reliable 3. Promotes community awareness of the need to integrate services.	1. Illness- and victim-focused 2. Bias from fact that people seek available treatment, not necessarily treatment they need most 3. Cannot be used to estimate population prevalence rates
Surveys	1. Most representative 2. Can be used to identify early adopters	1. Can be expensive 2. Potential for "victim focus"

records) would simply be impossible to obtain through other means.

Although some sources of archival data are obvious, others depend on the intuition and experience of the health professional. In the former category, census data can characterize a region's population, whereas local, state, and national health agencies provide a wide variety of details regarding diseases and their outcomes—mortality and morbidity. Occasionally, these governmental agencies also provide information on the prevalence of specific health-related behaviors

collected through public surveys or by other means. Data from these sources are usually summarized in reports but may also be available on computer files.

Other sources of archival data will depend on the specific health issue, the orientation of the person conducting this research, and any gaps left by other N/RA efforts. Police and motor vehicle records, grocery store inventories, newspapers and organizational newsletters, and school attendance and other records can shed light on the issues related to a health promotion program.

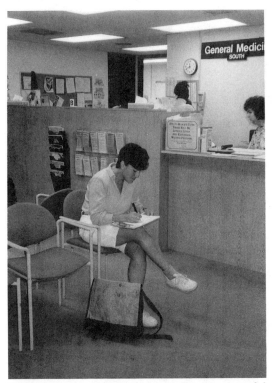

FIGURE 5-2. Patient records provide a useful source of data for health professionals conducting rates-under-treatment or other types of archive research. *Photo courtesy of Betsy Clapp.*

Often, these data may be in condensed forms: school district or chamber of commerce annual reports, or even general information from city hall or local libraries can save the person compiling the information valuable time.

Rates-Under-Treatment

Rates-under-treatment (RUT) assessment represents a special category of archival research which involves visiting local or regional hospitals and clinics and gaining access to reports, computer files or individual patient records. The purpose of RUT is to assess the number of people receiving treatment for various afflictions. Concurrent assessment of potential health problems other than the presenting one (e.g., high blood pressure or cholesterol) can also be accom-

plished asssuming such information is routinely charted. Like archival research, RUT may 'miss the mark,' compelling the researcher to sift through extensive information in order to locate small bits of relevant data. Additionally, RUT inherently is more illness-oriented than other approaches. In certain health promotion programs, however, such information may be necessary.

Table 5.1 summarizes the advantages and disadvantages of these N/RA techniques.

NEEDS/RESOURCES ASSESSMENT ORGANIZATIONAL STRATEGY AND APPROACH

Anyone who suggests that research is "value free" is probably not in touch with his or her values. Needs and resources assessment research is probably even more subject to influences of the values of the researcher than the more "scientific" techniques discussed in the following chapter. As we have seen in chapter 4, the entire ONPRIME sequence gains its flavor from its initial grounding in locality development, social action, or social planning strategies. The relative emphases these receive will also influence the manner in which the N/RA is approached.

Just as there is probably no "pure" community organizational strategy, individuals conducting N/RA with similar resources and targets will for the most part go about their jobs in equivalent fashions. Nevertheless, question content and N/RA approaches may vary according to organizational philosophy, as shown in Table 5-2. The tone of N/RA effort will be relatively paternalistic, democratic or activist if based in social planning, locality development, or social action, respectively.

THE PROJECT SALSA NEEDS/ RESOURCES ASSESSMENT

Project Salsa is a nutritional health promotion program for the largely Latino population of San Ysidro, California. "Salsa's" strategies are based primarily in a locality development model, selected because of the perceived sense of powerlessness among the population of this community.

One of the first activities of the Project Salsa advisory committee was to establish specific needs and resource assessment study objectives.

TABLE 5–2

Special Features and Types of Questions of Needs and Resource Assessment by Type of Organizational Philosophy

	Key Informant Interview	Archival Research	Rates-Under-Treatment	Surveys
Locality Development	Potential for involvement in program or "permission" for access to population	Community's history of self-help	How: referral sources, payment methods, follow-up rates	Membership in community groups; personal problem-solving approaches
Social Action	"Friend or enemy?"	"Investigative reporting," or more background on health issue	Who gets served—and who doesn't	Anger/emotion felt about issue; willingness to enlist in cause
Social Planning	Recruitment into planning group or acceptance of program	Mortality and morbidity patterns	What: enumeration of reasons for referral and other risk factors noted in medical records	Health behaviors, risks, and illness patterns

While the Salsa staff conducted the N/RA for the community and its nutritional problems, the advisory council helped determine the N/RA priorities. They discussed the need to identify specific community leaders, media sources, nutritional information, and other factors not typically thought of in the needs or resource assessment related to a specific health promotion problem. The Salsa staff then carried out the N/RA working within the study objectives established by the advisory council.

The needs and resource assessment consisted of key informant interviews, community forums, surveys, social indicator assessment, and other archival research. Key informant interviews were semi-structured discussions with key individuals (as identified by the advisory council) in the community with respect to their opinions of the community's health and general problems. These political and civic leaders then identified additional individuals whom they felt might be appropriate for such interviews. Subsequent individuals identified by two or more of the initial key informants were included on the list of people to be interviewed. The data collected from the key informant interviews were largely qualitative in nature. This gave the staff a good idea of the power structure in the community, who should be invited on the advisory council, and specific information related to the nutritional and health problems of the community. Equally important was the information gathered about what existing resources were being used to address these problems.

The specific key informant interview questions were as follows:

1. "What, in your opinion, are the 3 most important issues in order of importance related to San Ysidro (the community in which Project Salsa was based)?"
2. "Where do you rank nutritional health issues on the community agenda? Why?"
3. "How do you rate your organization's level of involvement in San Ysidro affairs?" (1 = very inactive; 5 = very active)
4. "In what ways is your organization most involved?"
5. "What major issues has your organization been involved in recently?"
6. "What types of organizations has your orga-

nization worked with in San Ysidro in the past 1–2 years?"
7. "Are there any groups with which your organization has had difficulty working? Why were there problems?"
8. "Briefly, in your opinion, what types of approaches will be effective in dealing with nutritional health issues in San Ysidro?"
9. "What kinds of regional or local resources exist which could be useful in dealing with nutritional health issues?"
10. "Who, in your opinion, is a champion of change in San Ysidro?"
11. "In what ways could we reward those who give assistance to Project Salsa?"
12. "In what ways can our groups work together?"

Results of the key informant surveys among political, religious, and other community leaders showed the most pressing problems of the community to be (1) economic issues such as lack of jobs (ranked first by 20 percent of the informants); (2) educational issues, especially the need for bilingual education (17 percent); (3) health issues, especially a lack of services and access to them (11 percent); and (4) powerlessness vis-à-vis the political process in San Diego and elsewhere. When prompted, 16 percent ranked nutritional health "high," 34 percent "in the middle," and 42 percent "low" on the community agenda, indicating a need to position nutritional health promotion within the context of the other more highly ranked issues. However, the most important result of the key informant interviews was the acquaintance ships developed with them by project staff (few of whom were from the community).

An additional group of key informants targeted for this phase of the N/RA were grocery store owners and managers. They reported that the bulk of their clients were Spanish-speaking Latinos, though many drove vehicles with Mexican license plates (indicating residence in neighboring Tijuana). Although they perceived that their customers were very concerned about nutritional issues, they reported no nutritional health promotion activities. Anticipating trends toward healthier eating and Salsa's potential for accelerating such changes, all stores indicated an interest in participating with the project. These expressions of interest turned out to be valid; many stores even provided funding and other resources for various project activities.

A Salsa-sponsored community forum was initially planned whereby individuals could represent themselves and speak publicly regarding health or civic priorities. Instead, given that the community was already actively involved in their monthly school board meetings, the project staff decided to be regular visitors at the school board meetings in order to "keep their fingers on the pulse of the community." Visits to these meetings indicated opportunities for a variety of intervention opportunities, particularly those oriented toward children. Participants in the meetings were unexpectedly vocal in their concerns about administrative and academic issues, indicating possible sources of contention or conflict for interventions requiring the cooperation of visible school officials. (Indeed, this proved to be an issue. A variety of the school district's administrative and nutrition personnel who initially supported Project Salsa quit or were forced to resign during the course of the project's implementation).

Archival and rates-under-treatment assessment were then used to define the more global problems of the community. Reviews of various newspaper articles, police records, immigration records, and other sources showed that crime and drug use were perhaps more pressing problems from the community's perspective than was nutrition per se. Using these data, Project Salsa staff decided to participate in activities which addressed these issues as well as nutritional problems. By reviewing county and state records to determine specific morbidity and mortality data, health clinic data, food stamp information, and other public access information, Salsa staff were able to learn even more about issues pertaining to nutritional needs of the community. Additionally, literature searches on the nutritional health of Mexican-Americans provided a more global picture of the health-related problems of this Latino community.

This phase of the Project Salsa N/RA was greatly facilitated by the preexistence of two documents: *Adelante! San Ysidro*, a study commissioned by the San Ysidro Chamber of Commerce; and a *primary health care profile* developed by the San Ysidro Health Center, which serves the bulk of the disadvantaged population of this community. The former document focused on eco-

nomic issues and approaches to improving the commercial and financial well being of the community. However, it also provided insight into a variety of other long-standing issues and realities affecting the city. First, it noted that freeway construction over twenty years has split the community apart to the point where it has lost its former identity. Second, the community is highly dependent not only on the health of the U.S. economy but also on that of Mexico, as many Mexicans cross into U.S. border communities to shop. Nevertheless, whereas San Diego and Tijuana realize many economic benefits of being border communities, these benefits seem to elude San Ysidro. Third, the city of San Diego has focused housing project development in relatively remote and unempowered San Ysidro, bringing a variety of "outsiders" from other ethnic and linguistic groups into the community. Finally, this study pointed out a widely known fact to Southern Californians and Mexicans alike: tens of thousands of undocumented migrants cross the border northward annually, many of them through this area.

The Health Center's data emphasized patients' profiles and needs. With over half of the community living at or below poverty and nearly 60 percent having no health insurance, subsidized care is clearly needed. Indeed, from 1978 to 1988, the Health Center's service demand increased 225 percent. Demands for pediatric services are 50 percent greater than typical for the national population. Among adults, hypertension, diabetes, and cardiovascular disease are the most typical diagnoses.

Surveys of the community residents were developed to determine statistically the health-related practices and problems of the community. Given the inexpensiveness and apparent receptivity of the community to this technique, Project Salsa staff decided to use a random digit dialing telephone survey followed-up by in-house surveys to obtain further detail. These data were the most statistically reliable and representative of the various needs assessment techniques used, although an extensive amount of staff resources were required to conduct this survey (in both English and Spanish).

The Salsa phone survey emphasized not only eating habits per se but also the shopping, food preparation, and other nutritional decision-making and related behaviors among the homemakers of the community. More general questions about health interests, social networks, and other issues were also asked. Two variables shed light on the kinds of responses attained. In terms of shopping habits, 86 percent of the respondents reported looking for sales when they shopped and 76 percent before they shopped; 72 percent reported reading food labels; and 56 percent shopped with discount coupons. In terms of program interests, 70 percent reported an interest in cholesterol screening; 70 percent in diabetes screening; 67 percent in blood pressure screening; and 51 percent in taste-testing new foods. Although additional formative research (of the nature described in chapter 10) was required to design the actual interventions, these data demonstrated the potential payoff for devoting part of the project's resources for a grocery store-based intervention.

The next step in the community organization plan was to analyze, summarize, and report the data to the advisory council, in order for them to set priorities. The council looked at the health problems, ranging from pregnant women to the elderly, and determined which problems were the most pressing and needed to be addressed first. Whereas the staff had initially thought that heart disease and cancer prevention in adults would be an initial priority, the advisory council decided instead to place the initial emphasis on breast feeding and nutritional health promotion for

school children. The staff then selected specific community organization, social marketing/communication, and motivational strategies to meet these goals and objectives established by the advisory council. When there was some doubt as to the best way to proceed, additional formative research through small studies or focus groups was conducted, while ongoing programs were evaluated using "quality assurance" research to ensure the achievement of appropriate results.

SUMMARY

In summary, the N/RA research tool kit is an important part of any health promotion effort. Effective community change efforts may indeed prove impossible without it, even for professionals highly familiar with a target community.

The process of priority setting will depend largely on the organizational strategy and philosophy being followed, while the priorities themselves should be based on the specific N/RA results. Variations in the process of priority setting are presented in Table 5–3. Regardless of the process followed, the end product should be specific, attainable goals and objectives, characteristics of which are amplified in Chapter 7. But first, Chapter 6 will present health promotion research strat-

TABLE 5–3
Priority Setting Process and Examples, by Organizational Strategy

Strategy	*Process*	*Example*
Locality Development	Sharing information with public; democratic or consensus-based decisions made by population or its representatives	Coalition for a Healthy California placed "Proposition 99" on the ballot, a resulting 25¢ tax increase for cigarettes (Chapter 17)
Social Action	Priority or strategy selected based largely on its emotional appeal	MADD's emphasis on punishing drunk drivers
Social Planning	Priorities established by health experts	U.S. National High Blood Pressure Education Program

egies appropriate for filling in any gaps in knowledge identified in the N/RA phase.

ADDITIONAL READINGS

Those needing an additional resource should consult:

L. Green, M. Kreuter, S. Deeds, & K. Partridge. (1980). *Health education planning: A diagnostic approach.* Palo Alto, CA: Mayfield.

EXERCISE

In teams of three or four, design and conduct a "mini" N/RA for a health problem in your community. After designing instruments, select and interview a few key informants and community residents. Review existing data. Integrate findings from these diverse sources and present a summary.

ENDNOTES

1. Wahreit, G., Bell, R., & Schwab, J. (1977). *Needs Assessment Approaches: Concepts and Methods.* Rockville, MD: U.S. Department of Health, Education and Welfare, pp. 12–13.

Chapter 6

Health Promotion Research

At the end of this chapter, the reader should be able to:

1. Define the following terms with "real-world" examples:
   - "AB" research designs
   - "ABA" or reversal research designs
   - covariance
   - epidemiology prevalence
   - false negative
   - false positive
   - focus group
   - gatekeeper review
   - incidence
   - in-depth interview
   - longitudinal studies
   - multiple baseline designs
   - negative association
   - positive association
   - pre-testing
   - prevalence
   - prospective cohort studies
   - reliability
   - retrospective case control studies
   - test marketing
   - true negative
   - true positive
2. Describe the roles of epidemiology and the scientific method in public health promotions.
3. List the Henle-Koch Postulates.
4. Given a research problem, determine whether to use a cross-sectional or longitudinal research design.
5. Given research data, compute relative risk coefficients.
6. Compare and contrast incidence and prevalence.
7. Given data from screening efforts, compute sensitivity and specificity.
8. Develop a focus group interview guide.
9. With supervision, conduct a focus group.
10. Develop an in-depth interview guide and conduct a simulated in-depth interview.

INTRODUCTION

Throughout the ONPRIME sequence, the public health promotion specialist functions as both a scientist and a practitioner.[1] These two hats are not generally worn concurrently, however. During the organizational, priority setting, and inter-

93

vention phases, the health promoter is primarily a practitioner; during the needs/resources assessment, research, monitoring, and evaluation phases (as well as during the formative marketing research aspect of the intervention phase), he or she functions more as a "scientist." Nevertheless, while the hats are not necessarily worn concurrently, they are changed frequently, as can be seen by the alternating nature of scientist and practitioner roles in the ONPRIME sequence. Research skills and knowledge areas emphasized by ONPRIME phase are presented in Table 6–1.

Research skills and resources will vary widely among health promoters, as well. Health promoters may include anyone from laboratory scientists gradually moving into the public health arena after years of bench research, to health educators recently leaving undergraduate work and embarking on their careers; from computer hacks to math whizzes; and from individuals located in research centers — rich in data analysis, library, and personnel resources — to others working in rural or underdeveloped areas with virtually no contact with the day-to-day research world. In the field of health promotion, however, a common call is issued to all health promoters. Research sophisticates must be able to define their technology or results in consumer-friendly terms, while research neophytes need to meet minimal requirements to respond to research priorities set by an organization and conduct basic formative research, monitoring, and program evaluation efforts. More importantly, all health promoters must be critical consumers of existing literature and data which can be used to plan programs and select health promotion interventions. The purpose of this chapter, therefore, is to define a common logic and terminology for understanding, communicating, and carrying out basic health promotion research.

TABLE 6–1
Research Knowledge and Skills Emphasized by ONPRIME Phase

Organization	General knowledge of epidemiological and health promotion research related to health issue
N/RA	Design and implementation of surveys, health services research, familiarity with epidemiological and health promotion data and research designs, especially case-control designs
Priority Setting	Familiarity with epidemiological data
Research	(See other ONPRIME steps)
Interventions	Time-series and control group (especially cohort) designs, formative research techniques, behavioral observation
Monitoring	Time-series methodology
Evaluation	Surveys, experimental designs and quasi-experimental designs

EPIDEMIOLOGY

Definitions

Epidemiology is the scientific flagship of public health. It offers formal training in research methods and the development of new applications of causal logic. Epidemiology has evolved because it leads to the collection and interpretation of more accurate information than typically true of casual or clinical observations. Such accurate information provides a better estimate of the public health risk for any given problem as well as what the best control procedures may be. Use of epidemiological research methods guide public health practitioners in the identification of true causal factors for disease and the application of *effective* prevention or treatment services. In turn, we are provided with a mechanism to increase our accountability.

Epidemiology has been defined as the study of the distribution and determinants (i.e., causes) of disease frequency in human populations.[2]

Within this definition we can identify two principal words: determinants and distribution. We are seeking to find out not only what are the patterns of disease and other problems in various populations, but also what factors cause these problems and how they might be changed.

The precise recording of the distribution of disease is very important for actuarial purposes and the provision of preventive or treatment services. Disease distributions tell us who and how many people have a disease, when they have it (e.g., flu season), and where it is contracted (e.g., southeastern U.S.). These data allow scarce and expensive medical and public health services to be channeled to the people in need.

Epidemiology parallels the concepts of behavioral observation, which in turn emphasizes two factors. First, we may quantify the frequency, duration, or other specific behavioral dimension. In other words, in an individual person we may be interested in the specific patterns or "distribution" of a particular behavior. For instance, observing the rate of smoking cigarettes will allow the behavior analyst to determine whether an individual engages in a risk activity, how often, and perhaps when and where. As in populations, this information can help determine whether the individual needs professional assistance and, if so, the nature and amount of service needed to reduce the risk of disease.

As a second step, we use narrative recording to determine antecedents and consequences related to the occurrence or non-occurrence of behavior. In other words, we seek to identify the "determinants" of behavior. Analogously, epidemiologists attempt to accomplish the same purposes in entire populations, focusing more on diseases than behaviors.

The emerging field of behavioral epidemiology looks at specific risk factors and other behaviorally-related phenomena using epidemiological techniques. In other words, those of us using behavioral epidemiological techniques seek to discover the distribution patterns of health-related behavior and their causes within given populations.

Four central concepts relating to the development of the field of epidemiology can also be applied to the subdiscipline of behavioral epidemiology. These concepts are as follow:[3] (1) human disease and health-related behaviors are in turn related to their environment; (2) the quantification of disease, behavioral and environmental phenomena may serve to advance people's health; (3) "natural experiments" can be used to investigate disease and behavioral phenomena; and (4) experiments conducted specifically for the purposes of modifying or further studying these phenomena can also be applied in certain cases.

Epidemiology, therefore, emphasizes studies of diseases and their determinants either in "natural" or "experimenter-initiated" studies. Natural studies are primarily observational in nature, emphasizing the examination of phenomena that are currently underway in the environment. Many times, however, the investigator will want more control over such phenomena or will be unable to study these phenomena in the natural setting. In such cases, the experimenter may actually want to develop his or her own study in order to be able to conduct a well-controlled examination of a particular cause-effect (or stimulus-response) relationship. In order to carry out either a natural or controlled experiment, the investigator will need to follow strict rules of causal logic and precise scientific procedures.

Illustrations of the Scientific Method

The rules of causal logic in epidemiology were originally established in **the Henle-Koch Postulates.** Although different authors emphasize slightly different "postulates" (rules for determining causality), the following are the basic rules which should be met in order to conclude that a given event causes a specific disease or behavior:

- Two or more events (also called variables) must be *associated;*
- The association must be *reliable* (i.e., occurs consistently);
- The presumed "causal" variable must be known to have *preceded* the "caused" variable (this is known as causal temporal order);
- All *alternate* possible causes must be known not to have caused the event in question (related to the concept of experimental control).

The scientific method is a system of procedures involving both deduction and induction and following the rules of causal logic. Anecdotal or clinical observations often become the basis for

Variable I
(Income)

		Present	Absent
Variable II **(Access to** **Medical** **Service)**	Present	A More Cases	B Fewer Cases
	Absent	C Fewer Cases	D More Cases

inducing a possible causal relationship — a hypothesis.

In order to understand the scientific method fully, it is important to dissect each of the rules of causal logic. What does it mean to say that two variables must be associated? The answer to this question in its simplest form is very elementary. **An association simply means that two variables "co-vary" or change together in some way (although not necessarily in the same direction). This concept is known as covariance.** Covariance can be positive or negative. For example, a positive association exists between income level and medical services. The more money a person has, the more medical services they may access. More simply, **a positive association can be described when the** *presence* **of one variable (e.g., income) predicts the** *presence* **(or occurrence) of the second variable (e.g., medical services). For a** *positive* **association, the reverse is also true. The** *absence* **of one variable predicts the absence of the second.**

A negative association exists when the *pres-*

ence **(or occurrence) of one variable predicts the** *absence* **of the second.** For instance, the absence of vitamin C in the diet predicts (and, in this case, causes) the disease scurvy. Conversely, the presence of scurvy predicts the absence of vitamin C in the diet.

An association can occur in degrees or various strengths, but it is clearer when conceptualized as all or nothing. The 2 x 2 table above illustrates.

A positive association exists when Variables I and II are (a) both present, or (b) both absent, concurrently. To determine whether there is an association, one must know whether the variables occur together and whether they are absent at the same time. In other words, most subjects will be categorized in Cells A and D (with few in B and C) if an association exists. The same is true for a negative association, except the presence of one variable predicts the absence of the other.

The contingency table below illustrates a negative association. Note, here, too, one must have information about both the presence and absence of both variables to determine an association.

Variable I
(Vitamin C)

		Present	Absent
Variable II **(Scurvy)**	Present	A Fewer Cases	B More Cases
	Absent	C More Cases	D Fewer Cases

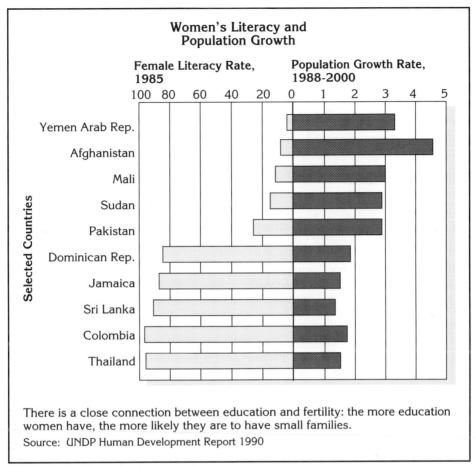

**Women's Literacy and
Population Growth**

There is a close connection between education and fertility: the more education women have, the more likely they are to have small families.
Source: UNDP Human Development Report 1990

FIGURE 6–1.   This chart demonstrates the strong negative association between women's literacy and population growth. Reprinted by permission of UNFPA.

The second rule of causal logic is reliability. **Reliability refers to the consistency of an observation or association.** If one were to observe salt consumption and find blood pressure to elevate above the level observed in absence of salt consumption, there would be evidence of an association.

However, one would need more information to assess reliability. The following sets of data show possible changes in blood pressure following salt ingestion for two individuals.

Table 6–2 shows two potential associations, one for each individual. Joe's blood pressure was observed to be higher after salt consumption. George's blood pressure, on the other hand, was no different after salt ingestion. This is evidence of an association between salt intake and increased

blood pressure for only Joe, with no association for George.

The problem with inferring a complete or perfect association in one case and none in the other is that an error may have been made in measurement. Or, other factors, such as antihypertensive medication use, might have masked the blood pressure-salt relationship in George's case.

One way to reduce the likelihood of conclusions based on error or misinformation is to collect more information—by obtaining repeated measures—and assess the consistency of the association among all observations. Table 6–3 shows repeated measures for Joe and George.

With repeated measures we note that Joe's blood pressure increased after each incident of salt consumption. Moreover, it increased by ex-

TABLE 6-2
Changes in Systolic Blood Pressure Following Salt Ingestion

| | Joe | | | George | |
Pre		Post	Pre		Post
110		120	106		106

actly 10mm of mercury. These results (which are hypothetical and probably unrealistic) illustrate a "perfect" association between salt intake and blood pressure increase. All of the four repeated trials showed the same direction and degree of change. This degree of consistency, especially if repeated ten or more times, would convince most observers that the association was reliable.

George's data show a different pattern. Here, the first trial did not result in any change in blood pressure—ergo, no association is present. The second trial resulted in lower blood pressure—a negative association. The final two trials showed increases in blood pressure—positive associations. Considering all trials, there is evidence of no association in 25 percent, negative association in 25 percent, and positive association in 50 percent. On average, 6 of the eight trials show positive associations. Thus, to conclude that there is no

relationship might be wrong. The variability (lack of consistency) is so great that one would conclude an unreliable association.

The strength and reliability of an association is determined mathematically by use of various statistics. Common examples include Pearson r correlation coefficients, chi square (X^2) coefficients, Students' t-tests and analysis of variance F tests. Each of these statistical tests answers somewhat different questions and employs somewhat different forms of data.

Regardless of the specific test, all of these statistical procedures are means to ascertain the strength and reliability of an association. The data in Table 6-2 could be used to calculate a Pearson r correlation coefficient. This statistic yields a number ranging from 0 to 1.0 and from 0 to -1.0 for positive and negative associations, respectively.

TABLE 6-3
Repeated Measures of Systolic Blood Pressure

| | Joe | | | George | |
Trials	Pre	Post	Trials	Pre	Post
1	110	120	1	106	106
2	115	125	2	110	100
3	112	122	3	108	118
4	110	120	4	106	116

In Joe's case, the correlation is 1.0, or a perfect association. There was no inconsistency. The correlation coefficient for George would be positive, but "very weak" (i.e., small), and difficult to interpret. It may be that there is no true association between salt intake and blood pressure increase in George's case. The Pearson r correlation coefficient can be judged in the context of the number of repeated measures, degree of variance, and average size of association. Then, using statistics, one can assess the probability that a given coefficient was truly different from zero. The p value provides this estimate.

If one were to measure George's blood pressure after salt intake for hundreds of trials, and the same results were obtained, this again would comprise evidence of a weak positive association. However, the degree of inconsistency in relation to the number of repeated measures would lead to a statistically significant r (that is, a p value of less than .05). This would mean that the association was reliable but weak. Such a result would imply that one or more other variables (perhaps unknown) were also influencing George's blood pressure. This result would lead many practitioners and scientists to search for additional causal variables, such as exercise or obesity. This would be an example of induction — creating a new research hypothesis based on the strength of an association observed.

The third rule which must be satisfied in order to conclude that one variable causes another is **temporal order:** the potential "causal variable" must be antecedent to the "caused variable" in time. The blood pressure and salt intake examples above were structured so that salt intake was known to have preceded the blood pressure change. However, this is not always the case. A common association in public health concerns wealth and health (or alternatively, poverty and disease). The poorer a person is, the more likely he/she is to be ill. This association is very often seen in **cross-sectional studies** where **a sample of many people** of varying degrees of health/illness and wealth/poverty are **studied at one point in time.** In such studies, the degree to which poverty causes disease or the degree to which disease causes poverty is unknown. The temporal order of these variables is unknown.

Studies which follow individuals over time are known as longitudinal studies. Longitudinal studies are necessary to determine the temporal order

of associated variables. As it turns out, when initially healthy poor people are followed over a period of time, they experience more illness than do wealthy people. This temporal order contributes to the conclusion that poverty might be causally related to disease.

Disease can be causally related to poverty, too. When individuals with a disease, such as AIDS, are followed over time, they become more impoverished than do their counterparts who have not acquired this disease. This observation has led to the "downward mobility" hypothesis.

These examples show that longitudinal analyses are needed to **determine the temporal order of associated variables.** They also illustrate how some associations may be due to reciprocal causal relationships. For some people, A precedes B; for others, B precedes A.

The fourth and most difficult rule to satisfy concerns the **elimination of all alternate explanations of causality** for a given association: no sources of bias (measurement error) and confounding (other causal variables) have caused the observed association.

Returning to the blood pressure and salt intake example, Joe had a reliable association between salt intake and increased blood pressure. The temporal order of salt intake followed by blood pressure change was known. However, many measurement errors or alternate causal factors might have accounted for this association. One possible source of bias might have been the observer. The observer recording blood pressure might expect an increase and either misperceive or falsely report them. Experiments which include precise measures and where the observers are "blind" to the intervention and hypotheses are relatively free of such sources of bias.

Other variables could have caused a true increase in Joe's blood pressure. Taking "medication" can be worrisome or quite frightening for some people. Anxiety is known to increase blood pressure. It is possible that adding salt tablets to the diet increased Joe's anxiety and, hence, his blood pressure increased. In this way, salt intake would be said to be an indirect causal variable.

This example also illustrates how a variable may be causal, but not in the way originally hypothesized. Implicitly, salt intake was thought to increase the body's water retention due to its chemical characteristics. To test this possibility completely, salt intake would need to occur for

Joe under conditions known not to cause him anxiety. This might require salt to be taken with regular meals or in some other unobtrusive manner.

Seemingly, causal relationships may be observed when, in fact, some unknown (not measured or observed) factor truly caused the dependent variable to change. Joe might have discontinued blood pressure lowering medication at the same time he began taking salt tablets. He might have increased his caloric intake and gained weight. Actually, there are numerous alternative possibilities.

To rule out all alternate explanations, a contrast or **control condition** must be part of the research design. This condition should be exactly the same as the "experimental" condition, except for the presumed causal (or independent) variable. Usually this is accomplished by comparing a group of people who are exposed to the independent variable with a group not exposed.

This type of study could be conducted by asking a group to take salt tablets, while a second (control) group does not take the tablets. If the group "exposed" to salt has a greater increase in blood pressure than the group "not exposed," we would conclude that salt intake was causally related to blood pressure. This logic is based on the assumption that the control group's experience was identical to that of the experimental group, with the exception of exposure to salt. Had the control group's blood pressure increased, we would know it was not due to salt. We would not know what caused the increase. It could be due to any one of a number of known or unknown factors. If the control group's blood pressure increased for reasons other than salt intake, we would suspect that the increase in the experimental group might have been due to the same unknown variable. We could not conclude that salt causes blood pressure elevation.

The process of conducting useful experiments is difficult. As noted earlier, the control condition should be *exactly* the same as the experimental condition, except for exposure to the independent variable. This standard is a goal to be worked toward but which might never be achieved.

Typically, random assignment of people to experimental groups is needed to establish equivalence. Based on probability theory, groups so constructed will be essentially identical most of the time. However, even when random assignment is used the groups may not be equal. More men than women may be randomly assigned to the experimental group, older people may be assigned to the control group, and so on. In such cases, differences between the groups may be due to the independent variable (e.g., salt intake) or differences in the two samples. Without random assignment, however, such differences in groups are much more likely. Hence, experiments without random assignment cannot rule out all alternate explanations.

Single case or small sample size experimental designs are discussed at the end of this chapter. These are alternate means of ruling out possible confounding variables. Depending on the experimental question and resources, either a group comparison or single case study design is the more reliable means of testing a causal hypothesis. The underlying principle is that some type of experimental evaluation is needed to rule out alternate explanations of causality.

Non-Experimental Studies

Non-experimental studies are generally either **cohort** or **case control.** In their simplest form, these studies look at the specific relationships between an exposure to a potential cause of a disease or behavior and the outcome of that exposure. Such studies may be accomplished either retrospectively, looking at individuals who have developed a disease or a health problem and tracking backwards to see what their exposure to proven or potential causal agents or risk factors had been previously, or prospectively, starting with the exposure and following a person for a period of time to determine whether s/he developed a disease or health problem. The former approach is most typically a case control study, whereas the latter is a type of cohort study. In the case control study, we might be interested in a variety of physical outcomes such as low birth weight among infants in a maternity ward, and then look "backwards" to see what sorts of prenatal exposures may have been related to this problem. As shown in Table 6–4, we could look at the total number of infants with low birth weight and the infants born with normal weight. The relative proportion of each of these groups who were exposed to maternal smoking is an indicator of association. The "odds ratio," as an

TABLE 6–4
Infants at Low Birth Weight

Maternal Smoking	Low Birth Weight Present	Low Birth Weight Absent	Total
Exposed	A	B	A + B
Not Exposed	C	D	C + D
TOTAL	A + C	B + D	A + B + C + D

estimate of relative risk compares the proportion of low weight infants (A) among all infants exposed to maternal smoking (A + B) to the proportion of low weight infants (C) among all not exposed to maternal smoking (C + D). The resulting ratio $\left(\dfrac{A}{A + B} \div \dfrac{C}{C + D}\right)$ is an estimate of the chance of acquiring the disease (e.g., low birth weight) if exposed to maternal smoking. We also, of course, need to examine the exposure of normal birth weight children to maternal smoking [B ÷ (B + D)].[4]

In a cohort (or "panel") study, we also study relationships between exposure and problem outcome. However, in this case we start with the exposure and track "forward" until we find the outcome. For example, we might want to examine the relationship between parental smoking and subsequent smoking of these parents' offspring during adolescence. Referring to Table 6–5, the "exposure" is smoking, identified in a large group of parents. Subsequently, we track whether or not the children of smokers and non-smokers take up the habit, following the logic of comparing the proportion of individuals exposed to a potential causal agent (in this case, parental smoking) and who develop the actual disease or behavioral problem (smoking). This ratio (A/(A + B)) is divided by the ratio of people who are not exposed to the causal agent and still develop the problem [C/(C + D)], a relative risk coefficient. The larger this coefficient, the greater the relative risk related to the specific exposure being studied.[5]

Incidence and Prevalence

Epidemiologists study both the **incidence** and **prevalence** of disease or problems in defined populations. Incidence refers to the actual onset or number of new cases of a specific problem, divided by the total population. This may refer to the beginning of an infection, the first trial of a cigarette, or the initial clinical confirmation of breast cancer. Prevalence, in contrast, refers to the proportion of people in a population who at a given point or period have a disease or problem. Analogously, we use prevalence statistics to describe the number of people with tuberculosis, the number of smokers, or the number of women with

TABLE 6–5
Relationship Between Parental and Adolescent Smoking

Parental Smoking	Adolescent Smoking Present	Adolescent Smoking Absent
Exposure	A	B
Non-Exposure	C	D

breast cancer in a defined group. Generally, infectious disease epidemiology places relatively more emphasis on incidence, whereas chronic disease epidemiology focuses more on prevalence statistics. This is because many infectious diseases are of relatively short duration, whereas the onset of chronic diseases can be more difficult to determine. However, both approaches are used in infectious, chronic, and behavioral epidemiological investigations.

Screening

A major tool in behavioral epidemiology and health promotion research (and interventions) is public health screening (followed by counseling and referral). Screening refers to any attempt to identify the onset or existence of a health problem in an individual. Therefore, one might be screened for high blood pressure, high cholesterol, tuberculosis, or any other problem potentially harmful to that individual or perhaps to others in his or her environment. For example, Figure 6–3 presents hypothetical results of data from a cholesterol screening in a community health center. In this screening, we determined that 50 of the 100 individuals who had their capillary blood tested for high cholesterol actually had high cholesterol, and 50 did not. Now let's assume we were able to retest these people with "gold standard" laboratory tests. These tests would have shown us that twenty-five of the fifty people we said had high cholesterol actually did. If we could have retested them, we would have also found that ten additional "true" hypercholesterolemic participants were not identified in our screening effort (Cell B). These incorrect classifications are referred to as "false positives" and "false negatives," respectively. In our study, we had twenty-five false negatives (Cell C), and ten false positives (Cell B). **The false positives, therefore, were people who actually did not have the problem but were told that they had it subsequent to our finger-prick screening. The false negatives, in contrast, were people who actually had the problem and yet were told that they did not have it (Cell C). The true positives (Cell A) and the true negatives (Cell D) were those who were correctly classified by our screening effort** (see Figure 6–3). Therefore, we had a total of sixty-five correct classifications (A + D).

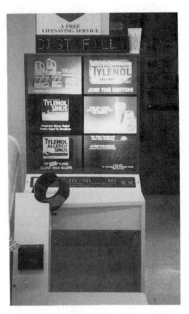

FIGURE 6–2. Although blood pressure machines in pharmacies increase access to this important screening service, the specificity and sensitivity of these machines has been questioned. *Photo courtesy of Betsy Clapp.*

Screening programs are generally evaluated on their **sensitivity** and **specificity.** Sensitivity refers to how many of the people who actually had the disease tested positive. In other words, we want to know how many true positives we detected divided by the total number of people who should have been classified as positive. The sensitivity rate in our example was $25 \div 50$ [A/(A + C)], or 50 percent. Specificity, by contrast, is the number of true negatives (D) divided by the number of true negatives plus the number of false positives, D + B, or $\dfrac{D}{D + B}$ which in our case was $40 \div 50$ or 80 percent. Specificity provides a "noise index" by showing how many people without the disease are being identified.

How do we use these results to determine whether screening is appropriate? First of all, we need to examine the potential problems caused by a false positive. In other words, if we tell someone they have a medical problem and they actually do not, we may have scared them away from future efforts at behavior change or health promotion or

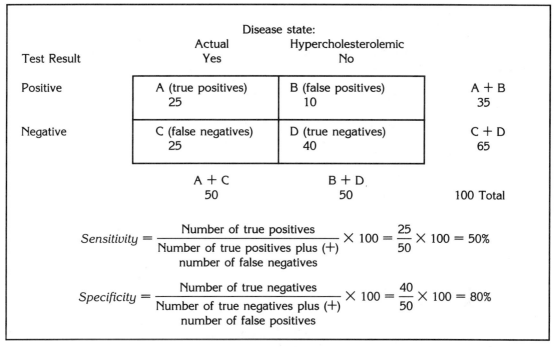

FIGURE 6-3. Hypothetical cholesterol screening results

caused them serious psychological distress. We also need to consider the impact of a false negative. By telling people they do not actually have a problem, we can give them too much confidence and make it less likely they will seek to have the problem detected in the future.

Another factor to consider in screening is the lead time that correct positive identification yields, as well as whether the disease is treatable. For instance, if we are screening for cancer, will we detect it far enough in advance to do something about it? This case may be hypothetically illustrated by the difference in screening for colorectal cancer and lung cancer. With appropriate lead time, the **case-fatality ratio (the number of people who have colon cancer compared to the number who die from it)** can be significantly reduced. Therefore, we are likely to continue to expand our efforts in colorectal cancer screening in the future (where early detection can lead to successful treatment). However, we are not close to this success for public health screening for lung cancer (where the case-fatality correspondence is extremely high no matter how early it is detected).

How can we extend the conceptual basis for evaluating screening technology to evaluating behavior change technology and health promotion? Assume we are setting up a reinforcement condition whereby clinics succeeding in vaccinating a certain percentage of their population are eligible for bonus payment from the Department of Health and a certificate congratulating this clinic and all of its staff on this accomplishment. As part of this organizational-level intervention (chapter 15), we need to establish a data system whereby we can determine whether this clinic had or had not met its criterion. We might want to look at clinic records, for example, or perhaps interview a sample of mothers in the community. Either of these techniques would be analogous to the screening device used in the cholesterol screening. However, like the cholesterol machine, we might not get "true positives" and "true negatives." In other words, our sample of mothers may have been biased toward women who had lived too far away from the clinic and therefore did not represent the overall catchment area, or our screening of charts may have yielded data which looked better than perhaps they should have, since the health workers who filled out the charts were aware of our reinforcement system. Therefore, we might fail to reinforce some clinics that should have received the award (false negatives) while reinforcing others that had not met the reward criteria (false positives). Again, the advisability of applying a certain reinforcement system would be predicated on the dangers associated with false positives and false negatives. Hence, a behavioral study using the concept of screening evaluation would estimate specifically the relative rates of a false positive or a false negative and evaluate the ramifications of each type of error.

RESEARCH DESIGNS AND TECHNIQUES

Threats to Internal and External Validity

In their classic opus, Campbell and Stanley[6] define **internal validity as whether the change observed in a dependent variable can actually be attributed to a specific causal factor, whereas external validity is the generalizability of the results of a study to other populations, settings, points of time, etc.** In Campbell's and Stanley's terms, internal and external validity roughly parallel concepts of reliability presented earlier in this chapter and generalizability, also important in behavioral psychological research and theoretical formulations.

According to Campbell and Stanley, specific "threats" (i.e., experimental factors which are problematic if not controlled) to internal validity include the following:

1. **History:** Things that happen between one variable and another (e.g., two measurements of a dependent variable) which were not controlled or perhaps even noticed by the investigator.
2. **Maturation:** Physical or other changes in subjects which could affect the data in some unplanned way.
3. **Testing:** Effects of taking a test (or going through an interview, etc.) on a second and subsequent testing period.
4. **Instrumentation:** Differences in calibration of an instrument (e.g., blood pressure cuff) or

readings made by the administrator of an instrument.
5. **Statistical regression:** The tendency of individuals with extremely high or low scores on a given variable to move toward an average on subsequent testing.
6. **Selection:** A bias created when subjects in different groups of a study are selected with different criteria (e.g., patients in a clinic versus non-patients).
7. **Differential dropout (or "experimental mortality"):** Higher rates of subjects dropping out of a study between experimental conditions (or groups).
8. **Interactions between two or more of the above biases:** (e.g., selection and maturation).

Four other factors which are potential threats to the external validity, or generalizability, of research results include:

1. **The reactive effects of pre-testing:** Individuals who have been pre-tested (or screened, etc.) begin to make changes based on this pre-testing, thereby making them different than the non-pre-tested population which might have similar risk factors or other characteristics.
2. **The interaction between selection and experimental variable:** A group selected for one experimental condition can be especially sensitive (or impervious) to a specific experimental intervention, whereas their comparison group does not have the same sensitivities. Such can often be the case when volunteers are used to study an intervention and non-volunteers serve as the backup comparison.
3. **Reactive effects of the experimental arrangements:** Something specific to the "artificial" nature of an investigation makes it an inappropriate representation of "reality."
4. **Multiple treatment interference:** A sequence of interventions is introduced and it is difficult, if not impossible, to evaluate the cumulative effects of later interventions, as the history subjects have with previous interventions is not "erasable."

These warning flags raised by Campbell and Stanley thirty years ago have guided much of social science and public health behavior change research ever since. Nevertheless, these principles do not necessarily imply that applied studies need to have laboratory-like purity in order to produce meaningful results. Indeed, the consumer-friendly research designs discussed in this section circumvent most of these threats to internal and external validity, while being fairly easy to use and understand.

Case Control and Cohort Techniques

Whether using direct behavioral observations or personal interviews, health promotion professionals emphasize different variables in research designs for planning or evaluating behavior change interventions. Typically, health promotion is intervention-focused; therefore, health promotion evaluation schema fall into the "investigator-initiated" category. However, much health promotion research emphasizes the determination of what behavioral strategies might best work. Case control and cohort research can be especially effective in helping plan an actual intervention program.

Health promotion specialists are specifically interested in behavior-consequence relationships and how these can be used to promote adaptive health behavior. Before designing a reinforcement intervention, for example, the behavior analyst attempts to determine what types of reinforcement strategies may be most effective, based hopefully on behavior-consequence relationships already defined. In this regard, it might be advantageous to compare "early adopters" with "later adopters." For example, why do some individuals get annual physical exams and others do not? A case control study might lead to interviewing the regular participants in physical examinations and contrasting these data with interviews from individuals who do not receive examinations. In this case, the "outcomes" are physical exam versus no physical exam. Subsequently, "exposure" questions would emphasize what reinforcers individuals who receive the exams get for obtaining the examinations, and what barriers or punishers are encountered (or expected) by non-users. This case control methodology is recommended for any health promotion program applying behavior change strategies which have not been thoroughly tested in previous investigations.

Practical Experimental Designs for Health Promotion

A frequent problem in health promotion research is that much of the research is conducted at an organizational, community, or other more complex level that does not enable a systematic controlled evaluation of program impact. In most cases, the resources are simply not available to conduct such studies. Also, in public health promotion, changes between a pre- and post-test in a rigorously-controlled setting is rarely possible. Often, any of a variety of factors may affect experimental outcomes, including (a) changes in the weather or other environmental factors, (b) changes in policy or law which may influence the health promotion effort, or (c) major news stories such as the death of a prominent community figure who had a known risk factor related to a particular health promotion program. While these events may have an effect on the outcome of the health promotion effort, we cannot "tease out" specific intervention effects. Therefore, behavioral research has often used time-series methodology to evaluate the impact of health promotion research efforts.

Time-series studies in behavioral investigations examine the "behavior" (or products of behavior) of interest over a period of time. This behavior is then graphed on a regular schedule to determine day-by-day or phase-by-phase fluctuations. In public health promotion, of course, we are not interested solely in the behavior of specific individuals. Instead, there is far more emphasis on the behavior or performance of groups, organizations, or entire communities. Therefore, we often graph the changes in attendance at clinics, accidents at the worksite, mortality due to dehydration in an entire region, or drunken driving arrests throughout a community. These are data resulting from the behavior of many individuals.

Figures 6-4, 6-5, and 6-6 are hypothetical representations of the three fundamental time-series designs we consider in our present discussion. They are the **baseline-intervention phases or "AB" research design,** the reversal or "ABA" design, and the multiple baseline design, respectively. **The AB design is a simple baseline to an intervention analysis of behavior change between phases.** Using our epidemiological terminology, these can either be natural or investiga-

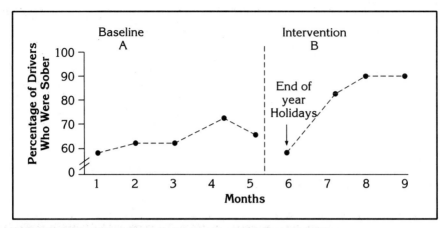

FIGURE 6–4. Hypothetical data to illustrate the AB design

tor-initiated studies. In the (hypothetical) natural study depicted in Figure 6–4, a highway patrol roadside check was established whereby drivers were randomly stopped to determine whether they were driving under the influence of alcohol on Friday and Saturday evenings. During the baseline period, drivers who were stopped and shown to be intoxicated were detained until someone could pick them up and drive them home. During the intervention phase, intoxicated drivers were given a night in jail and lost half of their points on their driver's license. As shown in Figure 6–4, this statute change had a dramatic effect on the percentage of stopped drivers who were sober, with the exception of the Christmas/New Year holiday season (month 6), where the percentage dropped substantially. We could assume that the effects of this type of intervention will be fairly powerful, although legal and political barriers would have to be overcome in order to implement this policy on a long-term or permanent basis. The use of time-series rather than pre/post data clearly demonstrates the impact of the holiday month on the intervention in effect. This impor-

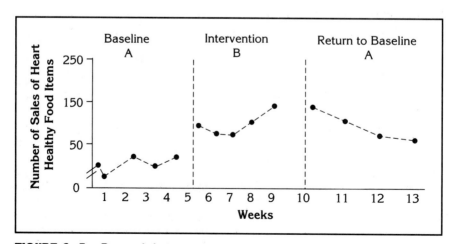

FIGURE 6–5. Reversal design

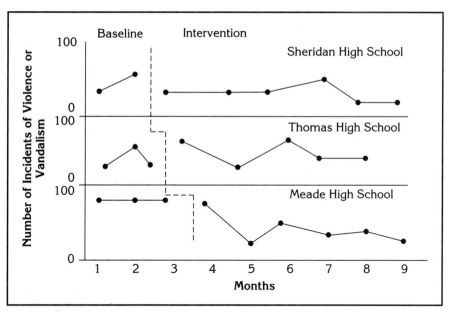

FIGURE 6-6. Multiple baseline design

tant finding would have been masked had just overall averages been presented on a pre/post basis.

Figure 6–5 presents the results of a hypothetical intervention for promoting heart-healthy food selection in a restaurant. This is an example of the "reversal design," which is a variation of the "AB" design discussed above. In the reversal or ABA design, we further demonstrate *experimental* or *functional* control by reversing an effect realized during the initial change from baseline to intervention. By being able to accomplish this reversal, we can show that other factors were not responsible for the observed intervention effect. Again, this approach reduces a need for a "control group," as the subject (or group of subjects) serves as its own control over time.

The reversal presented in Figure 6–5 is also called an "ABA" design. This hypothetical study evaluated the highlighting of heart-healthy menu items in a family restaurant with stickers indicating which items are relatively healthy. After five weeks of monitoring the sales of these items before the intervention, the stickers were placed on all of the menus and the sales of the heart-healthy items were tracked for another five weeks. Then, to demonstrate experimental control, the stickers

were removed after ten weeks while sales were monitored. This design gives more convincing evidence than the "AB" design that it was, indeed, the "menu marking" intervention that caused the changes in sales, rather than a change in some other variable such as seasonal fluctuations or customer demographics.

Unfortunately, the reversal design is often not practical in real-world interventions. Often, ample time is required to get someone interested in participating in a health promotion effort, and once participation occurs (and beneficial results are forthcoming), the prospect of reversing this effect may seem undesirable or even idiotic. The alternative design, which also uses subjects (or groups) as their own control and circumvents the problems of the reversal design, is called the multiple baseline design.

The multiple baseline design tracks the effects of an intervention replicated in a "staggered" fashion across different individuals or groups of individuals, behaviors, or settings. This design has, ideally, two or three replications of baseline followed by intervention. For instance, the multiple baseline design presented in Figure 6–6 tracks the effect of an intervention package for reducing school-ground violence replicated in three different high schools of a school district. This package might consist of briefly teaching students that there are alternative methods to being accepted by the group than by turning to violence. This could include working with other students to show them how to reinforce non-violent behaviors, and recruiting a popular musician to visit all classrooms with students demonstrating a substantial reduction in violence or vandalism. In our hypothetical study, we intervened at Sheridan High School at the end of two weeks, at Thomas High School at the end of three weeks, and at Meade High School at the end of four weeks. The initiation of this intervention was staggered across schools in order to demonstrate that seasonal or other non-experimental variables were not responsible for intervention impact.

As depicted in Figure 6–6, the intervention package was very effective at Sheridan and Meade High Schools, but less effective at Thomas High School. These data would indicate a need to determine why Thomas High School was less responsive than the other two and what can be done about these continuing problems in the future. When limited resources are a problem, this design's advantage over a control group design is that one can evaluate the intervention only in a selected group of schools, reducing the feasibility of a control 'group.' It is also superior to the reversal design in that we would not actually want to reverse our gains once they are initially realized. Since this evaluation was conducted with three groups of students in equivalent settings, it gives us an example of the "multiple baseline across subjects" design. The two other types of multiple baseline designs are across behaviors and across settings. In the former category, we may have sequentially targeted different behaviors (e.g., grades, physical altercations, wearing of gang insignia), whereas in the second setting, we may have examined schools, community parks, and sporting events. These three categories directly (and purposefully) correspond to the three categories of generalization described in chapter 8.

FORMATIVE RESEARCH

Social marketing and other intervention-oriented research frequently emphasizes formative or qualitative studies which allow program planners to obtain insight into the knowledge, atti-

tudes, practices, and motivational aspects of individual and group health factors. Generally speaking, **formative research[7] is evaluative research, conducted during program development. It includes the pretesting of programs, products, and materials through in-depth studies of small numbers of people,** whereas most other health research emphasizes brief enumerations of characteristics of large numbers of people. Specifically, such pretesting can:

- Assess the target audience's awareness of program materials, logos, mission statements, themes, etc.
- Assess recall of public service announcements, posters, and other promotional pieces.
- Identify specific strong and weak points of a program component.
- Determine the personal relevance of a message.
- Measure how controversial, sensitive, pleasant, or aversive a certain intervention may be.[8]

A variety of techniques characterize formative research, including focus group research, in-depth interviews, intercept interviews, behavioral observations, and secondary (or archival) research.

Formative and qualitative research characteristics of health promotion should not be considered a substitute for quantitative research. Small sample sizes, selection biases, and data subject to different interpretations by different researchers lead to a greater probability that erroneous conclusions could be drawn from qualitative research. However, a variety of advantages are unique to the latter form of research. Generally speaking, formative research is less expensive than quantitative research in terms of time, effort, and level of sophistication required to carry it out. Second, formative research is audience driven rather than researcher driven: it allows the researcher to share experiences with representatives of the target audience on a more natural basis. Formative research generates ideas for subsequent quantitative research or program design, and serves as a tool for exploring reactions of the target audience to stimuli intended to increase awareness, knowledge, acceptance, or behavior change.

In summary, formative research may be used at any point in the planning-implementation-evaluation cycle, helping to: (a) frame the context of research and planning (e.g., finding out local slang

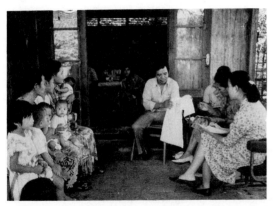 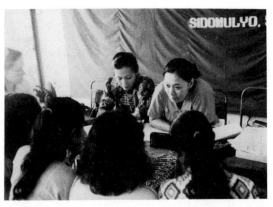

FIGURE 6–7. Formative research may be used to select reinforcers as well as marketing and health education approaches. Here, Indonesian health authorities show special T-shirts with symbols denoting health workers' community service to a group of mothers. In the second photo, health workers listen to various radio spots to choose which one they think would best reward them for their many efforts in village health promotion. The data from the mothers and health workers were used to design the reinforcement and maintenance system for village health volunteers. (See also pages 176–177). *Photo courtesy of John Elder.*

used for various sexual activities before designing a survey instrument to assess STD risk in a community); (b) solicit desired responses to various products, materials, and other program stimuli (e.g., pretesting an anti-smoking poster which uses fear appeal versus one which uses sarcasm directed against the tobacco industry); and (c) understand why certain results were not forthcoming (e.g., interviewing individuals living very near a clinic who have not used that clinic's services).

The in-depth interview and focus group are two common health promotion research techniques which incorporate similar question formats and presentation and probing styles. **A focus group is a type of research in which a moderator leads about eight to ten people in talking freely about a topic. An in-depth interview is a form of research consisting of an intensive interview to find out how a person thinks and feels about a given topic.** In general, focus groups are used to take advantage of group dynamics, whereas in-depth interviews are used when group dynamics can be counterproductive to obtaining valid information. For example, to research problems in a community related to racism and what to do about them, an in-depth interview would be preferable. Additionally, highly sophisticated or professionally trained individuals (such as physicians) often prefer to respond through the in-depth interview process. In rural areas where it may be difficult to

arrange a meeting of a larger number of people, in-depth interviews are more feasible than focus groups.

On the other hand, focus groups are especially desirable when the researcher wants to observe the group interaction as part of the formative/qualitative assessment. For example, in smoking prevention research, we are especially interested in the effects of peer pressure (and peer support) with respect to acquiring the smoking habit. In this context, focus group responses are likely to be more valid. In other cases, we want to see the group share ideas with one another rather than simply record two-way communication between interviewer and respondent. Focus groups are also preferable when time and resources are limited, as many more individuals can be studied through a format which gathers eight to ten people at a time. Focus groups may be especially effective in idea generation, a process whereby one group member may build on or modify ideas presented by another group member.

Conducting Focus Groups

After establishing research objectives, the steps in focus group research are as follow: setting up the group, writing the interview guide, selecting and preparing the moderator, and running the group.

Setting up the Group. A variety of issues need to be addressed when setting up a focus group, including determining the number and size of groups needed, deciding who should be represented in each group, organizing the logistics of transportation, finding a room, etc. Many of the decisions will be "judgment calls," depending on the specific topic and the target audience. In general, focus groups should represent key characteristics of the target audience. With a heterogeneous target audience, each group should be relatively homogeneous. For example, if both men and women are being questioned regarding a new teen pregnancy prevention campaign, male-only and female-only groups are desired.

Generally, eight to ten respondents is the maximum recommended size for a focus group, depending on the topic discussed and the characteristics of the individuals in the group. The group setting should be comfortable, easily accessible, and reasonably private. As in any research, a sufficient sample size (or in this case, the number of groups) should take into account the variability between groups. Therefore, the greater the variability in group responses, the greater the need to assess a larger number of groups. When variability in responses is relatively low, two groups per major theme or variable should be sufficient.

Developing the Interview Guide. As in any research, specific research objectives need to be specified before embarking on focus group work. The focus group interview guide consists of a general question-by-question outline, giving the moderator considerable flexibility in how to ask the questions. Since a period of time might be needed to establish rapport, questions should proceed from the general and non-threatening to the more specific and potentially controversial. The moderator begins by introducing the rationale behind holding the focus group and conducting any "warm-up" activities needed (e.g., having partici-

---

EXHIBIT 6–1
Focus Group Tricks of the Trade

Mary Debus lists a variety of "tricks of the trade" which focus group moderators can apply to optimize the constructive output of communication focus groups,* including:

- Probe for the specific context from which individuals are giving their opinions. What has been their experience with the behavioral product?
- "Man from the Moon" routine: e.g., "I'm from the moon and I have never heard of alcohol or the need to moderate my use of it. What do I need to know about this product? Is it something I want? Why should I limit my use of it? How do I go about doing that?"
- Benefit chain: e.g., "This product says it's low in fat. What's the benefit of that?" (Answer: It has fewer calories.) "What's the benefit of fewer calories?" (Answer: You won't gain as much weight.) "Why is it important not to gain as much weight?" (Answer: You will look better.) "And what's the benefit of that?" etc., etc.**
- Sentence completion and extensions: "The ideal birth control method is one that _____." "The best thing about this birth control product is that ____ ____ ____." "The birth control method I use makes me feel ____ ____ ____."

These and numerous other techniques can stimulate focus group discussions. Remember to use the method which best stimulates discussion without either threatening an individual group member or allowing other group members to dominate the discussion.

---

*Debus, Handbook for excellence in focus group research, pp. 32–33.
**This style of questioning is similar to Pablo Freire's consciousness-raising technique, except he works backwards from a present problem through the causal chain for that problem.

pants chat for a few minutes in pairs and then introduce one another to the entire group).

Figure 6–8 presents an example of a focus group guide used with Hispanic sixth graders in the Project Salsa school nutrition component.[9] The purpose of the school nutrition component was initially to increase the quality (e.g., lower fat, lower sodium) of school lunches and breakfasts. Since many students in the target community came from families of very modest means, school breakfasts were a potentially important part of the overall nutritional intake. However, after an initial assessment showed a severe deficiency in this important service, it was deemed important by project staff to begin with increasing the number of students participating in the school lunch and breakfast programs. Improving the nutritional quality of the food was targeted later, since usage rates were so low that proceeding conversely would not have proven meaningful. Therefore, school nutrition task forces sought to obtain information from the students themselves about why use rates were low and what could be done to improve them.

As can be seen in Figure 6–8, the introduction and warm-up are followed by the general questions, which in turn lead to more specific and pointed questions. The focus group ends with an invitation to participate in future student groups for continual work on changes in the cafeteria. Moderators were allowed the flexibility to track spontaneous issues as they arose. As you examine these questions, note how the five "Ps" of marketing (see chapter 10) are woven into this guide.

Selecting and Preparing the Moderator. The best moderators feel comfortable interacting with others, put others at ease, are enthusiastic, have good listening and reflective skills, and generally match the personal characteristics of the respondents (e.g., in dress, language, gender).[10] The moderator should be thoroughly informed about the project in order to guide the discussion appropriately and occasionally respond to inquiries of group members. Most importantly, the moderator must be able to obtain information from the respondents without biasing them in any way or leading them to give an answer they think the moderator is looking for.

At the end of the focus group discussion, the moderator and any observers are debriefed by the researcher. Then, the focus group results are summarized in written form.

The In-Depth Interview

The most common alternative to communications pretesting in focus groups is the **in-depth interview. The in-depth interview is a hybrid of focus group and survey techniques, combining the qualitative nature of the former with the one-to-one format of the latter.** It is generally less complicated logistically and technically than the focus group (although it may require more time to complete), and it can be done in the respondent's home or other "natural" setting. The in-depth interview may be more appropriate for obtaining reactions to partially completed products, alternative versions of products, or final testing, whereas the focus group is more appropriate for initial concept testing. The in-depth interview is especially useful when a behavioral observation of the respondent's use of a product is important.

The researcher may use techniques similar to those for focus groups in developing the interview guide, selecting and training interviewers, and selecting respondents for the in-depth interview. Depending on the needs and resources of the research program, however, the in-depth interview may take on a more scientific flavor than its counterpart. The interviewer might begin the interview with some quantitative survey questions and then continue with the qualitative in-depth interview or may weave them in throughout.

This combination of quantitative and qualitative items in an interview/survey tool is used frequently in social marketing to determine the cultural, institutional, and behavioral characteristics of various social groups. In contrast to the other qualitative techniques described elsewhere in this section, pre-testing surveys are generally conducted with a random sample of the population. The specific approach to contacting these individuals may be through household surveys, telephone surveys, and other techniques. A variety of questions might be asked during the interview, including the following questions assessing general characteristics of the target audience:

- What is the typical nature of their household and friendship groups?
- Where do they eat out and shop for groceries?

Materials Used: Tape recorder, audio cassette tapes, extension cord, snacks

I. Introduction to Project
   A. Background of Project Salsa
   B. Specifically, we want to make school breakfast more nutritious and more fun to eat.
   C. Children should be reminded that we want their honest opinions and we don't personally care if they think the current school breakfast is good or bad. We need to know exactly what they think.

II. Warm-up Icebreakers
   A. Each kid tells something about him/herself.
   B. Some of the following questions should be selected for further discussion as "icebreakers": What is your favorite food? What is your favorite food that your mom cooks? Do you like vegetables? Do you like chili? What is your favorite vegetable? What is your favorite fruit? What would be the best dessert for you—cake, fruit, or ice cream? Do you ever cook? What do you make? How often do you eat out? Do you think school is fun? If you get a present, what would you rather get: a surprise, something you already know about, or something you picked out? Would it be food? What do you want to be when you grow up?

III. Specific Focus Group Guide (If children give ambiguous answers to any of the questions below, ask a more specific question. Probe questions. However, try not to prompt for specific responses, but instead let children generate their own ideas.)
   A. Children's perceptions regarding the importance of breakfast: "Who can tell me what breakfast is?""Is one piece of fruit or one glass of juice a 'breakfast'?"
   B. "Who here eats breakfast?" (Have them raise their hands.)
   C. "What do you usually have for breakfast?"
   D. "If you eat breakfast every day, stand up."
   E. "How important is breakfast?" "Why?"
   F. "How many of you eat breakfast at _____ (name of school)?"
   G. "How many of you eat breakfast at some place other than home?" "At home?"
   H. "What are your two favorite breakfasts at school?"
   I. "What two school breakfast do you not like at all?"
   J. "What do you do when they serve a breakfasts you don't like?"
   K. "Do you have enough time to eat breakfasts at school?" "If not, why not?"
   L. Children's perceptions regarding food service workers: "What do you like about the ladies that work in the cafeteria."
   M. "What can I do to make you like them more?"
   N. Children's ideas for changes in breakfast program: "If you could change anything about breakfast at school, what would you change?" (As probes and prompts, use examples recorded from previous responses, including the actual food content, the cafeteria workers, or other/miscellaneous.)
   O. "Would you like to be in a group to help change the food program?"

FIGURE 6–8. School nutritional focus groups used by Project Salsa.

- Where do they get their health information?
- What do they like or dislike about the health behavior or product of interest?
- What outcomes would they expect from changing health behavior?
- What kinds of health behaviors (both health-promoting and health-damaging) are they actually engaging in now, as compared to the recent past, and what might they expect to be doing in the future?

- What money, time, or other "costs" would they be willing to expend to improve their health?
- Where do they receive media-based information (radio, television, newspaper, etc.)?
- Where are the most credible sources of health information and general information?
- What reinforcement would induce them to take healthy actions? What reinforcement are they receiving for unhealthy behavior, and what would it take to get them to forego that?

Archival Research

Both health promoters and social marketers rely heavily on archival (or "secondary") data (e.g., county health records) and previous research in a specific area or with a specific population (see chapter 5). Archival data are accessed in order to determine the types of activities successful in the past, the specific needs and attitudes of the target audience, the morbidity and mortality patterns among the audience, and related information. Of special interest to the communications researcher is previous *marketing* research accomplished for a given target area or population and already in the public domain. Radio and television stations, advertising firms, newspapers, retail chains, and others can contribute by sharing their previous research on audience segmentation and behavioral and product preference.

Often, archival research saves a considerable amount of time (and data processing resources) through finding out what relevant research has already been done.

Behavioral Observation

Behavioral observation may make important contributions to the effective social marketing of health behavior change.[11] Such observations can allow one to determine the functional relationships between behavior and environmental variables, leading to the definition of current consequences maintaining or inhibiting behavior. Indeed, one of the important contributions the field of behavior analysis makes to social marketing is the analysis of behavioral factors related to health and marketing strategies.

Due to practical constraints, behavioral assessment is often limited to self-report data but, in principle, nothing short of objective measures of the target behavior and the environmental stimuli (antecedents and consequences) which might be controlling the behavior are considered valid measures. When such measures are available, more precise manipulation of cues and reinforcing consequences may be possible.

Behavioral observations (see chapter 3) can be conducted unobtrusively (e.g., an observer standing at the end of an aisle in a grocery store watching shoppers examine shelf goods) or as a participant (e.g., a program staff member attending a PTA meeting, observing the overall process while occasionally participating). An advantage of this form of research is its superior validity: rather than having people describe what they have done or might do, we are watching them in action. Also, behavioral observations can be conducted in conjunction with other pre-testing methods, such as focus groups and in-depth interviews.

On the other hand, since we do not control the situation in which people are unobtrusively observed, a considerable amount of time is spent observing them engaging in behavior irrelevant to our purposes rather than controlling the pretesting stimuli as is the case in the in-depth interview and focus group. Also, the presence of an observer (especially in participant observation) may alter the behavior of the subjects.

Intercept Interviews

Intercept interviews are another important form of marketing research. Specifically, **individuals are *intercepted* at the point they are most likely to have been exposed to promotional material or engage in a health-related behavior (e.g., near a cigarette machine, in a supermarket, in a clinic waiting room, at the point of leaving a parking lot where people generally buckle their children in child safety seats).** These interception points should also be "high traffic" areas, allowing researchers to contact large numbers of respondents in a short period of time.

The procedure for the intercept interview involves approaching potential interviewees, asking them some questions to determine whether they match the characteristics of the target audience or consume the target product, showing them the products or materials being researched (either at the point of interview or at a nearby interview "station" set up for this task), and questioning them about the products. Alternatively, exit interviews are conducted with people who (might) have been exposed to a promotion or product. Combining brief, close-ended (or multiple choice) versions of questions developed for focus group and in-depth interviews with some behavioral observation techniques, intercept interviews allow for contacting people in an efficient manner who are engaging in or avoiding a target behavior. However, these interviews must be very brief, and researchers can expect a high rate of refusal. Permission from (and payment to) property managers or public authorities is often necessary before setting up the pretesting effort. In urban settings, health promotion programs may use survey companies who specialize in this type of research rather than attempting it with project personnel.

Figure 6-9 summarizes an exit interview conducted at an intercept point outside of a grocery store in San Diego County (California). This was part of a pre-test (similar to a test marketing procedure; see below) of the Comida da Vida ("Food Gives Life") program, which used a variety of point-of-purchase strategies to promote healthier shopping selections.

Gatekeeper Review

It is often cost effective to find **gatekeepers — a group of expert individuals who, through their positions of power in a community and/or as representatives of segments of the target audience, can "speak for" the audience.** (Approaches to selecting and interviewing these gatekeepers are described in chapter 4.) The researcher is, as always, cautioned that gatekeeper responses might not represent those of the target audience; this procedure should be used only in conjunction with one of the other more proven pre-testing methods. At a minimum, the gatekeeper contact represents a courtesy which proves valuable at subsequent points in time.

Test Marketing

Test marketing gives the researcher opportunities to explore any remaining questions through a real world test of products or materials. Test marketing is the introduction of a product into a carefully (and usually narrowly) defined market, with immediate tracking of audience reactions through intercept interviews, surveys, or other techniques. These data are then used to modify the product or promotional campaign, launch the campaign on a mass scale, or cancel it altogether.

Test marketing (or "formative pilot research") is especially useful when scant resources exist for extensive qualitative research, when a product is non-controversial or already proven in other markets, or when there may be a need for a success story to build upon before a full promotional effort is undertaken. It should be backed by more extensive qualitative research when a new or potentially controversial product is being introduced and the price of failure can be excessive.

Readability is the combination of visual layout and reading level.

Table 6-6 summarizes the advantages and disadvantages of these eight pre-testing methods.

How Much Pre-Testing Is Needed?

There is no firm rule for determining how much pre-testing is needed. The time and resources you have available to prepare and implement a program will in turn tell you what you can afford in terms of the quantity of pre-testing. The following factors should be considered within whatever flexibility available in deciding upon the pretesting effort(s):

- *What is the cost of a less-than-perfect product?* The production costs of TV ads render mistakes prohibitively expensive. Major health promotion research trials often do not allow for modifications in the "independent variable" once the study is underway. In contrast, radio PSAs are relatively easy to change, and occasional problems in small group face-to-face health promotion efforts are not likely to cause much damage.
- *How new or controversial is the program?* The less something has been tried in the past and the higher the "risk" associated with the target behavior, the more pre-testing should be used to optimize the potential for success (or at least prevent a disaster!).
- *How heterogeneous is the target audience?* The greater the number of subgroups, the more research needed. At least some pre-testing of people who have already changed the target behavior ("early adopters") should be undertaken.

Date: _____   Interviewer: _____

Language: ____ Spanish ____ English

Introduction: "Hello, my name is _____
and I work with the Comida Da Vida Project, which is a community nutrition program. Could I ask some questions about your shopping habits? This interview will only take a few minutes."

Beef

1. Did you buy beef in this trip? Yes ____ No ____
2. (If yes) Which type of beef? (circle appropriate cut) Eye of round/top loin/round/tip tenderloin/ground beef/top round/sirloin/other.
3. Did you see the television and video in the meat section? Yes ____ No ____
4. If yes, did you watch the video? Yes ____ No ____

_____
_____

5. If yes: can you describe what it is about? _____
6. What did you think of the video? _____
   liked it ____, didn't like it ____, neutral ____
7. (If the person bought meat low in fat and saw the video) Were you thinking about buying this meat before seeing the video? Yes ____ No ____
8. Did you take one of the recipes located in the meat section? Yes ____ No ____
9. Did you take an information card located in the meat section? Yes ____ No ____
10. Did you notice anything else concerning healthy shopping selections in the meat section? Yes ____ No ____
11. If yes, what did you notice?

_____
_____

Personal Characteristics

1. How frequently do you shop in this store? ____ times per ____ (day/week/month)
2. For how many people do you shop, including yourself? ____
3. How many of these people are less than 18 years old? ____
4. How many years of schooling have you completed? ____
5. How old are you? _____
6. How do you describe yourself? White, non-Hispanic ____, Hispanic, Latino, or Mexican-American ____, African-American ____, Asian ____, Filipino ____, Native American ____
7. Record gender: Female ____ Male ____

"That concludes this interview. Thank you very much for helping." (Also entered in the interview were questions regarding fresh fruit and vegetable selections, cooking and processing demonstrations, and other information pertinent to the Comida da Vida protocol.)

_____

*R. M. Delapa, J. A. Mayer, et al. (1989, March). Food purchase patterns in a Latino community: Project Salsa. Paper presented at the 10th annual meeting of the Society of Behavioral Medicine, San Francisco.

FIGURE 6-9. Comida da Vida exit interview (English/abbreviated version)*

TABLE 6–6
Advantages and Disadvantages
of Pre-Testing Methods

Method	Purposes and Advantages	Disadvantages
Focus Group	1. Group interaction can enhance creativity. 2. Opportunity to observe group dynamics as it relates to subject matter. 3. Economy of time and effort. 4. Good for testing of initial concepts.	1. Individuals may be intimidated or embarrassed to give opinion. 2. Higher possibility of biased responses. 3. Requires skilled researcher.
In-Depth Interview	1. Good for testing sensitive issues. 2. Allows observation of person in natural setting. 3. Can be combined with survey. 4. Good for testing of partially completed products.	1. Time-consuming and expensive. 2. Accessibility to homes may be difficult. 3. Security issues should be considered.
Archival Research	1. Very cost- and time-efficient. 2. Yields potentially valid data. 3. May require skilled researcher.	1. May be difficult to access data. 2. Information may be dated or not directly applicable. 3. May require skilled researcher, depending on form data are in (e.g., on computer disks).
Behavioral Assessment	1. Allows direct and potentially more valid assessment of behavior than does self-report. 2. Can be used with (and to validate) other methods.	1. Presence of observer may bias responses. 2. May be time-consuming. 3. Behavior observed may be irrelevant to research. 4. Requires experienced observer.
Intercept Interviews	1. Time-efficient both with respect to interview and analysis. 2. Respondents may be accessed at point where they engage in behavior.	1. Limited time available with each respondent. 2. Sampling bias possible. 3. High refusal rates possible. 4. Permission needed from authorities.
Gatekeeper Review	1. Highly efficient. 2. Person selected may be knowledgeable about larger group of target audience. 3. Scores "p.r." points.	1. Bias and invalid opinions very possible. 2. Some risk associated with not incorporating suggestions.
Test Marketing	1. Affords the most valid approach to researching communication. 2. Staff gain valuable experience before full-scale marketing begins.	1. Risky if little is known about product or audience, or if product is controversial.
Readability	1. Efficient.	1. Only provides a small part of pre-test data needed.

- *How consistent are the results?* The more variability between and within results stemming from various pre-testing methods, the more information is needed to clarify reasons for this variability.

SUMMARY

Health promotion professionals often have neither the resources nor time to conduct research for planning and evaluation. However, the health promoter needs much more than a passive awareness of research techniques. The best health promotion program is one evaluated on a timely and reliable basis. Be they individual clients, boards of directors, or scientific editors, consumers are more likely to be influenced by data derived from studies that are logically designed and well controlled. Intervention refinements depend heavily on such studies. Behavioral epidemiology and practical research designs comprise an ideal set of tools for individuals working in public health promotion.

Yet more central to typical health promotion practice is formative (or qualitative) research. Formative research assesses target audiences' awareness and understanding; their recall of message; strong and weak points of a health promotion program; and potential controversy related to an intervention. Focus groups, in-depth interviews, intercept interviews, behavioral observation, archival research, gatekeeper reviews, and test marketing are among the more frequently used formative/qualitative techniques.

With the community organized, needs and resources assessed, priorities set and appropriate research conducted, we now turn to specific techniques used in health promotion interventions.

ADDITIONAL READINGS

Keep these books (with a calculator and graph paper) next to the scientist's hat on your shelf:

1. D. Barlow, S. Hayes, & R. Nelson. (1984). *The scientist practitioner.* New York: Pergamon Press.
2. D. T. Campbell & J. C. Stanley. (1963). *Experimental design for research.* Chicago: Rand McNally.
3. D. Dooley. (1984). *Social research methods.* Englewood Cliffs, NJ: Prentice-Hall.

EXERCISE

Select a health promotion topic and test one or two promotion concepts (e.g., a "family-oriented campaign to combat drug abuse"). Divide the class into groups, with one group of four to five responsible for designing materials and procedures for a focus group, in-depth interview, and other pre-testing assessments. The rest of the class should take on varied roles as members of a particular target audience. Each role should be indicated on a placard or name card (e.g., "farmer," "seventh grader with disciplinary problems," etc.). Carry out the various pre-testing with different individuals and small groups of the "target audience." Have all class members discuss the results and critique the pre-testing questions and process.

ENDNOTES

1. Barlow, D., Hayes, S., & Nelson, R. (1984). *The scientist practitioner.* New York: Pergamon Press.
2. Ibid.
3. Campbell, D. T., & Stanley, J. C. (1963). *Experimental design for research.* Chicago: Rand McNally.
4. Mausner, J. & Kramer, S. (1985). *Mausner & Bahn Epidemiology: An Introductory Text.* New York: W. B. Saunders Co.
5. Although not necessarily implied in the present writing, cohort studies can be prospective or retrospective. Retrospective cohorts refer to tracking the outcome of an exposure that occurred in the past progressively to a present or future point. In terms of the timeframe, therefore, the retrospective cohort is similar to the case control study. However, the exposure is being identified first and the outcome tracked subsequently.
6. Campbell & Stanley. *Experimental designs for research.*
7. In this text, we will be using the words "formative" and "qualitative" research interchangeably. It should be noted, however, that formative research can include quantitative data, as well. Conversely, qualitative research could be used for summative as well as formative evaluation.
8. U.S. DHHS, *Making health communications work,* p. 39.
9. J. Candelaria. Personal communication, 1992.
10. Debus, *Handbook for excellence in focus group research,* p. 36.
11. J. Graeff. Personal communication, August 1992.

Chapter 7

Intervention I: Educational Objectives

OBJECTIVES

By the end of the chapter the reader should be able to:

1. Define the three major categories of educational objectives according to Bloom.
2. In selecting objectives for a health promotion campaign, ask appropriate questions for assessing the target populations' specific needs, abilities, and resources.
3. Identify the three main purposes of setting educational objectives.
4. Discriminate between goals and objectives.
5. Write a set of goals and objectives for a health promotion campaign.

INTRODUCTION

The next four chapters of *Motivating Health Behavior* address major, fundamental techniques for promoting health behavior change. Specifically, these are education, training, motivation, and marketing. As Glanz, Lewis, and Rimer note, "[t]heory-driven health education programs and interventions require an understanding of the components of health behavior theory as well as the operational or practical forms of the theory".[1] Health behavior change programs include, but go far beyond, more traditional health educational approaches to changing knowledge and attitudes. Educational objectives establish the cognitive, affective, and psychomotor endpoints we hope to reach with our health promotion interventions and thus guide the development of our intervention strategies. Fundamental to all four intervention approaches is the need to establish specific goals and objectives which allow us to know not only where we are headed, but also when we get there.

A generation ago, the field of health education drew a distinction between knowledge change and behavior change, placing increasingly greater emphasis on the latter. What once was known as "health education," therefore, has been subsumed by the broader concept of health promotion and its constituent technologies. Nevertheless, much of modern health promotion remains heavily influenced by traditional health education, especially in areas such as community development (see chapter 4) and the specification of educational objectives for health promotion intervention.

In his groundbreaking work, **Bloom described a taxonomy of educational objectives which included three major categories, namely, "cognitive," "affective," and "psychomotor."**[2] This taxonomy operationalized the knowledge-behavior distinction. **The cognitive domain emphasizes specific intellectual processes and tasks, typically referred to as "knowledge," "understanding," "memorization," etc. The affective domain includes the feelings and attitudes people experience with respect to certain information, health topics, other people, etc. The psychomotor domain consists of specific behavioral skills, whether they are related to athletic performance, technical ability, or the ease and efficiency by which one performs a particular task.**

Using this classification system, instructional technologists have developed much of the innovation and refinements underpinning the current "state-of-the-art" in education. They have also influenced thinking in other fields, for example, the knowledge-attitude-behavior (KAB) model which defines the context of many of health behavior research efforts. Although failing to give sufficient credence to motivational aspects of human behavior (see chapter 8), this "taxonomy of educational objectives" lends itself to specific operationalization of goals and objectives by individuals from a wide variety of areas. This taxonomy is especially useful in fields such as health promotion, where standardization is needed to coordinate and integrate the efforts of individuals from the various disciplines comprising this new field.[3]

Educational goals and objectives range from the very basic and easily measured to the complex and difficult. As behavior change specialists, we need to remind ourselves not to be overly "reductionistic" in our health promotion efforts by only emphasizing the simple and easily-measured objectives. Gronlund provides examples of the types of objectives we may consider ranging from the simple and straightforward to the more holistic and difficult.[4] Specifically, objectives from the cognitive domain include the following: (1) "identify," (2) "name," (3) "distinguish," (4) "define," (5) "describe," (6) "classify," (7) "order," (8) "construct," and (9) "demonstrate."

Table 7–1 gives examples of how Gronlund's "action verbs" may be used to operationalize and evaluate knowledge and skills related to oral rehydration of young children with diarrhea. Proceeding from the top to the bottom of the table, increasingly sophisticated levels of knowledge and skill are required to achieve the objectives presented in the left column. Each verb in the first column as well as corresponding words that begin the phrase describing performance (second column) are specific and observable verbal or physical behaviors. Using behavioral observation procedures, we can then evaluate whether our objectives have been met through procedures like those presented in the right column. Clearly, all of these cognitive domain objectives would not necessarily be addressed or sampled in one health promotion campaign. Target populations which have been extensively exposed to information in a given area may be ready for higher order objectives, whereas individuals having little or no knowledge about a particular topic may need to begin with identification and definition activities. Appropriate needs assessment and formative research enable the planner to determine at what level(s) to begin.

The selection of objectives depends on a variety of factors, including:

1. Are the objectives consistent with state-of-the-art health promotion? Can the objectives be generalized to other individuals and health problems?

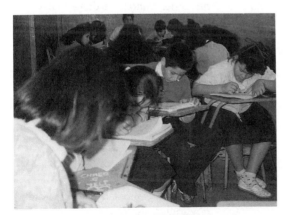

FIGURE 7–1. Traditional health education emphasized knowledge acquisition and attitude change. These Mexican sixth graders fill out workbooks on the effects of tobacco and drug use.

TABLE 7–1
Examples of How "Action" Verbs Are Used to Operationalize and Evaluate Oral Rehydration

Action Verb	Performance	Example of Evaluation Procedure (instructions to the respondents are in quotation marks)
Identify	Select, point out, or circle packet of rehydration salts	"Pick up the packet of rehydration salts," which is placed on the table next to a packet of table salt and sugar
Name	Label the product that is in the package	"What is this called?" with the teacher picking up the packet of oral rehydration salts
Distinguish	Tell which other products may be similar or different	Showing the respondent a packet of ORS produced by the World Health Organization, a locally produced packet, and packets of household table condiments and spices: "Which of these are about the same, and which are different?"
Define	Define or describe the meaning of the specific term(s)	"What does 'oral rehydration salts' mean?"
Describe	Expand on the definition by giving other important qualities or properties	"What are oral rehydration salts for?"
Classify	Group according to common functions or goals	"What other things are there that will keep your child from getting sick or dying?"
Order	Place in sequence by arranging or rearranging an incorrect sequence	Showing pictures of the different steps of oral rehydration therapy, "Place these pictures from left to right to demonstrate how a mother rehydrates her child."
Construct	Make, design, prepare	Handing the woman a glass of water, packet of oral rehydration salts, and measuring cup, and asking, "Show me how you mix the oral rehydration solution."
Demonstrate (model)	Perform procedures with or without prompting	"Show your neighbor how to use oral rehydration therapy."

2. Are the objectives attainable by the target population? In other words, do they have the general educational and skill background to engage in the learning process necessary to achieve these objectives? Are the potential participants sufficiently motivated and are there sufficient reinforcers available to maintain target performance (see chapter 8)?

3. Are the objectives appropriate for the particular domain? For example, although extensive resources may be put into developing a set of objectives for oral rehydration skills using prepackaged salts, many members of the target population may already be using appropriate home remedies (such as soups) for dehydration. In this case, the complicated auxiliary approach might actually be inappropriate and unnecessary.

4. Are the objectives consistent with those developed by others for similar target populations and health behaviors? Such external validation is especially important when developing a novel program or working with this population for the first time.

Health professionals must give careful attention to developing a list of appropriate educational objectives for health promotion efforts that promote knowledge and behavior change. Again, it is necessary to incorporate complex as well as basic objectives, because the former are more likely to promote the generalization of learning to other problems. By using appropriate educational procedures in combination with skills building and motivational approaches (see chapters 8 and 9), education can result in a significant public health impact.

THE PURPOSE OF EDUCATIONAL OBJECTIVES

Educational objectives have three basic purposes:

- to provide explicit or implicit direction for how to carry out the teaching;

- to provide criteria for evaluating effectiveness of the education; and

- to clarify the goals of the educational effort to both educators and students or trainees.

Objectives are stated in such a way that "students" grasp the specific outcome expectations. Although teaching methods are also implied, the target population could figure out a way to reach the same goals and objectives through different means. In other words, the learning processes may differ depending on the background and inclination of the learners.

Educational objectives use "action verbs." Although coming from different theoretical and experimental perspectives, behavioral psychologists and educational technologists converge in their agreement on the necessity to focus on measurable behaviors and their products rather than hypothetical internal states such as "attitudes," "feelings," or other phenomena difficult to operationalize. Although educators are more likely than behaviorists to state general goals in terms of cognitive processes, their specific objectives almost always tend to reflect reliance on operational definitions.

Let's examine the following two objectives:

- understands the physical harm of cigarette smoking
- ranks cigarette smoking first among all preventable causes of mortality in the U.S.

The first statement is a general goal with respect to the knowledge of or attitude toward cigarette smoking. The second is stated more precisely as a learning outcome, which would be much more easily measured than the previous statement. On the other hand, "understanding the harm of smoking" denotes much more than simply being able to indicate that smoking is the number one killer in the U.S. Indeed, the instructor will list several operationalizations of this general goal, sampling from different levels of complexity as is appropriate for the target audience.

A second feature of instructional educational objectives is that they specify an outcome rather than a direction of change. Consider, for example, the following two statements:

- increase use of condoms
- use condoms during sexual intercourse

The first statement above implies a direction of behavior change, emphasizing a process, while at the same time assuming a criterion has not already been met. The second statement indicates a specific outcome and is more appropriate as an educational objective. Thus, the second statement is appropriate either as "acceleration goals" or "maintenance goals" (chapters 3 and 8). Regardless of whether the person is already using condoms or never has used them, maximum protection can only be achieved through consistent use in the future.

In writing educational goals and objectives, we generally start with a more general statement about what is to be achieved, followed by the specific operationalization of that goal or samples of what that goal could entail. For instance, consider the following objective from the affective domain:

"Appreciates the relationship between importance of physical activity and quality of life":

- chooses physical activity over sedentary activity in at least 25 percent of weekend leisure time
- suggests to spouse and children ways that they can become more physically active
- spends 5 percent of discretionary income on goods and services related to physical activity

In the above example, a more general goal is again followed by specific objectives. In this case, these objectives are behavioral manifestations or indicators of the goal of "appreciation." This is by no means an exhaustive list. Dozens of other objectives could be written ad absurdum. The educator simply has to be aware of the fact that he or she needs to sample from a variety of possible outcomes that best represent the goal, as well as the various levels of complexity in achieving the goal.

The following definitions of goals, objectives, and performance are adapted from Gronlund.[5]

- **Goal:** an intended outcome of education stated in sufficiently general terms to include a domain of student performance.
- **Objective:** an intended outcome of education stated in terms of specific and observable stu-

dent performance, which the students would be able to exhibit when they have achieved the goal.
- **Performance** (see chapter 3): any operationalized student behavior that is a product of learning.

Writing Educational Objectives

The following guidelines apply to writing effective educational objectives for health promotion programs:

1. State objectives in terms of the expected performance to be achieved by the end of the educational program.
2. The first word in each objective should be an action verb reflecting an appropriate operationalization of the goal.
3. State objectives in terms of only one, rather than multiple learning outcomes.
4. Goals and objectives should not be content-specific, but instead should be generalizable to other learning activities in a curriculum or educational sequence. For instance, state "identifies the physical effects of drug abuse" rather than "identifies the physiology of addiction to minor tranquilizers in terms of central nervous system activity." An emphasis on the former style will promote generalization of learning to other areas.
5. Objectives should be stated in terms of student, rather than teacher, performance. For example, the statement, "teach the correct use of blood pressure equipment" describes a teacher activity which may or may not entail student learning.

Taxonomy of Educational Objectives

Bloom[6] and Krathwohl[7] define specific levels of instructional objectives within the "cognitive," "affective," and "psychomotor" domains. These levels of objectives vary from the most simple and basic to the most complex and generalizable. Tables 7–2, 7–3, and 7–4 give definitions and examples of each of these levels.

Table 7–2 presents Bloom's knowledge-oriented "cognitive" factors ranging from the fairly basic to the more complex. Bloom's factors

TABLE 7-2
Categories and Examples of Goals and Learning Outcomes from the Cognitive Domain

Definitions	Examples of Educational Goals	Examples of Learning Outcomes
1. Knowledge: Remembering previously learned materials, the lowest level of outcomes in the cognitive domain.	"Knows common medical terms." "Knows specific behavior modification procedures."	"Defines positive reinforcement."
2. Comprehension: Understanding the meaning of material, as demonstrated by interpreting, explaining, summarizing, or predicting.	"Interprets statistical tables." "Predicts the effects of aversive control."	"Projects changes in mortality rates." "Predicts drop off in rate of behavior as a function of punishment."
3. Application: Applying learned material in specific situations.	"Solves problems," "adjusts to changes," "Applies behavioral concept to health promotion planning."	"Discovers appropriate training procedures to be used for health workers." "Solves interoffice communication problems."
4. Analysis: Breaking down material into its component parts so that its content may be understood.	"Recognizes gaps in health promotion material." "Evaluates relevance of promotional campaign."	"Differentiates between proven fact and assumptions in background information." "Notes lack of appropriate formative research in developing social marketing strategies for a specific target population."
5. Synthesis: Putting together the parts to form a new whole.	"Designs multicomponent health strategies."	"Integrates solid waste management procedures with behavior change techniques for child survival."
6. Evaluation: Judging the value of a given material toward meeting a specific goal. This is considered to be the highest level of the cognitive domain in terms of its intellectual demands.	"Determines the adequacy of summative findings." "Judges the appropriateness of the overall research plan."	"Critiques the use of experimental and quasi-experimental research designs." "Compares the use of formative process and summative evaluation data in the overall evaluation."

TABLE 7–3
Categories and Examples of Goals and Outcomes from the Affective Domain

Definitions	Examples of Educational Goals	Examples of Learning Outcomes
1. Receiving: Presentation attending to information, media, or other stimuli.	"Listens to presentation about prejudice in society."	"Asks appropriate questions about the presentation."
2. Responding: Interacting with material in a way which demonstrates interest.	"Shows interest in gaining further information about topic area."	"Volunteers to participate in a discussion about race and society."
3. Valuing: Attaching worth or importance to a topic area.	"Demonstrates beliefs in equal rights."	"Joins minority voter registration team."
4. Organizing: Synthesizing and integrating values.	"Develops a career plan in harmony with belief in racial equality."	"Challenges discriminatory hiring practices."
5. Value-based living: Values are consistent in different situations and over time.	"Consistently acts against racial prejudice at home, work and play."	"Challenges racism whenever it is evidenced by friends, relatives, or co-workers."

roughly parallel those proposed by Gronlund, yet are less behavioral than the latter. The examples apply to the different skills the manager of a health promotion program might need in order to carry out her responsibilities. Note that although these are cognitive factors, their evaluation entails behavioral criteria.

The "affective domain" of the taxonomy of educational objectives again focuses on cognitive factors, but in this case identifies those factors which may predispose one toward one behavior or against another. Just as educators may target the cognitive domain, marketers are likely to zero in on affective factors (chapter 10). Table 7–3 presents hypothetical goals and objectives from a cultural sensitivity workshop given in an agency evidencing racial tension among staff. The objectives again range from basic to more complex. Also, the learning outcomes are once again be-

havioral in nature, in spite of this being in the "affective" domain.

Finally, Table 7–4 gives the taxonomy approach to considering "psychomotor" factors (which *Motivating Health Behavior* shortens to "skills" and treats in detail in chapter 9). Here we have an atypical set of skills, that of "negotiating" with a sexual partner to use a condom, and putting that condom on. Not only do the skills in the psychomotor domain range from the basic to the complex, in this case they also combine verbal with motor skills in one sequence that results in safe sex.

SUMMARY

Motivating Health Behavior represents health education and health promotion as consisting of

TABLE 7-4
Categories and Examples of Goals and Outcomes
from the Psychomotor Domain

Definitions	Examples of Educational Goals	Examples of Learning Outcomes
1. Perception: Obtaining environmental input to guide behavior.	"Recognizes romantic overtures."	"Distinguishes between mere social conversation and a 'come on'."
2. Set: Readiness and willingness to take appropriate action.	"Convinces herself of the need to insist on protected sex if the situation continues to evolve."	"Explains in the conversation that she is someone who doesn't take chances."
3. Guided behavior: Use of imitation or appropriate trial and error, especially when skill is first being learned.	"Mentally rehearses phrases learned in sexuality course to be used in this type of situation."	"Uses a phrase identical to one learned in a course when sexual encounter begins."
4. Mechanical behavior: Routine and skilled performance of task.	"Places condom on partner without interrupting normal process of sexual encounter."	"Places condom on partner without making an error which would necessitate redoing it."
5. Complex behavior: Skillful performance involving complex movements and/or verbal behavior.	"Places condom on partner with him virtually not noticing it."	"Combines efficient physical movement with smooth verbal interaction."
6. Adaptive behavior: Modifying behavior to fit specific situations or problems.	"Learns to detect and deal with non-cooperation by partner."	"Discontinues sexual encounter when partner's non-cooperation is evident."
7. Original behavior: Creativity stemming from highly skilled behavior.	"Develops creative ways to ensure safe sex."	"Creates own phrases that are subtle yet clearly indicate expectation of safe sex."

four basic (and interrelated) technologies: education, motivation, training, and social marketing. Excellent texts on health education have existed for some time; therefore, the present text emphasizes the latter three technologies and their various applications. Nevertheless, all four intervention strategies begin by establishing basic educational goals and learning outcomes. Different levels of cognitive, affective, and psychomotor (behavioral) changes should be agreed upon and specified prior to the implementation of a health promotion intervention, which is described in the next three chapters.

EXERCISE

Break into groups of three. Each person should write on a piece of paper a general health issue or health promotion (e.g., "promote vaccinations"). Pass the paper to the person on your right. The recipient should then write down at least ten goals and learning outcomes, sampling from the cognitive, affective, and behavioral domains. Critique one another's responses.

ENDNOTES

1. Glanz, K., Lewis, F., & Rimer, B. (Eds.). (1990). *Health behavior and health education: Theory, research and practice.* San Francisco: Jossey Bass, p. xxi.
2. Bloom, B. (1956). *Taxonomy of educational objectives: Handbook I, cognitive domain.* New York: David McKay.
3. Gronlund, N. E. (1985). *Measurement and evaluation in teaching* (5th ed.). New York: Macmillan.
4. Ibid.
5. Ibid.
6. Bloom, *Taxonomy of educational objectives.*
7. Krathwohl, D. R. (1964). *Taxonomy of educational objectives: Handbook II, affective domain.* New York: David McKay.

Chapter 8

Intervention II: Motivation— The Technology of Modifying Behavior

OBJECTIVES

By the end of this chapter the reader should be able to:

1. Define the following terms:
   - applied behavior analysis
   - functional determinants
   - motivation
   - performance deficits
   - skills deficits
2. Explain three reasons for the absence of individual health behavior.
3. Define the ABC model of behavior modification.
4. Given a health behavior problem, devise an intervention strategy using the six different contingencies of behavior modification: positive reinforcement, punishment, negative reinforcement, response cost, response facilitation, and extinction.

INTRODUCTION

Individual health behavior may be absent for one of three reasons:

1. The person does not have adequate *knowledge* to perform the behavior;
2. The person does not have adequate *motivation* to perform the behavior; or
3. The person does not have adequate *skills* to perform the behavior.

The focus of the field of behavior modification is on the latter two categories, which behaviorists call **performance deficits (the person has the knowledge and skills, but not the motivation)** and **skills deficits (the person does not have the capability to engage in the behavior, regardless of whether the knowledge or motivation is present).** This chapter discusses methods for remediating performance deficits, and chapter 9 focuses on skills training and related procedures.

The technology of motivation, or more specifically, **behavior modification, refers to the identification and change of "functional determinants" of behavior in order to increase or decrease toward or maintain at an adaptive level.** Functional determinants can be any of a variety of environmental stimuli including people, things, and situations. **Behavior refers primarily to observable performance of any individual which** can be objectively defined, just as learning objectives are. Thus, we can easily define the behavior of smoking as, for instance, picking up and lighting a cigarette, putting it to the mouth and drawing in, and exhaling smoke. However, we cannot objectively define urges to smoke except by relying on the person's subjective report of these urges. Therefore, smoking is a behavior, but an urge is not (chapter 3).

In the U.S. as in most Western and former Eastern Bloc countries, heart disease, stroke, cancer, accidents, and alcohol abuse constitute the major threats to the health of the public. Malnutrition, infectious diseases, and overpopulation contribute to the excessive illness and mortality prevalent in developing countries. Finally, pollution, tobacco and drug use, and war threaten people everywhere on the planet. The common thread running through all of these problems is that human behavior constitutes a major factor in each health threat or disease.

Moreover, these problems can largely be alleviated through health promotion efforts involving increasing, decreasing, or maintaining certain behaviors. In other words, by getting people to do more of some things (e.g., exercising) and less of others (e.g., smoking) while maintaining healthy habits (e.g., regular medical checkups), we can prevent many of the health problems currently confronting our neighbors and ourselves.

A Definition of Behavior Modification

The concept of behavior modification as presented in this book is established in the following definition:

> **Behavior modification is the systematic application of principles derived from learning theory to altering environment-behavior relationships in order to strengthen adaptive and weaken maladaptive behaviors.**

The technology of behavior modification has been referred to by various terms, including "applied behavior analysis," "behavior therapy," and others. Our definition of behavior modification is similar to, although more general than, that of applied behavior analysis. *Applied behavior analysis* has its roots in behavioral psychology developed by B. F. Skinner, John B. Watson, and others, primarily through laboratory research in the first half of this century. In the past two decades the principles of behavior, identified by Skinner and others in their laboratories, have been increasingly applied to natural settings and problems of individuals and communities, hence, the term "applied" in applied behavior analysis. Additionally, applied behavior analysis focuses primarily on observable behaviors, such as those defined above. Particular experimental designs (described in chapter 6) characterize the work of applied behavior analysis.

The authors of *Motivating Health Behavior* have elected to emphasize the term behavior modification instead of applied behavior analysis for a variety of reasons. First, our goal is to reach a large number of health professionals and consumers with health-related concerns, many or all of whom will have had little or no contact with academic psychology. Therefore, the distinction between the more commonly used "behavior modification" and the more specialized term "applied behavior analysis" may prove confusing. Relatedly, as behavior modification has been vastly misunderstood and confused with a variety of other techniques,[1] it seems advantageous to clear up this misunderstanding. This text goes beyond the traditional subject matter of applied behavior analysis, which has primarily focused on individual behavior in areas such as mental health and child and parent training.

In *Motivating Health Behavior*, we use the term "motivation" interchangeably with "behavior modification." This reflects our emphasis on the technology of behavior change rather than its theoretical foundations in behaviorism. Functionally, our technological emphasis puts behavior modification among the other technical areas related to public health, such as waste management, health services administration, occupational safety, and even biostatistics. However, the theoretical and disciplinary roots of behavior modification, in contrast to those of other specialty areas, are in the behavioral and social sciences.

MOTIVATIONAL PROCESSES

Think for a minute about the word "motivation." What does it mean to you? Many see it as a subtle stimulus to act, while others think of it as an intrinsic characteristic that is generally advantageous to those who possess it. Most people have their own definition of motivation, and most of these definitions are based at least in part on subjective processes occurring within a person. For our purposes, however, a more objective and functional definition is required. Therefore, we are proposing the following: **motivation is the interaction between a behavior and the environment in such ways as to increase, decrease, or maintain that behavior.** This definition emphasizes the observable (and therefore objective) qualities of the motivational process. It also precludes the error of "blaming the victim" for seemingly maladaptive behavior.

Why do people sometimes seem to do things that damage their health and at other times fail to take measures to promote health? A variety of reasons may be involved.[2] The person may have insufficient knowledge or skills related to a health issue. Or, they may receive reinforcement for doing unhealthy things while being punished (or at least not being reinforced) for healthy behavior. The present chapter focuses on the latter two factors and on how motivational procedures may be used to overcome them.

Behavior modification is based on the assumption that behavior is a function of environmental events which precede and follow the behavior (i.e., antecedents and consequences). Understanding the concept of motivation is as simple as "ABC," representing a chain of "Antecedents-Behaviors-Consequences." This chapter (and the field of behavior modification) emphasizes the "B-C," or behavior-consequence aspects of motivation.

Taxonomy of Motivational Procedures. Behavior modification is based on a highly developed and sophisticated system which cannot be totally represented within any simple schema or shorthand. However, behavior modification is at the same time a fairly straightforward and economical technology which can be understood by the majority of people taking at least some time to closely study it. In keeping with the goals of the present book, a straightforward 3 x 2 taxonomy of behavior consequence relationships is presented.

There are two primary dimensions to our taxonomy: (1) the action with respect to the motivational procedure being used, and (2) the outcome with respect to the behavior.

Dimension #1: Whether a Procedure Is Implemented. Consequences for various behaviors may be altered in a variety of ways, which can generally be categorized as application, removal, or discontinuation.

Dimension #2: Whether the Procedure Strengthens or Weakens the Behavior. If behavior-consequence relationships increase or continue the probability of a behavior occurring in the future (i.e., accelerate/maintain), reinforcement has occurred. If a decrease in future probability of behavioral occurrence results, this contingency is defined as punishment.

General cultural definitions of "pleasant" and "unpleasant" give us clues of what consequences potentially act as reinforcers or punishers. For example, most cultures and their members would perceive gold coins, food, and balmy weather as pleasant; whereas personal criticism would seem unpleasant.

Our first two dimensions yield the following template for basic behavior modification techniques (Figure 8-1). This schema yields six different behavior-consequence relationships. Not all of them will ultimately be among the tools of the professional health promoter. Yet, understanding these relationships is nevertheless important, as they will allow us to understand why certain unhealthy behaviors occur while seemingly healthy ones do not. These six different contingencies are as follow:

1. *Positive reinforcement:* the application of a consequence following a behavior which strengthens (increases or maintains) that behavior. The consequence is generally perceived as pleasant.
2. *Punishment:* the application of a consequence following behavior which weakens (decreases or eliminates) that behavior. The consequence is generally perceived as unpleasant.
3. *Negative reinforcement:* the removal of an unpleasant consequence which results in the strengthening of a behavior.[3] The type of behavior reinforced with this procedure is called either escape or avoidance behavior.
4. *Response cost:* the removal of a consequence which weakens a behavior. Very similar to punishment, this procedure is generally perceived to be unpleasant, as the person has lost

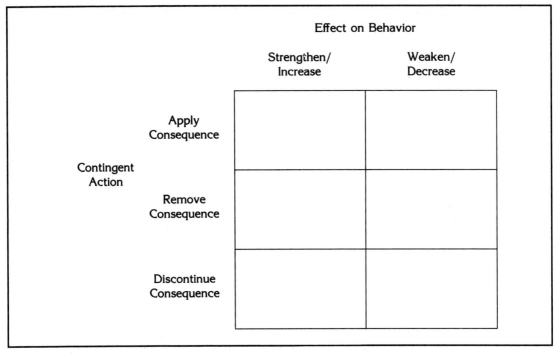

FIGURE 8–1. Effect of consequences on behavior

something of at least some value to him or her (e.g., a fine or the loss of a privilege).

5. *Response facilitation:* the reduction of barriers or the discontinuation of a punishment or response cost procedure which results in the strengthening or reappearance of a behavior.

6. *Extinction:* the discontinuation of positive reinforcement or the imposition of a barrier to receiving that reinforcement which, in turn, weakens the previously reinforced behavior.

As shown, there are essentially three behavior change procedures which produce two types of results: increasing (or maintaining) or weakening (or eliminating) the behavior. Our diagram can now be given more detail (Figure 8–2).

The cornerstone of behavior modification is a procedure called reinforcement, representing cells A and C of Figure 8–2. **Reinforcement is the process by which a response is strengthened, or the probability of its future occurrence is increased by the consequence that follows it. The consequence is called a reinforcer.**

Positive Reinforcement

Example #1. As part of the World Health Organization's "Operation Smallpox Zero" campaign, which successfully eliminated smallpox from the world health scene,[4] health workers in India were given a bounty as an incentive for detecting people in public places (open markets) who might have had symptoms of smallpox. These people were subsequently referred to health officers and, if actually diseased, were quarantined and treated appropriately. When correct positive diagnoses were made, the health workers received a reward payment equivalent to approximately one week's salary. This payment maintained high rates of vigilance on the part of the health workers in seeking out potential smallpox victims, and was part of an effective armamentarium of techniques responsible for the success of Operation Smallpox Zero in India.

In the program described above, the incentive announced to the health workers consisted of giving something (a reward) to the worker that re-

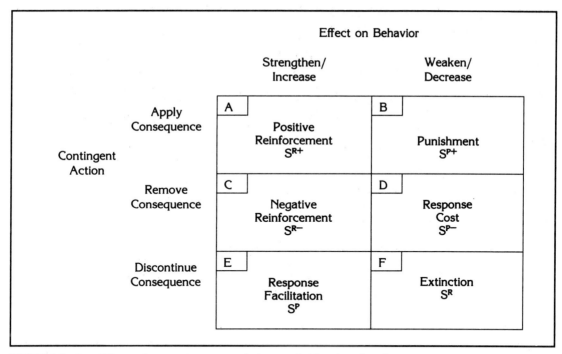

FIGURE 8–2.   Effect of consequences on behavior (with more detail)

sulted in strengthening of "vigilance" or surveillance behavior. These are the conditions that define positive reinforcement.[5] The term "positive" does not refer to the perceived value of the consequence, nor does it imply that the reinforcer is inherently "good." (For comparison, refer to the section on negative reinforcement.) It simply means that something was applied or added as the "environment's response" to the behavior.

Reinforcers may be characterized along a number of dimensions. Material reinforcers include tangible rewards, such as money, food, or lottery tickets. In contrast, social reinforcers refer to rewards of an interpersonal nature, including verbal praise, official recognition, or an affectionate hug. Activity reinforcers, such as taking someone out to a ball game for performing a job well, involves reinforcing a less preferred activity with a more preferred activity; this process is referred to as the

Premack Principle. It is important to remember that all of these rewards must be demonstrated to strengthen the behavior of interest before they can validly be labeled as reinforcers. Thus, reinforcement is defined by an effect on behavior.

Example #2.   Coates and Thoreson demonstrated that overweight adolescents who were given allowance money on a daily basis for progressive weight losses lost a significant amount of weight.[6] Thus, this money served as a positive reinforcer for increasing dietary (and perhaps exercise) behavior. The reinforcer in this example is a material reinforcer.

Example #3.   Low rates of handwashing by hospital staff are a major cause of hospital-associated infections. To address this problem, Mayer and her colleagues implemented a group feedback

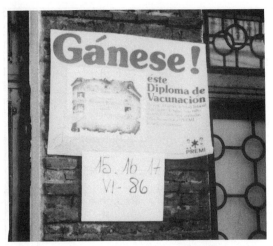

FIGURE 8–3.   Positive reinforcement may combine symbolic and material characteristics. This announcement outside a clinic in Ecuador promotes the "winning" of a vaccination diploma to parents with children under five years of age. *Photo courtesy of John Elder.*

system in an intensive care unit (ICU).[7] Specifically, each day of the intervention, the percentage of ideal handwashing for the previous day was posted in a central area on the ICU. This procedure increased staff handwashing from 63 percent to nearly 100 percent of the ideal level. The feedback strategy is an example of social reinforcement. (Note that this feedback could function as either positive or negative reinforcement; see subsequent section.)

Special Considerations in Using Positive Reinforcement.   In spite of the obviously compelling advantages to using positive reinforcement, a variety of considerations must be taken into account before implementing this motivational procedure.

1. One consideration relates to the **selection of the reinforcer.** Although it is easy to demonstrate that behavior modification works, it is important to select reinforcers that can be sustained over a long period of time. In our formative research, adherence to the principle of "inexpensiveness" is crucial if a given intervention is to be prolonged or to be useful to other individuals, organizations, or communities interested in the program. For example, Elder and Salgado demonstrated the short-

term effectiveness of a positive reinforcement system (e.g., weekly lotteries for bags of groceries) for increasing attendance at well-baby clinics in a Mexican community.[8] Only a few hundred dollars were required to maintain this intervention over a period of a few months. Nevertheless, a less expensive intervention was needed, because the host organization could afford only 25 percent of these costs over a longer period. Therefore, a "fading" procedure was used in which the number of lottery prizes was eventually reduced to 25 percent of the initial number, with no discernible drop in attendance.

In addition to being feasible for delivery over the long-term, reinforcers must be appropriate for and acceptable to the target population. It is important to remember that reinforcers will vary in effectiveness by demographic and cultural characteristics. Through formative research techniques (chapter 10), one can test the potential effectiveness of various reinforcers. This includes examining previous programs, interviewing potential consumers about how appealing they would find various reinforcers, and experimenting with these reinforcers for various behavior change efforts before making a commitment to a specific intervention approach.

2. A second consideration is the selection of reinforcers which are economically *feasible* and *appropriate.* By type of reward, we are referring to material reinforcers, including money, food, lottery tickets, or social reinforcers, such as verbal praise or an affectionate hug. Although at first glance social reinforcers may appear more economical than material reinforcers, they can be costly in terms of staff time. Second, to be effective, social rewards must come from credible and/or well-liked individuals. Finally, when working with a population deprived of basic quality-of-life elements (such as adequate food), the impact of social reinforcers may be relatively weak (and meaningless) compared to material reinforcers. On the other hand, social rewards can be cost-effective, particularly when they are delivered by supervisors, family members, teachers, or others who are a natural part of the interpersonal environment. Again, the issues of cost-effectiveness and appropriateness for the population based on cultural values and demo-

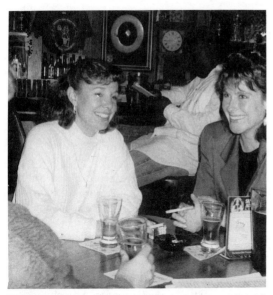

FIGURE 8-4. Professionals working in health promotion must contend with the fact that individuals derive substantial positive reinforcement from unhealthy behaviors. *Photo courtesy of LeAnn Swanson.*

graphic characteristics must be addressed when selecting the type of reinforcer.

3. Two other factors, *salience* and *delay of reward,* should be considered when planning a reinforcement-based intervention. First, in order for the reinforcer to be effective for the target population, there must be sufficient contrast between the reinforcer of interest and ongoing (or previous) reinforcers. This contrast, or salience, relates to both the size of the reinforcer and how frequently the population has been exposed to it. If, for example, the small amount of money used by Jezek and Basu[9] had been offered to American instead of Indian health workers, it obviously would have been insufficient to have produced any change in professional behaviors. Therefore, a technique involving social recognition and verbal praise may have been more effective in increasing, for instance, blood pressure screening activities on the part of American community health workers. However, if American health workers are working in a system where praise is commonplace, it is likely that additional praise would be relatively ineffective.

Therefore, another type of reinforcer which is more salient would need to be used.

Second, the time interval between the target behavior and reinforcement should be minimal. Positive reinforcement is most effective when delivered immediately after a target response. For example, if we want to reinforce small children for brushing their teeth, we need to do so (at least initially) immediately after or even during their tooth-brushing activity. Should we wait until the next day or later, the reinforcer may not be effective in accelerating tooth-brushing behavior. The behavior-reinforcement interval, however, can gradually be lengthened.

Negative Reinforcement

As mentioned in the previous section, the process of reinforcement consists of strengthening a behavior with a favorable consequence. In positive reinforcement, this consists of presenting a pleasant consequence following a behavior. A second method of reinforcing or strengthening behavior is to remove an aversive stimulus or situation as a result of the performance of the behavior (technically, escape behavior), or to avoid an aversive situation (avoidance behavior). This process is called *negative reinforcement.* For example, the alleviation of allergy symptoms after taking a particular medication will increase the probability that the medication will be taken again. In this example, the allergy symptom is the aversive situation, and medication-taking represents escape behavior which is negatively reinforced by the alleviation of the symptoms. If the allergic reaction is eliminated completely by the medication, then avoidance behavior was negatively reinforced. The word "negative" here refers to the "removal" of the stimulus and not to the characteristics of the stimulus itself. (Remember, when describing reinforcement or punishment procedures: positive = presentation of a stimulus; negative = removal of a stimulus; all reinforcement results in an increase in behavioral strength, punishment results in a decrease in behavioral strength.)

Example #1. In China, the use of various birth control procedures was fairly rare until approximately two decades ago. At that time, the government developed a "One Child Policy" whereby

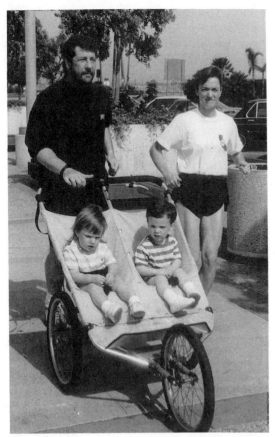

FIGURE 8-5. The positive reinforcement of a family outing and the negative reinforcement of not having to find a baby-sitter may both be powerful motivators for maintaining exercise behaviors. *Photo courtesy of Betsy Clapp.*

parents were strongly encouraged to plan families with no more than one offspring. This policy resulted in the need for more widespread use of birth control. In implementing this policy, Chinese government officials from the central to the neighborhood level used "threats" of loss of work benefits and preferential residential location to reinforce appropriate levels of birth control. Hence, negative reinforcement was being used in that parents were avoiding the loss of social benefits by maintaining their practice of birth control.

Example #2. Contingency contracts (see chapter 12) often involve making public the intentions of participants with respect to their behavior

change goals. For example, many weight loss programs involve a variety of public commitments, including commitments to exercise more frequently. In a sense, these commitments serve to remind individuals of the potential embarrassment should they not follow through appropriately. Therefore, the "threat" of being viewed by friends and family as behaving inconsistently with one's stated goals serves to negatively reinforce the exercise behavior.

Example #3. High rates of drug and alcohol use may be found in many impoverished communities, in spite of the fact that these behaviors seemingly exacerbate prevalent financial and social problems. Nevertheless, the pharmacological effects of the drugs may serve to buffer individuals from their aversive environment. Thus, the high rate of drug use is maintained through a negative reinforcement process whereby drugs serve as an escape from a dismal reality. Again, understanding the process of reinforcement is important for determining how problems come about as well as what to do about them.

Special Considerations in Using Negative Reinforcement. Guidelines for the use of negative reinforcement essentially parallel those for positive reinforcement. For example, the reinforcer must be sufficiently distinguishable from others in the environment to be effective. As an aversive procedure, however, negative reinforcement has a variety of ethical and legal problems not usually found with positive reinforcement. Therefore, an additional guideline is recommended regarding the use of negative reinforcement. If this procedure is used, plans should be made to maintain behaviors initially strengthened through a negative reinforcement process by changing to positive reinforcement. In other words, presentation of pleasant consequences should be substituted for removal of unpleasant consequences. Frequently, there is temporal overlap between these procedures, as illustrated in the following example.

Example #4. China's "One-Child Family Policy" employs rewards to complement negative reinforcement procedures for ensuring proper use of birth control procedures. For instance, in addition to escaping from the threat of losing job status, married couples may maintain or increase favorable benefits from their job by limiting their family to one child. Such benefits may include increased vacation days, additional or preferred schooling for their one child, or even promotional preference.

In China, as in many societies, large families help ensure that Chinese parents will have someone to take care of them in their old age. Since sons traditionally care for their elderly parents, they are even more highly valued than ever, due to this one-child policy, and daughters even more devalued. Female fetuses are most often aborted (only because of their sex) or are killed shortly after birth. Some villagers function as "spies" who report second pregnancies to government agents. The pregnant woman is subsequently badgered, bullied, and otherwise harrassed in an attempt to "persuade" her to abort the second pregnancy. Therefore, increased social security benefits are provided to couples with one child. These not only positively reinforce use of birth control but reduce some of the pre-existing incentives for having a great number of children (or just male offspring).

Punishment

Aversive control refers to the use of unpleasant consequences to control or modify behavior. One of the aversive behavioral procedures is referred to as punishment (cell B, Figure 8-2). Punishment refers to the method in which a stimulus (or "punisher") is administered contingent on a behavior. A punisher is therefore a consequence that weakens (i.e., decreases the frequency or future probability of) a behavior. Punishers are generally perceived as unpleasant, and have virtually no role for those of us planning health promotion or prevention programs. Punishment and response cost however, often comprise components of health policy and also play a role in suppressing behavior we would like to see occur. Therefore, it is important to understand these and other types of aversive consequence-behavior relationships.

Example #1. Cigarette smoking in coal mines is strictly prohibited, due to the possibility of igniting airborne coal dust or gases and causing a fire or explosion. Miners who have been injured in such explosions have experienced the "natural" punishment associated with this activity. Those who have been detected to be smoking subsequently may also receive punishment in the form of reprimands.

Example #2. An example in which punishment can be applied is in the area of contingency contracting for weight control, specifically in decreasing caloric intake. If a person consumes more than his or her caloric intake limit, the contract stipulates that they must perform a physical activity in excess of their usual daily activity at an intensity and duration that will equal the excess calories they consumed. The undesirable behavior is consuming an excess of calories and the aversive consequence (or "punisher") is caloric expenditure in the form of extra exercise routines. (Assuming the consequence results in a decrease in the undesirable behavior, this is an example of punishment).

Example #3. A lack of compliance among consumers receiving prescriptions for medications or health behavior change can stem from our inability to recognize the punishers they are encountering. Our insensitivity to the lightheadedness or sexual dysfunction occasionally attending the use of antihypertensive drugs may result in subsequent non-compliance with these drug prescriptions (i.e., compliance was punished by adverse side effects). Novice joggers who try to run several miles after not exercising for years encounter severe muscle soreness, which punishes their newly acquired interest in physical fitness. Careful formative research can help us (a) determine which punishers are suppressing target behaviors and (b) engineer solutions to circumventing or eliminating them.

At times, punishment-related techniques may be appropriate for the imaginative but careful health promoter. For example, the Nestlé Corporation was successfully "punished" for inappropriate marketing of baby formula to mothers in developing countries, which had suppressed adaptive breast-feeding behavior recommended by health professionals throughout the world. Public outcry against this marketing had no effect until accompanied by a punitive boycott of Nestlé products in the U.S. Similar national-level "punishment" has been proposed to curtail marketing conduct by American tobacco companies.

Many of the behavioral principles associated with punishers are similar to the principles associated with reinforcers. As with a reinforcer, a punisher can lose its effectiveness if it is applied too often. Effective punishers are contingent on

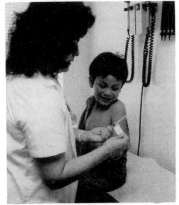

FIGURE 8–6A.

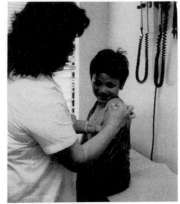

FIGURE 8–6B.

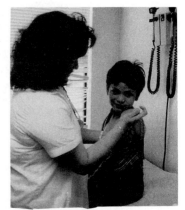

FIGURE 8–6C.

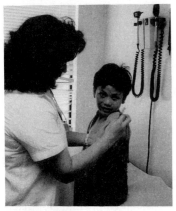

FIGURE 8–6D.

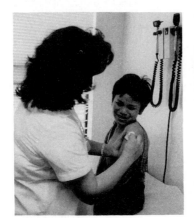

FIGURE 8–6E.

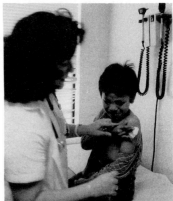

FIGURE 8–6F.

FIGURE 8–6.   Tragically, many parents do not have their children vaccinated because of the punishment (the child's pain and discomfort) and cost associated with the vaccination. *Photo courtesy of Betsy Clapp.*

the behavior, follow the response immediately, and are of sufficient magnitude.[10]

In practice, the use of punishment is fraught with problems and generally cannot be considered for use in public health promotion. Punishment can create a variety of undesirable side effects, such as resistance to or sabotage of a program, and raises a variety of legal and ethical issues. The term "punishment" itself may be unacceptable to health professionals due to its negative connotations. However, familiarity with the *concept* of punishment is critical, as adaptive health-related

behaviors may be naturally suppressed, a condition which may require our attention and understanding of punishment (see section on "Facilitation").

Response Cost

Response cost is the procedure whereby something desired is taken away as a consequence of the occurrence of a certain behavior. The withdrawal of the reinforcer weakens (produces a decrease in the rate of) the behavior. For example, a fine or loss of money may result in the decrease of the behavior for which the fine was received.

Example #1. Across northern Europe, the tradition of heavy drinking is under stiff challenge by governmental and health officials in a number of countries. Almost all of these countries have enacted strong laws concerning drinking and driving. Individuals caught with a minimum or greater amount of alcohol in their blood while driving a car stand to lose a substantial amount of money or even their freedom.

The former Soviet Union under the Gorbachev regime was much more concerned with public drunkenness and the lack of productivity among drinking workers than they were about auto accidents in a country where few automobiles are privately owned. Therefore, Gorbachev and his administrators raised the price of vodka and other popular strong drinks to the extent where a typical worker could afford much less alcohol than before. In other words, purchasing behavior has a much higher cost. Both of these examples are types of response cost procedures woven into health policy. (It is noteworthy that these measures were extremely unpopular, and eventually helped undermine Gorbachev's support and even contributed to his downfall.)

Example #2. A more subtle example of response cost is provided implicitly in health education approaches to increasing the rates of smoking cessation. In addition to talking about punishers (e.g., ill health effects) related to smoking, recent media efforts have emphasized the loss of a variety of attributes, such as physical and personal attractiveness. Such messages emphasize smokers' bad breath, smelly clothes, and other characteristics which eventually result in a reduction of their social acceptability. To the extent that these consequences decrease smoking behavior, these are additional examples of response cost.

Functionally, response cost is equivalent to punishment. The difference is that punishment involves applying an unpleasant consequence following a response, which may result in a reduction of that response, whereas response cost involves taking away something of at least some value.

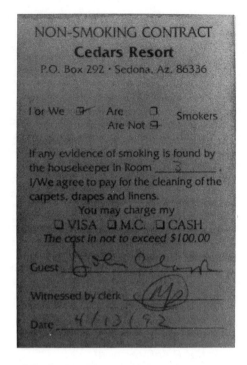

FIGURE 8–7. The possibility of response cost for smoking in a non-smoking room is used by this resort hotel to keep its rooms smoke-free.

Response cost is also functionally equivalent to extinction in that the procedure will result in a reduction of the probability of future occurrence of the behavior. However, extinction is a discontinuation of a person's ability to gain reinforcers whereas response cost takes away previously acquired ones. In practice, the distinction among these three procedures becomes somewhat blurred. At a minimum, it is important for us to distinguish among the three in order to design effective policy and procedures for eliminating obstacles for adaptive, healthy behavior.

All of the above approaches to decelerating behaviors have some problems inherent in them. All of the procedures mentioned here can be met with strong public resistance or unpopularity. Therefore, they should be considered only after (1) an acceleration target representing a positive health behavior is defined and targeted, (2) the target group or community agrees with and helps develop the procedure, and (3) the target behavior for deceleration is deemed sufficiently noxious or dangerous for such procedures to be used.

Perhaps a most important reason for being familiar with these types of contingencies is that health professionals often need to determine why certain adaptive health behaviors are not occurring. For example, health professionals might investigate whether response cost, punishment, and/or extinction are naturally occurring in the environment and what can be done about these problems. For example, children who begin using drugs could have been previously punished by their peers for prosocial behavior, such as achieving good grades in school or engaging in frequent exercise. If such punishment is a "naturally" occurring phenomenon, one intervention strategy should be to reduce the aversive consequences for these activities as well as to provide additional positive reinforcers for them (see section on "Facilitation").

Differential Reinforcement

Guadalcanal Playground is frequently vandalized, littered, and otherwise rendered undesirable by neighborhood parents and their children. Smoking rates continue at an unacceptably high prevalence in a midwestern blue-collar city in spite of the fact most smokers have indicated they want to kick the habit. In a region of a developing country where the indigenous population is frequently at odds with the political party in power, sewage disposal and laundering contaminate unprotected supplies of drinking water, resulting in frequent outbreaks of bacterial infections.

How do we approach the supplanting of these problematic behaviors with more adaptive (i.e., healthy) ones? Theoretically, punishment or response cost procedures would be implemented in an attempt to reduce the frequency of these problems. However, these aversive control procedures could at best lower the incidence of these problems without replacing them with adaptive behaviors to protect or promote the health of the target population. Second, punishment procedures could be ineffective by causing severe undesirable repercussions, such as avoidance behavior or sabotaging of the entire behavior change program.

What culturally acceptable (and potentially far more effective) alternatives do we have to punishment or response cost? Differential reinforcement is a behavioral procedure in which a desired behavior is reinforced while other maladaptive behaviors which normally occur in place of the desired one are extinguished. **Differential reinforcement may be defined as any procedure that has these characteristics: (1) two or more different behaviors can occur in one situation; (2) one**

> **BUDDY-UP** and have a **WILD** day at the *SAN DIEGO ZOO* for free!
>
> <u>**SUNDAY, DECEMBER 13**</u>
>
> **10,000 FREE TICKETS are available to school age children (up to age 15) WHO COME WITH SOMEONE FROM ANOTHER RACIAL, RELIGIOUS OR ETHNIC GROUP.**
>
> We want to show the world that San Diego kids don't judge people by their **skin color**, or **religious views**. Having <u>*friends*</u> who look and think differently from us makes life *interesting.*
>
> For ticket infor, CALL 233-1234 EXT 736 from Nov. 20–Dec. 10. And <u>hurry</u>, it's first come, first served. (Oh yes, your parents are cool, bring them along at half price.)
>
> *Hosted by the San Diego Coalition for Equality Youth Associates & The Zoological Society of San Diego*

FIGURE 8–8. Differential positive reinforcement can be used to promote cross-ethnic socializing.

behavior is reinforced; (3) while the other maladaptive behavior, often the primary target of the program, is extinguished.

Differential reinforcement can be used to increase the rate at which a desired behavior occurs while weakening those behaviors closely related yet unwanted. For example, an instructor teaching lab technicians phlebotomy techniques may use differential reinforcement to reinforce the proper procedure for accurate, painless blood draw while not attending to mistakes made in analogue practice.

Example #1. A World Health Organization health program director in an Indochinese refugee camp noted that mothers treated their babies' diarrhea with a folk method which was always ineffective and sometimes deadly. This was an

important problem, as diarrheal illnesses are among the major causes of infant deaths in these areas of the world. To encourage utilization of medical services at the camp, extra rations of fish and rice were offered to mothers who brought in their infants with diarrhea. Within one week, the number of infants with diarrhea seen at the clinic tripled. Here, mothers were reinforced for seeking medical help instead of employing (in this case, dangerous) home remedies. In other words, clinic attendance was differentially reinforced while the home remedy approach was ignored—and presumably extinguished.

The challenge for any health professional faced with the necessity of weakening or eliminating maladaptive behaviors is first to consider whether it is possible to reinforce differentially an alternative behavior which would "compete" with the

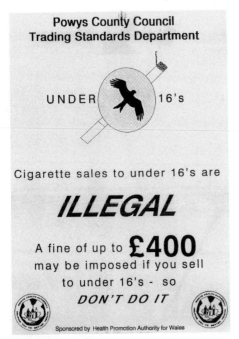

FIGURE 8-9A.

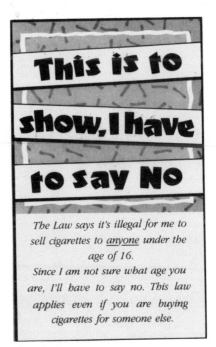

FIGURE 8-9B.

FIGURE 8-9. The Wales Health Promotion Authority combined negative reinforcement and response facilitation to motivate merchants to not sell cigarettes to minors without appropriate I.D. The flyer on the left announces to merchants the fine that they may receive if they sell to children under the age of sixteen (the legal age of purchase in Wales), while the leaflet on the right is what the merchant is encouraged to hand to the young person who is trying to buy cigarettes. With this device, the merchant avoids being forced into the awkward position where they have to verbally challenge the youth. Reprinted by permission of Wales Health Promotion Authority.

maladaptive target, thereby resulting in the latter's reduction. The use of differential reinforcement may have limited potential only when (1) no realistic adaptive alternative exists (e.g., in the case of an alcoholic who spends all of his waking hours drinking) or (2) when the maladaptive behavior is so "toxic" that it demands immediate attention (for example, we may eventually be able to change the abusive parents of a two-year-old by teaching them parenting skills, but the child's immediate needs dictate that we take immediate, even aversive, action).

Facilitation

We now turn to two motivational techniques which involve the discontinuation of behavior-consequence relationships or procedures which in turn result in a change in the behavior being af-

fected by that relationship. **Facilitation is the re-emergence of a behavior that had previously been suppressed by barriers or through response cost or punishment.** In essence, recovery of the behavior occurs with the elimination of barriers to health-related behavior, which, in turn, results in people engaging in behavior.

Example #1. Women in a rural Andean mountain region heard on the radio that their children's lives could be saved by periodic vaccinations given at a local health post. They were, of course, interested in protecting their children and initially came in large numbers to the health post on vaccination clinic days to have their children immunized. However, the trek through the mountain pass to the health post was a formidable one and attendance rates eventually declined. After visiting a few villages, health workers discovered the trips were simply too hard for the mothers to

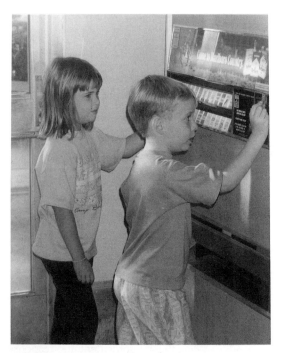

FIGURE 8–10A.

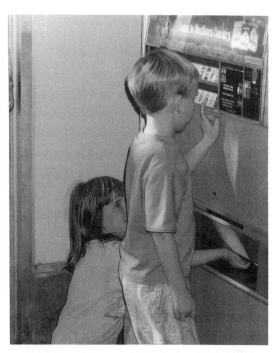

FIGURE 8–10B.

FIGURE 8–10.   Katie and Philip, ages 6 and 7, demonstrate how tobacco purchasing is facilitated by easy-to-use and accessible cigarette machines. (In this ten minute photo session in a state-owned building, only one adult passed by, and he paid no attention to their use of this machine.) *Photo courtesy of John Elder.*

take, given their many duties at home and the difficult terrain. In other words, the barriers (or "punishment") associated with clinic visits were sufficient to suppress this behavior. Eventually, the health workers decided to get the necessary equipment to visit the villages for many vaccination campaign days and reduce the amount of effort that each mother had to make to have her child vaccinated. This facilitation resulted in immediate *recovery* of the health promotive behavior.

Example #2.   Jimmy was a fifteen-year-old who frequently stopped at a local convenience store on his way home from school to buy a pack of cigarettes, from which he smoked two or three in the half-hour walk home. After a health promotion campaign aimed at retailers lax in enforcing the rules regarding tobacco purchase, the owner of the convenience store insisted on identification to verify age before he would sell tobacco to young people. The embarrassment of not being able to appear to be older and the corresponding barriers to purchasing tobacco led Jimmy to avoid this store on his way home. However, the ownership of the convenience store changed hands, and

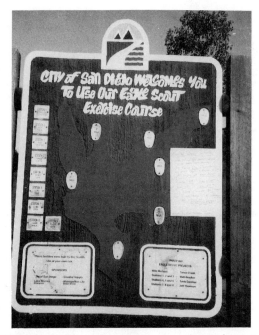

FIGURE 8–12.   Changes in the physical environment, such as through the construction of exercise courses, can facilitate healthy behavior. *Photo courtesy of Betsy Clapp.*

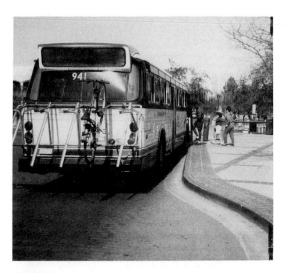

FIGURE 8–11.   Governmental offices, such as transportation authorities, can facilitate physical activity and protect the environment by encouraging the use of bicycles. *Photo courtesy of Betsy Clapp.*

Jimmy tried once more to buy cigarettes from the new manager, who sold them to him without any hassles. Jimmy's behavior of after-school cigarette purchasing recovered in full force.

The phenomenon of facilitation can work for or against health. The health promoter's job, then, is to first assure that all reasonable attempts are made to remove barriers to behaviors before elaborate health promotion efforts are undertaken in the face of these barriers. Second, we must keep in mind that some barriers to health damaging behaviors are appropriate. Efforts in this case should emphasize policies or procedures which maintain or reimpose these barriers.

Extinction

Extinction is used relatively infrequently (if at all) in health promotion. However, it is important to be familiar with this process, as, again, it can help us identify why certain health behaviors are

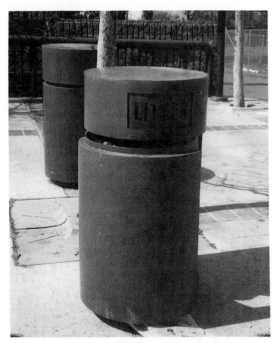

FIGURE 8–13. Although we can make it more convenient for adaptive behaviors to occur, this environmental intervention (providing a labeled trash can) by itself may be insufficient to promote behavior change. *Photo courtesy of Betsy Clapp.*

not occurring. Technically, extinction is the discontinuance of a reinforcement procedure— usually through the imposition of a barrier— resulting in the weakening or "extinction" of the previously reinforced behavior. In the applied behavior analysis literature, extinction is frequently taught to parents and teachers who are having trouble determining what to do with children who continually demand attention through inappropriate means. Parents or teachers are taught to ignore their children's inappropriate behavior (and perhaps to reinforce them later when they are acting more "appropriately"). Given that much of health promotion involves the reinforcement of healthy behaviors or the weakening of health damaging behaviors which usually cannot be ignored, extinction is seldom found as a component of formal health education or promotion programs. However, knowledge of this process is important in situations like those described below.

Example #1. A heart disease prevention program offered a multiple risk factor screening and counseling service to all residents of a community. Although the entire array of risk factor screening procedures was available, the residents were especially interested in the finger-prick cholesterol screening instrument and learning their serum cholesterol levels. Initially, the response to the weekly free screenings was very strong. However, at several consecutive screenings the cholesterol machine was not functioning correctly, and therefore, only blood pressure, height/weight, and carbon monoxide tests were available. Attendance at the screenings dropped off, as the interest in the cholesterol screening was extinguished through use of a dysfunctional machine.

Example #2. An energetic staff training coordinator at an urban hospital put together a series of workshops for the hospital's nursing staff. She was convinced the learning experience would be optimized by having each participant write a brief essay between each of the weekly sessions. She promised to respond in writing to each of the essays in order to "reinforce" the nurses for their attention. Agreeing with her logic, the nurses initially turned in their weekly essays and received written feedback. However, the staff trainer did not anticipate how much work responding to each of the essays would be and became more and more tardy in her feedback. Naturally, the nurses gradually stopped turning in their essays and eventually attended the staff training less and less regularly.

The "moral" of these hypothetical examples is that we must always be able to sustain reinforcement at maintenance levels. Once a behavior extinguishes, it may be very difficult to re-establish it.

Stimulus Control

Stimulus control may be defined as the linking of responses to antecedent stimuli. In other words, stimulus control is the development of the Antecedent-Behavior, or AB, rather than BC, relationship. Stimulus control is enhanced in applied situations by (1) designing environments to make behavior change convenient and comfortable; (2) adding reminders (e.g., signs saying "do

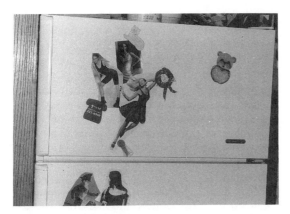

FIGURE 8–14. Stimulus control procedures prompt people to perform or avoid certain behaviors, such as avoiding the consumption of high calorie foods. *Photo courtesy of Betsy Clapp.*

not smoke," buzzers for orienting one to safety belt use); (3) announcing particular incentives and disincentives for the target behavior; (4) obtaining written or verbal commitments from consumers to engage in the behavior being targeted; (5) having health educators, opinion leaders, and others demonstrate the behavior; and (6) presenting slogans, demonstrations, and educational materials to ensure consumers have the requisite skills for engaging in the behavior.[11]

Traditional health education and much of the field of marketing (see chapters 7 and 10) may be viewed by behaviorists as efforts which emphasize antecedents to health behavior changes. Those educators who endeavor to impart knowledge in order to change behavior are in a sense attempting to establish cues for pro-health behaviors. That is, knowledge can result in verbal reminders, demonstrations, written messages, or signs that prompt health behaviors. Such cues might not actually lead to behavior change, however, until the message is accompanied by effective consequences (e.g., peer disapproval for smoking). Recently, health educators have begun to emphasize the importance of consequences in their antecedent strategies (e.g., education, public service announcements, demonstrations). For example, in their development of the widely acclaimed PRECEDE model,[12] Green and his colleagues delineated a variety of techniques for examining causal links among health behaviors, reinforcement, and related factors in reaching "educational" and "behavioral diagnoses." Experimental community heart disease prevention efforts both in this country and abroad have developed novel combinations of communication, educational, and behavioral strategies for fighting the greatest health problem in the Western world. Given that risk factors for disease are largely behavioral, approaches to their prevention and early treatment may be designed best via synergistic combinations of antecedent and consequence strategies and technologies.

An example of stimulus control is the "tip-sheets" developed by the Stanford Heart Disease Prevention Program[13] to summarize risk factor reduction strategies in a few words on a colorful piece of paper. Tip-sheets for how to select food lower in fat and sodium are placed on the consumer's refrigerator in order to bring the selection of healthy food under the stimulus control of the tip-sheet. Several types (and colors) of tip-sheets may be rotated in and out of use in order to maintain the salience of these antecedent stimuli.

Summary of Motivational Procedures

In summary, six different motivational procedures can accelerate/maintain or decelerate

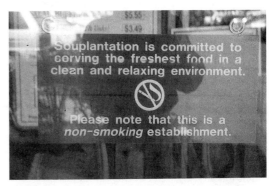

FIGURE 8–15. Stimulus control and other antecedent procedures announce the potential for reinforcement or possibility of punishment to different individuals. This sign indicates that non-smokers will find the atmosphere of this restaurant reinforcing, whereas smokers attempting to light up can expect problems. *Photo courtesy of Betsy Clapp.*

healthy or non-healthy behaviors. Three involve non-aversive procedures (including "facilitation"), whereas three include relatively aversive ones (including "extinction"). A seventh procedure, differential reinforcement, is the application of non-aversive motivational procedures to indirectly decelerate a behavior.

Figure 8–16 presents an algorithm which may be a useful reference for selecting the most effective, appropriate, and ethical motivational procedure for a given health-related behavior. This algorithm prioritizes the selection of acceleration targets and non-aversive procedures. In other words, the reader is "steered" toward the left side and upper part of the figure and away from the restrictive or punitive measures in the lower right section. Although more factors (described in subsequent chapters) actually enter into program development decisions, the following examples show us how this decision-making process can be applied systematically to select a behavior change effort.

It will be useful to examine the following examples while tracking the decision-making processes outlined in Figure 8–16.

Example #1. A health educator in an outpatient clinic is running a weight loss group for four obese patients. Similar to most weight loss programs, her sessions focused on increasing exercise and consuming fewer calories. Her first participant had previously thought she needed to be a jogger or in other ways engage in vigorous exercise in order to lose weight. As a result, she occasionally attempted to go out for a two-mile run, even though her physical condition was not sufficient for this level of exercise. After these sporadic events she was sore for a week and unable to consider trying again for some time. The health educator wisely saw that this woman was being punished for exercise by trying to accomplish too much initially. By helping the woman decide on a plan of walking, followed by a run/walk, she was able to eliminate this punishing experience and the woman was able to exercise more regularly.

The second participant was a middle-aged single parent of two adolescent children. Although she was overweight, she was still physically able to exercise and enjoyed doing so. However, her children paid little attention to her efforts, and she had few friends living in her neighborhood with whom to exercise. Therefore, she often let her exercise practices lapse. The health educator perceived that the target behavior of exercise was not really being suppressed, and thus she helped the woman develop a contingency contract (see chapter 12) with her children whereby they would reinforce her exercise habits (and provide her more time for exercising) by doing housework on nights she wanted to exercise.

The third participant was totally uninterested in increasing her exercise behavior. Therefore, she and the health educator agreed that focusing on reducing calories was perhaps the only feasible approach to her losing weight. After a thorough behavioral assessment, they found the cause of the excess calorie consumption was the fact that the woman had difficulty relaxing and falling asleep at night unless she had eaten a rather large amount of food just before going to bed. In other words, the habit of excessive calorie consumption was being negatively reinforced by restlessness at bedtime. Therefore, a plan of systematic deep muscle relaxation and meditation was used to replace the negative reinforcement and potentially lead to a reduction in late night snacking.

The fourth participant felt he already was exercising at a sufficiently high rate. In addition to feeling no anxiety related to excess calorie consumption, he could think of no competing behaviors which would be appropriate alternatives to his eating. Therefore, a contingency contract was developed whereby the man agreed to give up $10.00 to his least favorite political candidate every week he failed to reach his weight-loss goal.

Example #2. A group of concerned citizens in a middle-sized city formed a committee to develop plans to deal with the city's drunken driving problems. The strategy they chose was to work directly with bartenders and managers of taverns and restaurants selling liquor to see whether they would be willing to keep a closer eye on which patrons were becoming "tipsy," refuse to sell them more drinks, and suggest politely but firmly that they go home. These plans were developed in response to the finding that a large percentage of drunken driving-related accidents and arrests came as a result of bars extending their happy hours.

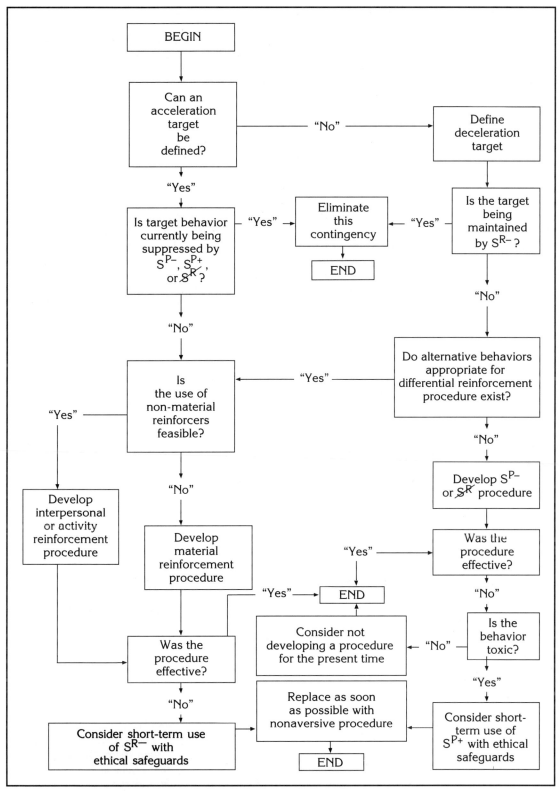

FIGURE 8–16. Algorithm for selection of motivational procedures

The first manager of a restaurant/tavern, Gil B., was somewhat reluctant to implement the procedure, as he made a big percentage of his profits from liquor sales in the restaurant. The committee thought about this genuine concern and decided to offer him public commendation through press releases and other media in hopes of offsetting any loss of revenue through favorable publicity. After some thought, Gil decided to implement the procedure on a trial basis until such time that he could evaluate whether expected revenues changed.

A second bartender, Tanga Ray, admitted that at times she served people who perhaps were too intoxicated to drive, but she felt "that was their business" and she simply did not want to get too rigid in her management rules for an establishment where people came to relax. Tanga did, however, agree to provide more food with the drinks and to consider implementing a "designated driver" system, both of which could serve to suppress the amount of drunken driving without punishing it directly.

A third bartender, Gene Erich, adamantly refused to reduce the amount of sales to anyone in his establishment, be they drunk or not. Since it was discovered that a relatively high proportion of drunken driving arrests came from patrons of this establishment, the committee decided that Gene's indiscriminant selling was indeed dangerous to the public and needed to be stopped, even if it meant the use of aversive procedures. They therefore sought to increase police surveillance in the area surrounding his bar as well as legal avenues to address this problem. However, they continued to communicate with Gene and assured him that they would be more than happy to replace their punitive strategy in the event that he became willing to compromise.

Example #3. A dentist, Dr. Ross, decided she wanted to figure out ways of encouraging her smokeless tobacco users to quit chewing and dipping, since she could clearly see this habit was leading to periodontal disease and mouth sores. She proposed the notion of cessation to each of her patients using smokeless tobacco. First, Dr. Ross determined that she was dealing with a maladaptive behavior. No amount of increased brushing or use of different forms of smokeless tobacco would result in risk reduction in any substantial way. Her first patient, a twenty-year-old man,

started using smokeless tobacco a few years previously with his high school friends. As he expressed some interest in quitting, Dr. Ross decided that a financial incentive for doing so, such as a reduction in her fees by a figure of 20 percent, might serve as an effective differential reinforcement program.

Her second patient had been using smokeless tobacco for a substantially longer period of time than her first patient. He indicated he would like to quit but felt he was addicted to the substance and could not quit without a lot of unpleasant withdrawal. Dr. Ross sought to help him eliminate this negative reinforcement contingency by making an appointment for him with a smoking cessation clinic which implemented methods to withstand withdrawal symptoms.

Her third patient said he simply was not interested in giving up chewing tobacco, which he thoroughly enjoyed. Dr. Ross tried to present all of the evidence regarding the health-damaging effects of this habit, but to no avail. Dr. Ross considered aversive methods such as frequent nagging or an increase in fees until such time as this man quit. However, she realized she was on shaky practical and ethical grounds with such procedures and decided not to do anything at all for the present.

Example #4. An international donor agency specialized in health promotion in underdeveloped countries. It embarked on a program to help host governments promote the use of condoms and safe sex to decrease the spread of AIDS and sexually transmitted diseases (STDs). One recipient country's government indicated the use of condoms was probably a feasible health promotion target, but condoms were simply too expensive and unavailable to rural areas. Therefore, the donor agency developed a plan to reduce cost and improve distribution within this country, hoping a reduction in response cost would increase use.

A second developing country indicated that condoms were readily available but simply not being used, because sexual partners were insufficiently motivated by fear or other contingencies to protect themselves. This country developed a campaign to encourage women to suggest the use of condoms to their sexual partners and socially reinforce them for using them. Similarly, a third country indicated that males in the society were ridiculed by friends and relatives for acting so "cowardly" when it came to sexual behavior, which negatively reinforced unsafe sex. Therefore, the social marketing campaign in this country emphasized the need for man-to-man interactions to reduce the promotion of unsafe behavior. Finally, in a fourth country the minority of couples who were monogamous had a much lower incidence of STDs than did the majority who were either polygamous or routinely engaged in extramarital sex. The health promotion campaign in this country emphasized differential reinforcement of monogamy, not as a social value but as a health protective behavior.

SHAPING

In their classic text on training health workers in developing countries, Werner and Bower warn:

> . . . if students are at (the primary education) level and you try to teach them from (a secondary or greater education) level, you will be talking over their heads. You will bore them and, in time, lose them. You will make them feel stupid. Start with the knowledge and skills a person already has and help him build on these.[14]

How can we ensure our motivational, educational, and other behavior change approaches are both efficient and effective, and avoid embarrassing, boring, or patronizing the intended audience? With the above advice we introduce the concept of **shaping, whereby new behaviors that did not previously exist in a person's repertoire can be developed and reinforced.** This is accomplished by (a) selecting a well-defined end-point or target behavior and (b) reinforcing a series of successive approximations to the selected target behavior. Successive approximations are behavioral elements or subsets, each of which more closely resembles the specified target behavior.[15]

The importance of the concept of shaping in behavior modification cannot be overemphasized. Many complex skills are acquired through shaping. For example, most complicated skills trained in academic courses employ the concept of shaping procedures, whereby successive approximations of end-point target behaviors are selectively reinforced throughout one or several semesters of study. Other examples of behaviors that have been shaped include speaking, walking, partici-

pating skillfully in a sport, reading, playing a musical instrument, and writing.

A good example of an exercise behavior that can be shaped is swimming. In order to learn to swim, a child (or non-swimming adult) must master a series of behavioral subsets or successive approximations before being able to jump in the water and swim effectively. In teaching a child to swim unaided by an adult, the sequence of successive approximations could include the following:

Step 1: Get the child to stand comfortably in the shallow end of a pool unaided by an adult.

Step 2: Socially reinforce any attempt by the child to move around in the water, but no longer reinforce merely standing in the water. Once the child is comfortable in the water, discontinue reinforcement for this step and proceed to Step 3.

Step 3: Reinforce any attempt by the child to dunk his/her head and hold his/her breath under water. Once the child can easily hold his/her breath and dunk his/her head, discontinue social reinforcement for this step and proceed.

Step 4: Reinforce any attempt to float with adult support and then without it. Once the child can float without support, discontinue reinforcement for this step and proceed.

Step 5: Reinforce any swimming motions made by the child while floating until the child can successfully swim for short distances. Then continue reinforcement only for longer and longer distances until the child can successfully swim with confidence.

The above does not detail all the approximations required to teach a child to swim. However, it briefly demonstrates the key points to remember about shaping, which again are (a) to specify an end-point target behavior (i.e., unaided swimming), and (b) to differentially reinforce a series of successive approximations to the target behavior of swimming. As the child becomes proficient at one step toward becoming a good swimmer, reinforcement for that behavior is discontinued and applied only to the next approximation.

Behaviors which do not approximate swimming (e.g., earlier behavior in the successive approximation sequence) are extinguished.

This example illustrates *intentional* shaping or the deliberate effort to create a new behavior. Shaping can also be unintentional. For example, consider the obnoxious behavior of some children. Suppose a mother often rewards her little boy with a candy bar for good behavior at the grocery store. Perhaps later at the dentist's office she reads some literature on the relationship between sugar consumption and dental caries. Hence, she decides to protect her child's teeth by cutting off his candy. Later that week at the grocery store the boy asks for his sweet treat, but the mother refuses to give it to him. At this point the child persists and the mother finally breaks down and gives the treat to him. At a later time the mother regains her resolve and again refuses the child's requests. This time the child is more persistent and more noisy and even obnoxious. Finally, in response to the child's cries and the disgusted faces of the shoppers around her, the mother gives in again. In this case, the mother has differentially reinforced first the request for a candy bar, then the more persistent requests, and finally the loud and obnoxious requests — each request being a successive approximation to the unintentional target of getting access to unhealthy food through pestering.

Another example of unintentional shaping comes from the problem area of excess drinking. Initially, a young executive first entering the work force stops off at the local bar on Friday evenings to have a couple of drinks with his fellow co-workers in order to get to know them better. His fellow employees seem to enjoy his company, and as the weeks go by they encourage him to stay later and "loosen up" more. This activity actually becomes his primary vehicle for socialization into the company. The executive eventually stops by the bar during weekday evenings, as well as Fridays, and stays later and drinks more. This gradually becomes his only meaningful access to interpersonal enjoyment, and before long, frequent and excessive drinking have been unintentionally shaped.

As shown by these examples, shaping may not only be either intentional or unintentional, but also adaptive or maladaptive. As health professionals we are mainly concerned with how to shape beneficial health habits. The following two examples examine further the use of shaping in the health promotion literature.

Example #1. In 1977, Pomerleau and Pomerleau designed a behavioral shaping procedure to help smokers quit their habit.[16] After establishing (and graphing) their baseline level of cigarette use, smokers conduct a form of narrative recording of cigarette smoking in which they determine situations where it would be the most difficult. For example, it might be relatively easy to quit smoking in restaurants with friends (some of whom smoke and some of whom do not), and while being busy and having lots of energy. Alternatively, other situations can elicit smoking, such as being bored in the office, being alone at home, or being with one or two other people who smoke. These situations would be the most difficult with which to cope without cigarettes. Over a five-week period, the smokers are reinforced for giving up cigarettes in progressively difficult situations. They may receive verbal or material reinforcement from their group leader or from themselves through a process known as "self-reinforcement" (see chapter 12). The ultimate goal of being a non-smoker is gradually shaped through successive approximations of this goal.[17]

Example #2. Shaping procedures need not always be as obvious as in the above example. Actually, interventions at all levels of complexity can employ forms of shaping. For example, policies which require employees to maintain a certain level of physical fitness, increases in sin taxes for alcohol and tobacco products, and mandated gender and race balance in community and institutional governing bodies all represent important changes which may be implemented incrementally over time. Positive (and negative) reinforcement for appropriate changes should be contingent on successive approximations of some ideal criterion (e.g., gender and race representation matching that of the population at large).

An actual example of shaping at the policy level involves federal and local requirements for mileage and emissions for automobiles. Following the oil embargo nearly two decades ago, the U.S. government demanded that U.S. auto manufacturers produce fleets with increasingly higher fuel efficiency. Because of the chronic air pollution problems in the Los Angeles basin, regional authorities are placing even higher demands on the

U.S. and foreign auto industries, ranging from gradual improvements in emissions to percentages of sales representing vehicles using less polluting fuels. Both of these indices are expected to show annual improvement over the next ten years. (The former federal effort has met with only partial success, due to intense lobbying by the auto industry; it remains to be seen whether Southern California will achieve its ambitious pollution reduction goals.)

When using shaping to change behavior, keep in mind the following guidelines:

1. Select and define the end-point target behavior as carefully and clearly as possible, and maintain an emphasis on this goal throughout the shaping process.
2. Carefully select a reinforcer that is available, effective, and immediate. What acts as a reinforcer for one person does not necessarily act as a reinforcer for another. Try to understand something about the person(s) with whom you are working before designing a reinforcement procedure.
3. Select a starting behavior that already exists in a person's repertoire and resembles the target behavior as closely as possible.
4. Continually record results and reevaluate the program. If a person has difficulty moving from one approximation to the next, perhaps the step is too difficult or the gap is too large, in which case a new intermediate step should be created. Conversely, if steps are moved through too quickly, your program is perhaps boring or inefficient and suggests too many successive approximations are included and steps could be "larger."

GENERALIZATION

Instead of confining behavior change to only certain situations, **generalization training aims to promote the spread of a specific behavior from one situation to another.** Generalization in this sense refers to a behavior occurring "across situations" (i.e., stimulus generalization).

Generalization can also occur "across behaviors" (i.e., response generalization, or the spreading of the training to different behaviors) and "across people" (i.e., interpersonal generalization,

or the same behaviors spreading from one person who has learned them to others in his/her environment). An example of stimulus generalization is provided by a housewife's responses to the promotion of "heart healthy" foods in her favorite supermarket. As she became more accustomed to purchasing groceries low in sodium and fat, she eventually began to choose fish, poultry, and vegetarian dishes when she and her family went out to eat (i.e., her "purchasing behavior" generalized from the supermarket to the restaurant setting). She then sought to promote her cardiovascular health by exercising with the assistance of an aerobics video three times per week (an example of response generalization from nutritional to exercise behavior). Finally, her healthy behavior generalized to other people when she got her teenage daughters involved in her exercise program. These three types of generalization are described in more detail below.

Stimulus Generalization

Stimulus generalization training is the procedure in which a behavior is reinforced in a variety of related situations. Such generalization training encourages the repetition of a behavior to other stimuli within the same stimulus class. A stimulus class is a set of conceptually related stimuli, such as graduate students, New York City residents, textbooks, or blue objects.

An example of stimulus generalization training is provided by various "psychosocial inoculation" smoking prevention programs.[18] In the psychosocial inoculation process, adolescent students are taught to refuse offerings of cigarettes by classmates in analog role-playing situations. Clearly, the specific situation (being offered cigarettes in the classroom) is not particularly problematic, but represents a class of events (being offered cigarettes by same-or-older-aged peers or siblings on playgrounds, at home, and elsewhere). Instructional and role-playing procedures are therefore designed to encourage the generalization of desirable behaviors learned in class to other stimulus conditions.

Generalization training and stimulus generalization are essential to effective health promotion. Without them our students would have to learn separately how to refuse cigarettes in each new situation they encounter, thereby making it impossible to prevent adolescent smoking. However, generalization training needs to be carefully structured. We would not, for example, want refusal skills to generalize to various prosocial, normal peer instructions. Should our "inoculated" students begin refusing invitations to play or attend slumber parties, they could soon become socially isolated and suffer unpleasant consequences. These instances are referred to as overgeneralization.

Response and Interpersonal Generalization

Generalization of behavior change to other behaviors in a similar "response class" is referred to as *response generalization*. By spreading intervention effects to various health behaviors, response generalization serves to improve the effectiveness and efficiency of our health promotion efforts. For example, Ludwig and Geller[19] found significant increases in the use of vehicle turn signals by pizza deliverers after these employees of a pizza franchise received an effective intervention program to increase the use of vehicle safety belts.

Another example of response generalization was provided by the Pawtucket Heart Health Program's (PHHP) stress management course.[20] The staff at PHHP was initially reluctant to offer such classes as part of its worksite heart health promotion effort, which although popular were dubiously related to heart disease risk reduction. A compromise was reached whereby the stress management course included modules on exercise, weight management, and smoking cessation as well as references to blood pressure control. In this manner, increases in stress reduction behaviors (e.g., use of deep muscle relaxation and time management procedures) generalized to other behaviors which were less directly related to "stress" but more directly associated with risk of heart disease. By presenting the interrelatedness of such behaviors, however, PHHP was able to address heart disease risk reduction more directly through its stress management courses.

The principles for maximizing response generalization include: (1) specifying the stimulus condition under which such behaviors will be rein-

forced; (2) defining the expanded response class, either conceptually (e.g., all are aspects of social behavior, such as conversation and hand gestures), or functionally (e.g., the intake of dietary sodium and saturated fat, both of which are related to heart disease risk); and (3) reinforcing the generalization of behaviors within the expanded response class (e.g., smoking cessation group leader reinforces participants for exercising more, as well).

Finally, and of primary importance to public health promotion, is interpersonal generalization. An important departure that public health takes from medicine is in the former's emphasis on efficient large scale rather than one-to-one or small group change. Although media and marketing, staff behavior management, and organizational and community level interventions all contribute to greater efficiency and effectiveness, the spread of behavior change from one target person to others can also help accomplish these goals.

Returning to smoking prevention programs, most of these emphasize assertive refusal skills such as simply saying "no" or "no thank you, I don't like cigarettes." Recent adaptations of this approach, such as Project SHOUT,[21] not only train students to say "no," but also train a "point-counterpoint" skill. Specifically, students are trained to tell the offerer that not only are they not interested in smoking, but they are concerned about their friends' habits and would like to help their friends quit. In this example, the non-use of cigarettes may be generalized from confirmed non-users to friends who are experimenting with or regularly using tobacco.

How do we promote the generalization of behavior change to others? No simple answer exists, but a variety of "rules-of-thumb" are available, including: (1) initiate behavior change with a highly visible and/or credible model or opinion leader, a person who is more likely to be listened to or observed; (2) through the model or some other method, specify the conditions under which reinforcement is likely to occur, and define the nature of the reinforcement; (3) establish a system for appropriate shaping and reinforcing the model's outreach behavior (e.g., through public recognition or other rewards); and (4) finally, "advertise" the success of the model through various formal and informal media channels which you should have at your disposal.

This concludes our initial presentation of principles and procedures for motivating health behaviors. After exploring the additional intervention technologies of training and social marketing, we revisit these motivational procedures in Section III.

SUMMARY

Motivational procedures can be broken down into six basic categories. Positive reinforcement, negative reinforcement, and response facilitation can strengthen or increase behavior. Punishment, response cost, and extinction weaken or eliminate behavior. Professional health promoters are encouraged to target behaviors which can be increased or strengthened through non-aversive techniques (e.g., positive reinforcement). Sometimes, however, we are left with no choice other than to attempt to reduce or eliminate behaviors which place people directly or indirectly at risk. Differential reinforcement procedures present a non-aversive method for indirectly zeroing in on a "deceleration" target.

Behaviorists view a lack of behavior as stemming from either performance deficits or skill deficits. Motivational procedures address the former problem, while training, our next topic, is used to build skills.

ADDITIONAL READINGS

Reinforce your quest for more knowledge about behavior modification with these sources:

1. L. Keith Miller. (1980). *Principles of everyday behavior analysis*. Monterey: Brooks/Cole.
2. Beth Sulzer-Azaroff & G. Roy Mayer. (1977). *Applying behavior analysis procedures with children and youth*. New York: Holt, Rinehart & Winston.

EXERCISE

Self-Change Activity. Now you're ready to begin. Select one or more motivation procedures along with any additional training you may need (chapter 9) to acquire new skills. Use a "contingency contract" if you feel it would be helpful.

Remember to graph your data on a regular basis. Good luck!

ENDNOTES

1. Krasner, L. (Ed.). (1980). *Environmental design and human behavior: A psychology of the individual in society*. New York: Pergamon Press; and Geller, E. S., Johnson, R. P., & Pelton, S. L. (1982). Community-based interventions for encouraging safety belt use. *American Journal of Community Psychology, 10,* 183–195.
2. Academy for Educational Development. (1987). *Communication planning for child survival programs.* Washington, D.C.: Academy for Educational Development.
3. Note that the "positive" and "negative" which precede "reinforcement" refer not to how pleasant these stimuli were, but to whether they were applied or removed.
4. Jezek, Z. & Basu, R. N. (1976). Operation smallpox zero. *Indian Journal of Public Health, 22,* 38–63.
5. Although technically different, we will interchange positive reinforcement and its synonym, "reward."
6. Coates, J. & Thoreson, C. (1978). Treating obesity in children and adolescents: A review. *American Journal of Public Health, 68,* 143–150.
7. Mayer, J. A., Dubbert, P. M., Miller, M., Burkett, P. A., & Chapman, S. (1986). Increasing handwashing in an intensive care unit. *Infection Control, 7,* 259–262.
8. Elder, J. & Salgado, R. (1987). The well-baby lottery: Motivational procedures for increasing attendance at maternal and child health clinics. *International Journal of Health Services, 18,* 165–171.
9. Jezek & Basu. Operation smallpox zero, op. cit.
10. Miller, L. K. (1980). *Principles of everyday behavior analysis.* Monterey: Brooks/Cole.
11. Green, L., Kreuter, M., Deeds, S., Partridge, K., et al. (1980). *Health education planning: A diagnostic approach.* Palo Alto, CA: Mayfield.
12. Ibid.
13. Farquhar, J., Maccoby, N., Wood, P., Alexander, J., et al. (1977, June). Community education for cardiovascular health. *Lancet,* 1192–1195.
14. Werner, D. & Bower, W. (1977). *Helping health workers learn.* Palo Alto, CA: Hesperian Foundation.
15. Miller, *Principles of everyday behavior analysis.*
16. Pomerleau, O. & Pomerleau, C. (1977). *Break the smoking habit: A behavioral program for giving up cigarettes.* Champaign, IL: Research Press.

17. Alternatively, the procedure may be considered an example of "fading" situations in which smoking is allowed.

18. Evans, R. I. (1976). Smoking in children: Developing a social psychological strategy of deterrence. *Preventive Medicine, 5,* 122–127; see also Perry, C. L., Maccoby, N., & McAllister, A. L. (1980). Adolescent smoking prevention: A third year follow-up. *World Smoking & Health, 5*(3), 41–45.

19. Ludwig, T. D. & Geller, E. S. (1991). Improving the driving practices of pizza deliverers: Response generalization and moderating effects of driving history. *Journal of Applied Behavior Analysis, 24,* 31–44.

20. Elder, J., McGraw, S., Abrams, D., Ferreira, A., Lasater, T., Longpre, N., Peterson, G., Schwertfeger, R., & Carleton, R. (1986). Organizational and community approaches to community-wide prevention of heart disease: The first two years of the Pawtucket Heart Health Program. *Preventive Medicine, 15,* 107–117.

21. Elder, J., Wildey, M., de Moor, C., Sallis, J., Eckhardt, L., Edwards, C., Erickson, A., Golbeck, A., Hovell, M., Johnston, D., Levitz, M., Molgaard, C., Young, R., Vito, D., & Woodruff, S. (1993). Long-term prevention of tobacco use among junior high school students through classroom telephone interventions. *American Journal of Public Health, 83* (in press).

Chapter 9

Intervention III: Training

OBJECTIVES

By the end of this chapter, the reader should be able to:

1. Determine when skills training is needed.
2. List the six essential skills training components.
3. Give a specific example of a skills deficit, and outline a skills training program for its remediation.
4. Plan a training-of-trainers intervention using behavioral training methods.
5. Explain ten principles for effective training.

INTRODUCTION

The previous two chapters presented methods for motivating behaviors which already exist and for establishing new behaviors through shaping. Skills training, the generic name for remediating skill deficits, subsumes the concept of shaping and expands the technology of establishing new behaviors to include the entire antecedent-behavior-consequence relationship. Skills training is especially appropriate for working with larger groups of individuals in a variety of health promotion settings, where people can learn not only from one another, but can also directly practice interpersonal behaviors relevant to a health skill or problem.

A complete skills training format consists of six essential components: (1) instruction, (2) modeling, (3) practice, (4) feedback, (5) reinforcement, and (6) homework. The first two components are frequently found in a variety of health education or promotion efforts. However, whenever skills deficits are involved, it is unlikely the effort will be effective without the direct behavioral steps of practice, feedback, reinforcement, and homework. Specific descriptions of each of these steps are presented below.

1. Instruction. Most training programs and individual sessions begin with an activity equivalent to traditional "teaching" which we call instruction. Instructions generally prepare the trainee by including a rationale for the behavior or skill to be trained, whether it be in terms of becoming more socially or technically skilled or simply healthier. Second, the skill is verbally described by the trainer, which further orients the learner to the new behavior (and may even be sufficient for the learner to give it a try). Additional information imparted during this initial phase includes when it is appropriate to apply the skill, and what behaviors if any can be used as alternatives to the skill. For example, refusal skills trained in drug and tobacco use prevention programs should be used specifically for offers of drugs, alcohol, and tobacco and not for invitations from peers to engage in non-harmful behaviors. In other words, the training teaches the adolescent not to overgeneralize to non-target situations and thus lose friends. In contrast, other students in the groups may be too timid to refuse offers effectively. For these students, simply walking away from the situation may be an appropriate alternative covered by the ideal training program.

In Summary.   The trainer should develop a rationale for the skill and a good verbal description of it, for what situations it is and is not appropriate, and what alternatives may be substituted.

2.   Modeling.   Following instruction, the trainer models or demonstrates the skill behaviors. Modeling is used to clarify the description of the behavior given in the Instruction phase. There are many variations in modeling procedures (see Table 9–1), including the following:

- Modeling may be used to demonstrate various levels of quality of the behavior. For example, it may be appropriate for the instructor to begin by making a mistake in demonstrating the skill. This gives better definition to what is *not* appropriate, and might get the group more involved by having them try to catch and point out the purposeful mistake. Many trainers dispense with this aspect of training and proceed directly to demonstrate the skilled behavior.
- The trainer may elect to do the modeling him or herself, or ask a member of the group to demonstrate the skill as well as possible. While the former approach may be more instructive, the latter may appear more realistic to fellow learners and, therefore, have more appeal. Meichenbaum calls this distinction "mastery" versus "coping" models.[1] Either or both can be effective, depending on the nature of the group and the skills being taught.
- A model need not always be present, but may be presented through audiovisual or print media

or symbolically. To increase instructive attention, the trainer may ask the participants to think about a neighbor, someone else they all know, or even a media celebrity (for young children this may even be a cartoon character).

Recent *innovations in modeling* include the use of videotape and audiotape models and implicitly suggest the preferability of using group settings for interventions emphasizing modeling. In essence, participants can be shown videotapes of individuals or groups engaging in appropriate behavior and then be prompted to imitate this behavior. Given the current wide availability of videotape technology, the use of electronic media is becoming increasingly common in training. Webster-Stratton (1981) developed a set of parent training guidelines applicable to the use of any videotape modeling program.[2] These guidelines include the following:

- Participants should be told the models presented in the videotape are individuals coping with the same problems (e.g., parents, school children in similar schools). To assure viewer identification with the models, the models should be appropriately matched for race, gender, etc.
- The models presented in the videotape should be shown receiving appropriate positive reinforcement for engaging in the target behavior. As much as possible, this reinforcement should be a natural consequence of their behavior.[3]
- The videotape should be stopped frequently in order for the participants to "discover" the correct behaviors being modeled and discuss the applicability to their own situations.

In Summary.   The trainer has to decide who is going to be the model, whether the model will be present, and whether mistakes should be programmed into the demonstration.

3. Practice.   In the practice (or "role playing") segment, as many participants as possible try their hand at performing what they were taught. Through either prior investigation or information provided by the participants in the group session, the role plays are set up to approximate as closely as possible each participant's real world environ-

TABLE 9-1
Factors Which Can Influence the Effectiveness of a Model

I. Factors enhancing acquisition and retention
  A. Characteristics of the model
    1. Similarity of sex, age, race and attitudes
    2. Prestige of the model in the peer group, organization
    3. Competence of the model in performing the skill
    4. Interpersonal warmth
    5. Reinforcement the model receives and its "value"
  B. Characteristics of the observer
    1. Capacity to process and retain information
    2. Uncertainty about what to do in various situations
    3. Level of anxiety, with very high or low levels having deleterious effects
  C. Characteristics of the modeling presentation
    1. Live or symbolic (e.g., "Think about what Superman would do in this situation.")
    2. Multiple models
    3. Mastery versus coping (e.g., "we try harder") models
    4. Graduated modeling procedures, going from less to more difficult skills and situations
    5. Instructions by the model, trainer, or other "actor"
    6. Summarization by the observer
    7. Rehearsal by the observer
II. Factors enhancing performance
  A. Factors providing motivation for performance
    1. Vicarious reinforcement (reward to the model)
    2. Vicarious extinction of fear of responding (no negative consequences to the model)
    3. Direct reinforcement to the observer
  B. Factors affecting quality of performance
    1. Rehearsal and feedback
    2. Participant modeling
  C. Transfer and generalization of performance
    1. Similarity of training setting to everyday environment
    2. Repeated practice
    3. Incentives for performance in natural setting
    4. Training a class of behaviors rather than single ones
    5. Provision of variation in training situations

ment and problematic situation. (One variation of this approach is to give the participants a few minutes to write their own scenarios and allow them to be their own directors as their turns come up.)

Again, the participants themselves should describe the who, what, when, and where of the role-play scenario, selecting the trainer or other participants to perform other roles as needed. Watching the role plays, the other participants have the opportunity to learn vicariously through imitating their peers or learning from their mistakes.[4] Thus, the trainer may decide that a sufficient amount of practice has taken place before all participants have actually been involved in a role play. A fairly technical or complex skill, such as cardiopulmonary resuscitation (CPR), should be practiced once or multiple times by all participants. For purposes of efficiency, participants may be paired or put in smaller subgroups for additional practice.

Two examples of role plays developed by seventh graders involved in Project SHOUT[5] are presented below. First, the general scenario is described, followed by prompts the "confederate" (the person who plays the part of someone else) gives. Below each prompt are listed three responses representing "aggressive," "passive," and "assertive" behavior on the part of the trainee for that particular skit. Although either of the former responses might be appropriate in certain situations and is deemed better than accepting the offer of tobacco, the SHOUT program, like all in this genre, attempts to train participants to the "gold standard of the *assertive* response.

Project Shout Skit #1: At a Friend's House Watching TV. Scene: One of the guys from class has invited you and some other boys and girls over to his house to watch *Police Academy 5* on TV. His parents are out for the evening and you've got the whole house to yourselves. Everyone is sitting on the floor having cokes and popcorn. You're having a great time, waiting for the show to start.

- **Confederate:** "Here — I've got some snuff. Take a pinch and pass it on."
  —[Aggressive: "No thanks, Jerk. I don't dip snuff."]
  —[Passive/ignoring: "Hey — did you see *Police Academy 1* and *2*? I really liked them."]
  —*[Assertive: "No, I think I'll pass on this one."]*
- **Confederate:** "Come on, I said take some and pass it!"
  —[Aggressive: "Hey, I said I didn't want to and I mean it. If you're going to dip, then just get out of here."]
  —[Passive/ignoring: "Why don't you just pass me some popcorn and soda?"]
  —*[Assertive/broken record: "No, I think I'll pass on this one."]*
- **Confederate:** "Just a little won't hurt you."
  —[Aggressive: "No way, stupid."]
  —[Passive/ignoring: "Move over some, the movie's started."]
  —*[Assertive/broken record: "No, I think I'll pass on this one."]*

Note that the "assertive" responses to the second and third offers are repeats of the first response. This "broken record" technique is used to counter interpersonal pestering and negative pressure without either ignoring the "pest" completely or getting into an argument.

Project Shout Skit #2: Football Game. Scene: You and a good friend decide to go to the local high school football game together. At half time, your friend drags you out of the bleachers to find some of her friends from the other team's school. You find a group of kids behind the bleachers. You're having fun meeting the kids from out of town. You notice a cigarette is being passed around the circle. Everyone else has taken a drag or two, including your friend.

- **Confederate:** "Here you go, have a drag."
  —[Aggressive. "No way, guys. I don't want to, so just lay off me!"]
  —[Passive/ignoring: "What do you think of the game so far? That last touchdown was awesome."]
  —*[Assertive: "No thanks. I don't like the smell of the stuff."]*
- **Confederate:** "Sure, one drag won't hurt you."
  —[Aggressive: "Why don't you shut up, Jerk? You guys are going to get into big trouble."]
  —[Passive/ignoring: "Has anyone tried the hot dogs here? Are they pretty gross, or what?"]
  —*[Assertive/broken record: "No thanks, I don't like the smell of the stuff."]*
- **Confederate:** "Come on, we're waiting. Let's see how much older you look when you're smoking."
  —[Aggressive: "Well, you'll be waiting a long, long time. Got it?"]
  —[Passive/ignoring: "I think half time is about over. The band just stopped playing."]
  —*[Assertive/broken record: "No thanks, I don't like the smell of the stuff."]*

As can be seen in both of these role plays, the Project SHOUT format assumes that "just saying no," at least just once, will be insufficient to resist negative pressure as it occurs in the real world. Therefore, all students are trained to anticipate and respond to multiple offers.

In Summary. In the practice phase, the trainer works with the participants to set up the most realistic role play possible, and decides how many participants to engage in the role play before all have had adequate opportunity to acquire the skill.

4. Feedback.   Just as participants may serve as models and design their own practice scenarios, they should also be involved in providing one another feedback as to the quality of performance in the practice session. Often, the trainer first asks the performer to indicate what she or he thought of the practice. In some settings, this can be done after reviewing a videotape or audiotape of the performance, a very effective training tool, especially for interpersonal skills.

It's important for the trainer to explain that feedback should refer to the behavior and *not* the person (e.g., in a CPR training, "you did a good job of placing your hands correctly and compressing the mannequin's chest," rather than "you're really good at this — you should be an EMT!"). Guides for giving feedback on complex behaviors, such as interpersonal responses in difficult social situations, may be useful to the trainer and participants giving the feedback (see the SHOUT role plays, above). Also, there should be an accentuation of the positive — all participants should take note of at least one commendable aspect of the practice in order to avoid discouraging the participant. The theme is to "catch them doing something good," which sets the stage to shape even the most humble behavioral beginnings into skillful performance. This does not preclude the need for corrective feedback on any errors made. One should be as positive as possible, emphasizing how to correct the error: "next time, look the other person in the eye and speak up when refusing to take a hit on his joint," rather than "looking down and mumbling — boy, you sure screwed that up!"

Generally, the trainer will solicit feedback from the participants and then provide some of his or her own. By giving personal feedback, the trainer (a) has the opportunity to correct any of the comments made by the other participants, including excessive negativism, and (b) demonstrates a "personal touch" to the performer, who probably expects at least some input from the trainer.

In Summary.   Feedback on the in-session practice performance should accentuate the positive and be specific to the behavior and not the person. Both participants and trainer should be prepared to offer the feedback.

5. Reinforcement.   In terms of its ultimate effect, reinforcement is often functionally equivalent to rewarding feedback — hearing from others that the performer did a good job will make it likely that skill will occur again. We should ensure our verbal feedback includes some reinforcing qualities. Contrast the following two statements:

"You lost two pounds last week, and your records indicate you've been sticking to your 2200 calories per day limit."

"Wow! You lost the three pounds we would expect from your calorie reduction, and you're looking great!"

Although both statements were specific and constructive, the latter included a tone and phrasing that is potentially far more reinforcing. Reinforcement may include more than just an adjunct to the feedback, however. Diplomas, intra- or inter-group competition, letters of commendation from the trainer to parents, or even hugs may be appropriate, depending on the type of group, the setting and target skills, and the style of the trainer.

In Summary.   Reinforcement is presented in conjunction with feedback. It generally takes a verbal form, but may also include other forms of interpersonal or material rewards.

6. Homework.   Finally, guided behavioral assignments, or "homework," promote the practice of the new skill in the real world. Often, this practice takes place between sessions, with the subsequent session leading off with a discussion of the participants' experiences in carrying out their homework. In some cases, training may be restricted to a single day or session, in which case the trainer should arrange for some sort of follow-up with each participant to troubleshoot or reinforce, as appropriate.

The specific type of behavioral assignment will vary as a function of the nature of the participants and the target behavior. Drug or smoking prevention program participants may be asked to note only the occurrences of offers and their reactions to these offers (if there were any). Health workers learning individual counseling techniques may be asked to be proactive and seek to conduct a health education session before the next meeting with the other trainees. Professionals learning other highly technical skills over a long period of time will progress through a shaping process from basic to complex assignments. Smokers might be assigned a daily reduction target of five cigarettes and urged to practice the coping skills to combat each temptation to smoke (at the same time they may also be instructed to write down descriptions of these urges and coping responses). Mothers learning oral rehydration skills would probably just be asked to remember what happened.

In any case, information provided by the participants is feedback to the trainer; therefore, participants must be urged to be totally honest and avoid simply trying to look good for their instructor. Are training objectives being met? If not, is the pace too fast or slow? Are the participants progressing at equivalent rates? Is there reinforcement in the natural environment using the skill? Are there barriers?

In Summary. Homework is essential for ensuring the skills learned in a training session generalize to the real world. It is also the primary source of feedback to the trainer with respect to how well he or she is doing in teaching the skills.

Table 9–2 briefly summarizes each of the six steps of training and gives the lay terms for these steps.

Training as Reinforcement

Health professionals constantly seek out new information, challenging professional opportunities, interaction with colleagues, and other rewards associated with training. Taking advantage of this motivation, training itself can be used as a reinforcer for a job well done or, more directly, for successful applications of previous training. In resource-poor environments, training may be one of the few reinforcers a manager has available. Through training, the skilled manager can continuously update staff skills while maintaining motivation.

Training-of-Trainers

Effective training may be conducted on a one-to-one or small group basis, but a public health impact is achieved when we train "change agents" (or "multipliers"), who in turn train, counsel, or provide services to others. This pyramiding approach is known as "training of trainers."

TABLE 9–2
Brief Summary of the Six Steps of Training

Behavioral Term	Lay Term	Description
1. Instruction	Teaching	Trainer gives rationale for and describes target skills or behaviors.
2. Modeling	Showing	Trainer or participant demonstrates example (sometimes including an incorrect one) of the behavior.
3. Role playing	Practice	Participants practice the behavior in realistic scenarios.
4. Feedback	Feedback	Participants receive behavior specific assessments of how well they did from all participants (as well as through self-assessment) and from the trainer.
5. Reinforcement	Reward, "attagirls/attaboys"	Trainer and participants give verbal and other reinforcement, as appropriate.
6. Guided behavioral assignment	Homework	To create the potential for generalization to other situations, participants are given inter-session assignments and report back at the next session.

Emergency Medical Training. For example, training is frequently used by managers to enhance the skills of health workers. However, such training must be carefully designed and implemented or problems may ensue. For example, despite extensive training, it is questionable whether certified emergency medical technicians have actually mastered essential CPR skills. Previous studies suggest a need for more extensive practice and follow-up to this practice. Seaman compared a standard training approach for CPR with behavioral skills training.[6] In standard training, the instructor modeled the steps of CPR using a mannequin, after which trainees practiced on the mannequin and then received feedback from the instructor. In the behavioral training condition, the trainer continued to work with the subjects who had received standard training and commented on each specific step of the CPR with respect to whether the trainee had performed it correctly or incorrectly (e.g., opened patient's airway, established breathlessness, ventilated patient, established pulse, activated EMS system). The trainer also used charts to present feedback publicly to each trainee. Participants who received this additional behavioral training performed more effectively than those receiving the standard package alone. Additionally, the skills were maintained over a longer period of time.

Family Planning Motivators in the Philippines. Some very compelling examples of training-of-trainers come to us from the health promotion literature in developing countries. In such areas with minimal or no primary health care services, it is sometimes necessary or even preferable to work with traditional healers and other individuals recognized in the community as having expertise in health. In the rural Philippines, for example, a project was undertaken to train traditional birth attendants as family planning motivators.[7] Nearly 500 traditional birth attendants (TBAs) underwent a one-week training program. Subsequently, some of the TBAs received additional supervision (focusing on their family planning behavioral assignments), while others received supervision and a monetary incentive for family planning to bolster the recruitment activities of the traditional attendants. Following up the lecture, modeling, role playing, and homework with supervision increased the effectiveness of the traditional birth attendants in recruiting women to

family planning efforts. Interestingly, the addition of a monetary incentive did not increase this number beyond the effects of extended supervision alone. Thus, it appears that extended supervision was a sufficient reinforcer in and of itself to ensure application of the skills learned during training.

The Bangladesh Rural Advancement Committee. As it is in many countries, diarrhea is the major cause of morbidity and mortality in rural Bangladesh. The Bangladesh Rural Advancement Committee (BRAC)[8] developed a health message called "Seven Points to Remember" for teaching mothers to combat diarrhea. The seven points were as follow:

1. Loose stools and increased frequency of stools are the first symptoms of diarrhea, which result in loss of water and salt from the body.
2. The consumption of clean water and food will help prevent diarrhea. Flies should be kept away from food, while hands and mouths should be washed before eating. Breast milk is harmless, but dirty breasts may make children ill.
3. The only treatment of dehydration is to replenish water and salt loss. This is best done through oral rehydration.
4. Oral rehydration is made by mixing a pinch of salt with a fistful of molasses in water.
5. Oral rehydration solution should be administered immediately after the first loose bowel movement.
6. Children should be given oral rehydration at frequent intervals but not more than they want at any one time.
7. Regular nutrition should be maintained as much as possible during bouts of diarrhea. Increased amounts of water and food for at least seven days after recovery will also help prevent malnutrition.

These seven points were communicated to mothers through the use of female outreach workers who contacted 60,000 households during a one-year pilot phase. Subsequently (in 1980), an attempt was made to reach 2.5 million households (accounting for 14 million people) throughout Bangladesh. During home contacts the outreach worker introduced herself and engaged in friendly conversation. She gradually shifted the conversation to the "Seven Points," inviting questions as they went along. Once the initial knowledge was understood and accepted, the outreach worker modeled preparation of the oral rehydration solution mixture. In this modeling she focused on measurement of the liquids as well as the salt and sugar. She then asked the woman to practice it herself and subsequently reviewed the Seven Points one more time. Next, she asked the woman to identify any diarrhea cases in the neighborhood and visited those households, as well. These outreach activities were supported by visits to village chiefs prior to the home visits by "team chiefs" who were males (as were the village chiefs). The team chiefs organized diarrhea control campaigns complementing the home visit campaigns and organized meetings with local healers to teach them about the mixture and to elicit their acceptance.

A monitoring team visited a randomly selected 5 percent of the households to inquire about the Seven Points among women who were previously visited by the outreach workers. The women were also asked to prepare a mixture (which was taken back to a laboratory for analysis). They were asked if there was a recent diarrheal episode in the household and, if so, what treatment was used. Women were reinforced for using appropriate treatment and were given corrective feedback if inappropriate or no treatment was applied.

The outreach workers were paid strictly according to an incentive system. Each woman interviewed was graded according to her ability to answer questions regarding the Seven Points and to prepare an appropriate ORS mixture. An "A" was given if the woman remembered all seven points and made the mixture correctly, a "B" if she remembered most of the points and made the mixture correctly, a "C" if she remembered fewer points but made the mixture correctly, and a "D" if she could not make the mixture correctly. The outreach worker received the average grade which was multiplied by the number of houses she visited to determine her salary. Approximately twenty cents (U.S. equivalent) was paid for each household in Grade A, whereas ten cents and five cents were paid for B and C, and nothing was paid for D.

Attendants were carefully selected before becoming outreach workers. A preselection training period included three days in the classroom and two days in the field, allowing the supervisors continually to evaluate knowledge and skills re-

lated to outreach and health education ability. Tests included paper and pencil as well as role playing. Preservice training lasted at least two months for candidates passing the preselection training, and ongoing in-services were provided as well.

In the two and a half years of the program, over 1.5 million households were reached. A staff of 903 (over half of whom were outreach workers) accomplished this goal. The amount expended to teach a single household was approximately $1.00. Results showed that women maintained knowledge of the Seven Points over a six-month follow-up period. Usage of appropriate oral rehydration however ranged dramatically from 8 percent to 80 percent, depending on the area. This program showed that illiterate mothers are capable of understanding health messages delivered on a face-to-face basis, and that health workers can be appropriately motivated to accomplish this difficult yet challenging task. Specific behavioral assignments and material reinforcement were especially important aspects of this training-of-trainers success.

Indonesian Kader Training.   While mass and print media have been useful in increasing awareness and knowledge of oral rehydration therapy (ORT) for cases of diarrhea, face-to-face communication has been important for teaching mothers when and how to use oral rehydration solution (ORS) in the home. Village level health workers as well as clinic-based health workers, therefore, have become increasingly viewed as a valuable channel for helping mothers learn to use ORS appropriately.

The deployment of Indonesian village health workers, called "kader," is especially important in rural areas of Indonesia, where socio-economic and geographic barriers can prevent large numbers of individuals from obtaining professional health care. Underscoring their emphasis on the training and deployment of kader in the primary health care system, the government of Indonesia soon hopes to have nearly two million of these village health volunteers trained and functioning throughout this nation of 184 million people.[9] However, brief and infrequent training, lack of subsequent supervision and support, high dropout rates, and a corresponding lack of application of these services by villagers undermine this important approach to health care delivery and preven-

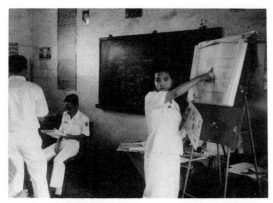

FIGURE 9–1A.

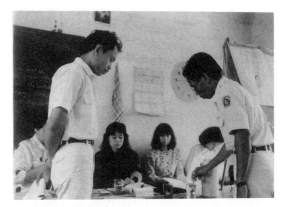

FIGURE 9–1B.

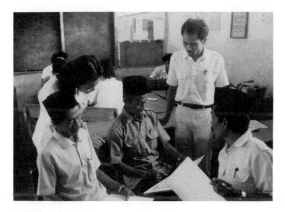

FIGURE 9–1C.

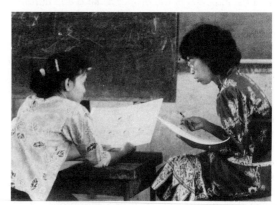

FIGURE 9–1D.

FIGURE 9–1.   In the above sequence, an Indonesian physician instructs community health volunteers in how to use counseling cards for mothers of children with diarrhea, while her two assistants role play the use of the cards. Next, the village health volunteers break out into groups of three and practice the use of the cards, as one plays the role of the parent, the other the health worker, and a third provides feedback (assisted by the health professionals). Finally, each village health volunteer is individually checked for his or her proficiency by role playing individually with a physician, who takes the role of a mother. Later, the physician (on the right) gives feedback to the volunteer. *Photo courtesy of John Elder.*

tion.[10] These problems limit the effectiveness of kader, especially when they are faced with tasks as complex as the control of diarrhea and the management of dehydration through ORT. These are relatively complex skills, requiring not only knowledge about how to diagnose and treat diarrhea and dehydration, but also how to communicate these strategies to the parents so they will use them with affected children.

In cooperation with USAID's HEALTHCOM Project, the West Java Department of Health car-

ried out an extensive research and development effort to produce effective job aids for the kader diarrhea control, as well as a training program to teach their use. A set of counseling cards were produced to provide kaders with tools to diagnose and treat diarrhea and teach the proper use of oral rehydration.

The idea for developing a set of counseling cards came out of research on kaders revealing that current materials were inadequate to help kaders advise mothers on diarrhea. West Java

Health Department staff launched an extensive effort to develop more "user friendly" materials for kaders and mothers.

Counselling cards were developed, field tested, and eventually refined into a single set of five 11" × 5" cards consisting of a diagnostic card and four treatment cards. The diagnostic card applies a binary algorithm that leads to a diagnosis of one of the five categories of diarrhea specified in the Ministry's case management approach. The categories of diarrhea are color-coded and numbered to match the four treatment cards. One side of the treatment cards contains specific advice and illustrations depicting the steps the caregiver should take. The reverse side of each card describes and depicts the proper mixing and administration of ORS.

In a formative research study, researchers assessed the cards' effectiveness through observations of kader performance and interviews with the mothers they had counseled. In the intervention group, fifteen kader underwent one day of training to use the cards when diagnosing and advising treatment for cases of diarrhea in their villages. The sixteen kader in the control group received comparable training and teaching posters, but not the cards. During a second training session, both intervention and control kader participated in role plays, during which they were evaluated on the accuracy and thoroughness of their diarrhea counseling. Each group of kader was also given a list of local mothers to counsel. Researchers then held follow-up interviews with those mothers to test their level of knowledge on diarrhea control and to observe their ability to mix ORS properly. Analyses of the data showed significant performance differences between the intervention groups of kader and mothers compared to the control groups. Although the kader in the control group did reasonably well, the intervention kader were consistently more accurate in their diagnoses and recommendations for treatment. Mothers counseled by the intervention kader also prepared ORS significantly better than the mothers counseled by the control kader. This training-of-trainers work with Indonesian kader shows how skills training, accompanied by a highly effective "portable supervisor" (the counseling cards) and specific behavioral assignments, produced dramatic changes not only in the kader, but also in the mothers they counselled.

SUMMARY

We close this important section with **ten guiding principles for effective training** developed by the Indonesian Department of Health:[11]

1. "We Teach the Same Way We Are Taught."   Participants trained through dry lectures by trainers with patronizing styles will go on to use similar training techniques and styles. Conversely, effective skills training can also be passed down from generation to generation.

2. "The Goals of Training Need to Be Clear and Understood by All."   Goals need to be well formulated (see chapter 7) and understood by each participant. "Tell them what you're going to tell them, then tell them, then tell them what you've told them." One way to ensure that this understanding takes place is to review what was covered at the end of each session.

3. "The Trainer Must be Credible."   Former smokers, qualified health workers, or top graduates from previous workshops can all become qualified trainers. The participants need someone with whom they can identify and trust.

4. "A Distinction Must Be Made Between Correct and Incorrect Behavior."   While emphasizing the positive, the trainer has precious little time with each individual trainee. In many cases, the last training session is the last face-to-face contact between trainer and student. Participants cannot leave this encounter with the impression that "anything goes." By using modeling in which participants are encouraged to detect the model's flaws, videotaped feedback of role plays, and other techniques, the skillful trainer can maintain an upbeat tone while at the same time ensuring the discrimination between skillful and incorrect behavior.

5. "Participants Are There to Participate."   From helping to set objectives to interacting in a give-and-take during the instructions, participating as models, designing their own role play scenarios, helping provide feedback, and completing and reporting on homework, active participation is both egalitarian and effective.

6. **"Use a Variety of Sensory Modalities."** Combining reading, acting, writing, and audiovisual presentations keeps everyone's attention.

7. **"Break Out into Small Groups Frequently."** Practice and feedback can be much better personalized in groups of three to four participants.

8. **"Master One Skill before Moving on to the Next."** This fundamental rule of shaping ensures that each skill will serve as a solid foundation for its successor. Breaking up the instruction between each skill facilitates remembering. To do this, a careful behavioral analysis of the skills involved is a prerequisite to the training.

9. **"Participants Measure Their Own Progress."** Grading their own pre- and post-tests, watching videos of successive role plays, and self-monitoring homework completion and other extra-group practice puts the participants in charge of their own skill acquisition efforts.

10. **"Practice, Practice, Practice."** Both in and outside of the group, repetition is a must; the more complex the skill, the more repetition is necessary. However, the trainer walks a fine line between the desire for perfection and the danger of boring the participants.

Being able to conduct effective health education and training as well as remediate performance deficits are fundamental health promotion intervention skills. We turn now to the final intervention topic of marketing, which integrates these techniques with others from communications and advertising to create public health behavior change.

EXERCISE

Take turns practicing training by role playing participants and a trainer. Decide the topic and persona each will assume beforehand. Videotape or audiotape the role play and critique the trainer. Trainers may purposefully "goof up" so the class can catch the mistake.

ENDNOTES

1. Meichenbaum, D. (1971). Examination of model characteristics in reducing avoidance behavior. *Journal of Personality & Social Psychology, 17,* 298–307.
2. Webster-Stratton, C. (1981). Videotape modeling: A method of parent education. *Journal of Clinical Child Psychology, 10,* 93–98.
3. Participants can thus receive "vicarious" as well as direct reinforcement.
4. For an innovative use of vicarious reinforcement through radio spots depicting health workers receiving praise, see chapter 10.
5. Wildey, M. & Edwards, C. (1990). *Project SHOUT Trainers' Manual.* San Diego, CA: San Diego State University.
6. Seaman, J. E. & Green, B. S. (1986). Behavioral system for assessing and training cardiopulmonary resuscitation skills among emergency medical technicians. *Journal of Applied Behavior Analysis, 19,* 125–135.
7. Fernandez, T. L., Estrera, N. O., Barba, C. V. C., Guthrie, H. A., & Guthrie, G. M. (1983). Reinforcing mothers for improving infants' diets with local available food. *Philippine Journal of Nutrition, 36,* 39–48.
8. The Center for Community Health Education and Program for Diarrhea Disease Control, Department of Health, Republic of Indonesia. (1989). *Communication Strategy for Diarrhea Control: Diarrhea Treatment in the Community,* pp. 24–25, Jakarta.
9. Ibid.
10. Ibid.
11. Ibid.

Chapter 10

Intervention IV: Social Marketing and Health Communication

OBJECTIVES

After reading this chapter, the reader should be able to:

1. Define the following terms:
   - advertising
   - broadcast media
   - display print
   - interpersonal channel
   - market analysis
   - mass media
   - print media
   - products
   - promotion
   - PSA
   - segmentation
   - social marketing
2. Describe the role of social marketing in ONPRIME.
3. Describe the steps of public health communications.
4. Propose a market analysis and segmentation strategy for a particular public health or health promotion challenge.
5. Select appropriate channels of communication for a particular public health problem or health promotion challenge.
6. Describe the similarities and differences between social marketing and behavior modification.

BACKGROUND

Social marketing is the "design, implementation, and control of programs seeking to increase the acceptability of a social idea or practice in a target population."[2] Although this definition of social marketing overlaps substantially those of the other elements of STEM (education, training, and motivation), there is one functional distinction that remains and probably will endure for the foreseeable future. Social marketing relies on mass media to a much greater extent than do other health promotion technologies. Mass media is usually considered to be newspapers, magazines, radio, and television using impersonal communication approaches delivered to large numbers of people. Actually, social marketing is currently the rage in health promotion: while few texts in related fields of health psychology or health education gave much attention to this topic fifteen years ago, nearly all contemporary texts in this area (including *Motivating Health Behavior*) have at least a chapter on it.

This burgeoning popularity of social marketing

can be attributed to a variety of factors. Consistent with its affiliation with the field of advertising, social marketing techniques sell well to public health planners and educators. We grew up with the mass media as our baby sitters and companions, and we continue to enjoy working with technologies and topics associated with marketing. Second, through its use of mass communications techniques, social marketing greatly enhances our potential for achieving a public health impact for our health promotion efforts, whereas more traditional strategies could be more appropriate for individuals or small groups. For better or worse, social marketing and its component discipline, public health communication,[3] have permanently altered the practice of health promotion.

Public health communication includes a variety of techniques, but specifically emphasizes: (1) a two-way flow of information; and (2) a few practical and simple messages through as many "channels" (see below) as possible. The success of a communication program is determined by a variety of factors, including: (1) how much access the target audience has to the information (e.g., Does a large percentage of the target audience own television sets and telephones?); (2) whether people were actually exposed to the media advertisement (e.g., If used in a billboard on a highway, did the billboard stay up long enough for people to see it?); (3) whether the target audience acquired sufficient knowledge and skills to perform the target behavior; (4) whether the target audience actually has the opportunity to emit the behavior (e.g., in the case of promoting jogging in northern cities with long winters); and (5) whether this trial and subsequent short-term adoption can be reinforced naturally through subsequent communication approaches. As can be seen, a substantial overlap exists between behavior modification and health education on the one hand and communications and social marketing on the other.

More than other health promotion techniques, however, communication is the process of sharing information between two or more persons via mass media, face-to-face exchanges, or other "channels" using words, pictures, music, and other audio-visual or symbolic approaches. Specifically, the uses of media for health promotion include:

- building awareness and promoting visibility of the health promotion program;

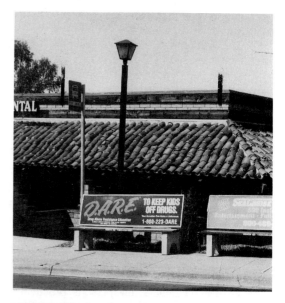

FIGURE 10–1. Print and other media may be used to convey a brief health message and provide information about program services. *Photo courtesy of Betsy Clapp.*

- adding the issue of health to the "agenda" of the community's various interests;
- promoting health behavior change directly; and
- recruiting people for special behavior change activities such as self-help groups, screenings, or health services.[4] Mass media has a low cost per person reached relative to more intensive behavior change efforts; however, it may be less effective than behavior modification approaches for individual change.

For purposes of this text, social marketing is defined as the application of communication and marketing concepts to the design, implementation, and management of social change programs, such as health and safety promotion.

Differences Between Marketing and Social Marketing

While marketing is the parent of social marketing, the two differ on several key dimensions. First, marketing generally involves the selection of a product by a consumer with no actual behavioral skills required. Social marketing, in contrast, promotes multiple behaviors which, at times, require high levels of skills.

Second, marketing relies on natural and immediate reinforcers. For instance, when we buy a new car or a bag of potato chips, we are immediately reinforced (albeit in different ways) for these purchases through our enjoyment of them. In contrast, health behaviors often have little, if any, immediate reinforcement associated with them. Social marketing, therefore, must overcome (directly or indirectly) the delay of primary reinforcement in order to be effective.

Third, to be a success, marketing requires one or very few purchases by a small percentage of the population. Social marketing for public health change, in contrast, requires high levels of response rates from large numbers of individuals in order to have sustaining influence on public health. For instance, the infrequent use of condoms or use by only a few persons practicing high-risk behaviors would do little to reverse the rate of the spread of HIV infection: only rates approximating 100 percent will suffice.

Comparing Behavior Modification and Social Marketing

The technology of behavior change is the main focus of this text. Behavior modification aims to identify environmental factors which, when systematically controlled, enables behavior change in desired directions. In other words, the behavior change agent is interested in establishing and maintaining certain target behavior(s) under appropriate circumstances.

Social marketing is a spin-off from the fields of advertising and communications. The goals of marketing are primarily to prompt individuals to buy some product or service and, thus, are quite different from those of behavior modification. Segmentation is designed to identify subpopulations most likely to buy a particular product, with an eye to the subsequent marketing of the product (or service) to those individuals. Most businesses need only to sell their product to a small proportion of the population in order to make profits. Thus, a marketing goal may be to change a few people only once or occasionally in order to make money. Although most commercial producers recognize the importance of manufacturing quality products (e.g., toasters that work) in

order to bring established customers back, they are not necessarily interested in sustaining a high frequency of individual behavior.

This illustration shows that marketing goals are often directed at recruiting new customers to buy a given product or service. As a company saturates its market, it must change its sales product or service, as when restaurants add new food items. These strategies enable businesses to continue selling products and services to make money.

Social marketing is a term which implies the use of marketing procedures to change social behavior. Its goal is not necessarily to sell a product or service, but rather to change the attitudes or behaviors of a population. When a political party is interested in getting a majority of voters to vote for its candidate, for example, marketing techniques might prove effective. The party might attempt to change the candidate choice for only 15 percent of the voting public. Advertising campaigns are designed to prompt a relatively small portion of the population to change one simple behavior (voting) at one time (on election day). For such short-term behavior change objectives, marketing may be very effective. Such techniques, however, may not sustain attitudes, voting, or other social behaviors

Marketing techniques are often held to be valuable and effective procedures for altering protective or risk-related behavior. Indeed, marketing strategies may be very useful in prompting an initial behavior change. However, marketing tactics should not be expected to sustain behavior change except where the new behavior is "naturally reinforcing" (i.e., is reinforced by consequences intrinsic to the task or available in the environmental setting). The use of advertising, for example, to get individuals to attend a community or social function can be effective in establishing long-lasting behavior. Presumably, once the process is set in motion, continued participation is maintained by the naturally occurring reinforcement inherent in the community or social activities.

As a rule, marketing techniques are relatively ineffective when the target behavior does not lead to "natural" reinforcement, and are even less effective when the objective is to stop undesired risk behavior already maintained by powerful reinforcers. Vehicle safety belt use may be illustrative. The use of advertising to prompt and sustain safety belt use has produced only modest effects alone, particularly because the use of safety belts can be inconvenient and physically uncomfortable (see chapter 19). The negative reinforcement potentially derived from surviving an automobile crash is too unlikely to be a reliable reinforcer. Advertising might prompt initial belt use, but such behavior is not likely to be sustained in the absence of passive systems in the automobile (e.g., interlock systems) or the individual's social network. Thus, even for a relatively simple protective behavior like safety belt use, advertising alone is probably inadequate to establish and maintain the behavior for a majority of the population.

Social marketing and behavior modification differ in other important features. Although both technologies entail measurement, they rely on different theoretical models and corresponding measurement procedures. Most marketing campaigns attempt to change the consumers' attention, attitude, knowledge, or beliefs. The theoretical assumption is that new cognitive processes will lead to "informed" decisions to buy the advertised product. Given this theoretical model, marketing research is often directed toward identifying people already predisposed to buy the target product. This usually involves collecting demographic characteristics of certain subgroups of the population. Expensive automobiles need not be advertised to low-income people, as they cannot buy them even if they want to. Once the major subgroups are identified, survey researchers ask target consumers about their preferences, knowledge, attitudes, and beliefs. This information is used to identify more precisely subgroups who may be most likely to buy the target product or service. These data are also used to design advertisement campaigns for changing the knowledge, attitudes, and beliefs of individuals who report attitudes not conducive to purchasing the target product. Again, the assumption is that changing an individual's beliefs will lead to a change in his or her purchase behavior. The tactics used to change knowledge, attitudes, and beliefs are largely antecedent-oriented educational procedures.

Marketing, as noted above, suggests media-based advertising. In turn, media can be used to enhance applications of motivational and training procedures. Learning theory research has illustrated the power of role models (see chapter 9) and the types of conditions which enhance the effectiveness of models for evoking target behavior. Unfortunately, the modeling for risk behavior seems to occur far more often than the modeling of healthy or protective behavior. (For example, Geller and his students documented disappointingly low [below 20 percent] safety belt use on television from 1984 through 1987, while coverage of sports events often includes a prominent cigarette or beer ad in the background.)

The use of media to provide models for healthy behavior might be exploited more completely for health promotion purposes. Legislation ensuring equal time for risk reduction ads might be one approach. Another might be the more aggressive use of dramatic arts. Why does it seem, for example, that actors have to display smoking or alcohol consumption as a component of an amorous relationship? Drama can certainly be entertaining when actors are practicing safe, protective, or health-enhancing behavior. For example, buckling a vehicle safety belt prior to a chase scene can add to the drama by cueing the viewer of an exciting vehicle chase. The systematic use of the entertainment industry to provide repeated models of health promotion behavior could improve public health dramatically and thus requires much more attention.

Marketing and Social Reinforcement

Marketing procedures might also alter the frequency and nature of social reinforcement and/or punishment for target behaviors. It is plausible that reported advertisements and models aimed at prompting new social interactions could establish new behavior which would be maintained by "natural" social consequences. The media can set in motion a snowball effect where a cumulative increase in the number of people imitating a given behavior can occur. If enough people try out a new behavior, they provide additional examples and socially reinforce one another (and others) for initiating similar behavior. Taken to its logical extreme, such an event may lead to new social norms.

Public opinion (i.e., voting support) of the Vietnam War was generally favorable in the early 1960s. However, as the news media displayed war horrors and protests, the public's opinion began to shift. This process took years, but ultimately culminated in the U.S. withdrawing from the war.

Such complex social shifts cannot be attributed solely to models as presented by the media. Failure to win a decisive and early military victory undoubtedly played a part. Nevertheless, extensive press coverage and ever growing numbers of protestors provided an increasing number of models for anti-war sentiment.

The same type of process is probably taking place presently with regard to smoking behavior (chapter 7). Increasingly, news, theatrical presentations, and signs sponsored by special interest groups (e.g., the AMA) advertise "no smoking" messages. Models are increasingly present for asking smokers to stop or at least not smoke in public buildings. As a result, more people (nonsmokers) assert themselves and ask smokers not to smoke, or insist on no-smoking sections in restaurants. As these assertions increase, so do the social reinforcers for such assertions. In fact, a nonsmoker increasingly reinforces another nonsmoker for asking a smoker to stop smoking.

Indeed, this process can accelerate to the point where the smoker may not only put out a cigarette, but express an apology (again, social reinforcement) for disturbing the nonsmoker. Media-based input to the community about smoking, its risks, and its distastefulness (as a social behavior) might have prompted these changes. However, relief from environmental smoke (negative reinforcement) and social support (positive reinforcement) for anti-smoking assertions may be the more important consequences for sustaining such behavior. It remains to be seen whether such social behavior change will be sufficient to increase the rate of smoking cessations or decrease the rate of smoking initiations.

These accounts illustrate how marketing might contribute to the initiation of behavior which is then subsequently reinforced "naturally." They are at best speculative. To be more certain of the power of these marketing techniques, systematic interventions should be tested. At any rate, mar-

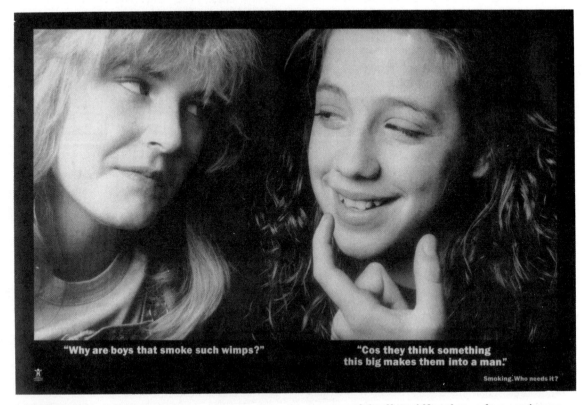

"Why are boys that smoke such wimps?"

"Cos they think something this big makes them into a man."

Smoking. Who needs it?

FIGURE 10–2.   Social marketing pieces, such as this one out of the United Kingdom, often use humor to make their point or deride an unhealthy habit. Reprinted by permission of Health Education Authority.

keting techniques will be increasingly relied on to engineer changes in social reinforcement which can sustain health protective behavior.

In summary, social marketing skills are valuable tools for the behavior change specialist and health professional. Although coming from very different conceptual and theoretical backgrounds, marketers can greatly enhance public health promotion efforts, especially given their sense of reaching large numbers of people for large-scale behavior change efforts. The behaviorist, in turn, can contribute to the effectiveness of a social marketing approach, especially regarding consequences necessary to enhance and maintain performance of health-related behaviors.

THE PROCESS OF SOCIAL MARKETING

Our discussion now turns to practical issues with respect to how social marketing can be integrated with the technology of behavior change for enhancing public health. Social marketing can serve a variety of purposes. Applied specifically to health promotion, it has been used to: (a) create awareness of a health issue, problem, or solution; (b) create demand for health services or support for individual or community action; (c) teach skills; and (d) prompt and reinforce the maintenance and generalization of beneficial behavior change.[5] In other words, social marketing can be used to target any of McGuire's "output variables" (see chapter 3), ranging from the initial stages of simply getting people's attention to long-term maintenance of change to the intervention and follow-up processes.

The Academy for Educational Development's Health Communication for Child Survival (or "HEALTHCOM") Program[6] is one of the most innovative approaches to the integration of communication, social marketing, and behavior modification for health promotion in developing countries. Their basic public health communications model (adapted for this text) is as follows:[7]

Step 1: Working within the general goals (or "mission statement") of the project, _plan_ the communications component of the health promotion strategy and _test_ the general concept of the intervention strategy.

Step 2: _Select channels_ of communication (print, broadcast, interpersonal, etc.). Also, _develop_ or select materials, "products" (e.g., medications, exercise equipment, specific health behaviors), and select change agents (a.k.a. "multipliers" or "intermediaries") and means of providing them training on how to use materials, perform the behaviors, etc.

Step 3: _Pre-test materials_, products and training by examining different ways to present the message, audience reaction (recall, understanding, acceptance, etc.), different formats, and various distribution approaches.[8]

Step 4: _Revise_ materials, products, and training according to the pre-test data.

Step 5: _Implement_ and deliver materials, products, and training.

Step 6: _Monitor_ and _evaluate_ audience reaction to the communication and corresponding behavior and attitude change, and modify the program accordingly.

As can be seen, a strong parallel exists between this model and the more general ONPRIME approach, with Step 1 embodying the _Organization_ and _Needs/Resources_ Assessment phases; Step 2 equating to the _Priorities_ component; Steps 3 and 4 comprising the _Research_ phase; and Steps 5 and 6 having direct counterparts in ONPRIME's _Intervention_, _Monitoring_, and _Evaluation_ phases.

PLANNING HEALTH COMMUNICATIONS

Concurrent with at least the initial phase of marketing research activities (see below), marketers develop a health communications plan which lays out in general terms how the marketing activities will be developed, implemented, and evaluated. This plan may consist of the following components: market analysis, market segmentation, marketing strategy (including lists of products/behaviors, message construction, creative approach, and marketing mix), materials and products distribution, a training plan, a monitoring and evaluation plan, a management plan and a timetable, and a budget.

First, a **market analysis is conducted to establish the market "boundaries" (i.e., who and what** are to be targeted and excluded), the geographic area encompassed, and whether the market size is growing or declining. Second, the market analysis obtains information about the wants, needs, perceptions, attitudes, habits and readiness for change, and satisfaction levels of the potential market (i.e., the target population). It also obtains basic demographic information. The important characteristics of targeted individuals or groups are derived from both primary data (gathered from questionnaires, focus groups, and interviews) and secondary data (obtained from archival investigation). This step is crucial for any marketing effort and provides the foundation upon which market segmentation and strategies are constructed.

If the plan is being developed by someone external to the organization, the analysis may also address the organization's financial, staff and managerial resources, and commitment. Also, a list of other agencies which are potential competitors can benefit the market analysis.

Market **segmentation is the partitioning of a potential market into homogeneous submarkets based on the common characteristics identified from the market analysis.** The purpose of market segmentation is to provide a basis for selecting target markets and developing optimal promotional programs for individual target segments. In public health promotion, high-risk market segments are often identified in the hope of achieving the "biggest bang for the buck," whereas at other times groups high in "readiness for change" represent ideal targets (see Figure 10–3).

Although this segmentation is rather straightforward in the field of advertising, it can be problematic in health promotion programs. Bloom and Novelli identified two specific problems that social marketers face during market segmentation.[9] Many health and social agencies resist segmentation because their egalitarian mandate or philosophy prohibits treating certain groups differentially or treating some groups while ignoring others. Also, self-report data may not be adequate to identify the market segments objectively. Nevertheless, in an era of limited resources for health promotion, some form of market segmentation is essential if any impact is to be realized.

After social marketers analyze the market and determine target segments, they develop a specific **marketing strategy** to achieve the desired behavior change in the context of the interests and characteristics of the identified targets. A specific, central communication message consistent with program goals is decided upon at this point. This message will be presented clearly and consistently in all subsequent promotion efforts, program materials, and products. Several other key elements of the marketing strategy are considered, including the development or diversification of the "product," backed by "promotion," and put in "place," "position," and at the right "price" — the five "Ps" of marketing.[10] The implementation of specific strategies depends on the novelty of experience with the product or audience (see Figure 10–4).

The products of health promotion programs generally comprise specific health-related behav-

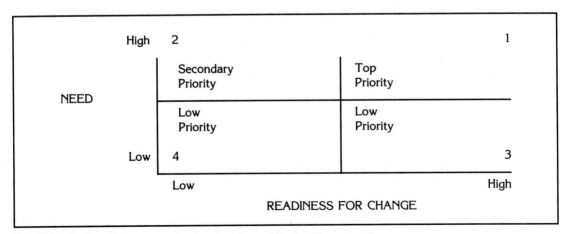

FIGURE 10–3.   Marketing segmentation for public health promotion

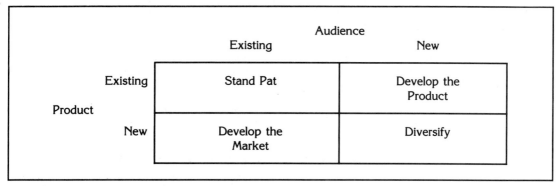

		Audience	
		Existing	New
Product	Existing	Stand Pat	Develop the Product
	New	Develop the Market	Diversify

FIGURE 10–4. Categories of marketing strategies

iors. While developing the product, the objective is to package the social idea in a manner which: (a) is desirable to the target audience, (b) makes the audience willing to "purchase" (in terms of attitude or behavior change), and (c) facilitates the social cause. For example, cancer prevention agencies must decide (among other things) if their "product" consists of behaviors which prevent the dreaded disease or the promotion of a healthier lifestyle in general. In many cases, no single product can achieve the desired social change; various products and marketing strategies that contribute to the social objective must be developed.

Product **positioning refers to the selection of a niche in the marketplace for a product or behavior, taking into account both the needs and wants of the consumer and whatever competition may exist.** For example, the promotion of oral rehydration solutions is done within the realization that mothers use home remedies and other products (some of which are dangerous) in response to their baby's diarrhea. Family planning, low-fat diets, exercise, and even waste recycling programs all face major competitors.

Another important factor to consider in product development is the price of the product. **The price represents the buyer's cost. Such costs may include monetary expenditure or time and energy spent..** For example, the costs of maximum automobile occupant safety may include: (a) the monetary charge for installing air bags; (b) the response or time cost of buckling and unbuckling the safety belt; and (c) the psychological cost of worrying about an accident while fastening a safety belt, or the fear of actually being better off

not using them in an accident, or of losing control when an airbag inflates.

Next, we need to determine where and in what situation (e.g., time of day/day of week), we can best reach our target audiences. Promoting breast self-examination on daytime television may be a good way to reach housewives, whereas women in the workforce may be more easily reached through print media at the worksite. Thus, **place refers to providing adequate distribution and response channels whereby the social idea can reach the relevant public.** A distribution network should be established that will: (a) permit implementation of the social change effort on a broad scale, (b) facilitate communication between the change agents and recipients, and (c) expedite the desired behavior change.

Finally, there is promotion: the publicizing and advertising of a product so it will be purchased and used. What should be our "creative approach" and "media mix"? The creativity of a marketing approach may greatly influence how much attention people pay to the message delivered. Within the findings of their research, marketers apply their creativity in developing:

- the *content* of the message;
- the *product position* (i.e., how this behavioral product compares to others being promoted or promoted in the past (see "product" section);
- the *tone* of the message—whether comforting or alarming, intellectual or emotional, or upbeat or angry (for instance, note the difference between messages which focus on AIDS prevention versus those which promote exercise);

- the *source* of the information with specific attention to his/her credibility regarding the issue (e.g., the Surgeon General vs. an alcoholic doing time in jail for drunken driving);
- the visual appeal, recognition value and meaningfulness of the *logo* to be used; and
- the *phasing* of the messages (i.e., determining how the message should evolve over time or, for instance, in a multiple risk-factor prevention program, defining what specific behavioral or content area should be addressed first and later).

Communication strategies and tactics that make the social idea familiar, acceptable, and desirable to the target audience describes promotion. Promotion can be accomplished through a "marketing mix" of any or all of the following:

- **Selling** — any form of non-personal presentation of ideas, goods, or services paid for by an identified sponsor (see "Step 2").
- **Personal selling** — any form of paid personal presentation or promotion involving direct face-to-face communication.
- **Publicity** — any form of unpaid non-personal presentation of ideas, goods, or services.
- **Sales promotion** — any promotional activity (other than those cited above) which stimulates interest, trial, or purchase of goods or services.

Distribution Plan.   The distribution of products, services, or materials must be given as much emphasis as the promotion itself, since promising and then failing to come through is a much more disagreeable outcome than never having made an effort in the first place. Most or all of the following distribution-related questions should be answered affirmatively before promotion is begun:

- Does an adequate number of materials exist?
- Is there sufficient transportation available to distribute these materials and transport staff, volunteers, and program participants?
- Is there an adequate "sales force" (e.g., trained facilitators) to carry out the program?
- Are contingency plans in place in case there is an excessive demand for the products or services?

Training Plan.   The complexity and difficulty of behavioral adoption will in part determine how much training, if any, is needed as part of the social marketing system. One can expect an incredible range in the degree of difficulty and amount of training needed from one health promotion program to another. For example, it may be fairly simple to train mothers to bring their children to the health clinic for immunizations, but much more difficult to teach them how to rehydrate children with severe diarrhea. Additionally, even in the immunization example, we might need to train health workers to promote immunization at the local level as well as to carry out the logistical aspects of the immunization program itself (e.g., cold chain, sterilization of needles, re-supply, and record keeping). Specific techniques for training have been described previously and can be applied with great success to the training needed in social marketing techniques. However, face-to-face training for public health programs may be somewhat difficult and expensive. Therefore, social marketers are often faced with the challenge of determining how to use broadcast and print media as efficiently as possible in order to conduct training on a mass scale. Again, training may be targeted at specific consumers of the information or intermediaries/behavior change agents (e.g., health workers) expected to deal with the ultimate target population on a face-to-face basis.

In the field of public health communication, we are interested in not only creating awareness and demand for "products," but also insuring that health professionals and other change agents, as well as actual members of the primary audience, have adequate training for using these "products" or facilitating health behavior change in others. Training is important whether these products are for personal use or for family members or friends.[11] Therefore, the type of training described previously (chapter 9) is a critical component of all public health communication programs.

SELECTING CHANNELS AND DEVELOPING PRODUCTS

Channels of message delivery include forms of mass and face-to-face or **interpersonal communication. An interpersonal channel involves face-to-face communication.** Interpersonal communication, central to the human experience, is as such an integral theme of health promotion. Since illness and health have their roots in social existence, the modification or mobilization of inter-

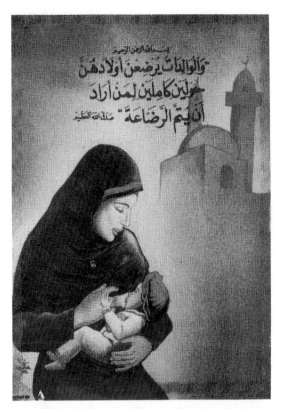

FIGURE 10-5. Social marketing strategies must work within the cultural norms of an existing target population. This print piece developed by UNICEF-Yemen cites Koranic scripture promoting the practice of breast feeding. Reprinted by permission of UNICEF.

personal forces is usually the direct or indirect objective of health promotion programs. Working through natural caregivers, family members, friends, teachers, or clinicians, the effectiveness of our programs can be generalized and maintained.

In spite of its appeal, the use of face-to-face communication in social marketing programs presents a major engineering and management challenge. Through a pyramiding approach, the effects of communication are multiplied through second and even subsequent generations of "multipliers," change agents who not only attempt to enhance their own health, but also that of people with whom they are in regular contact. For example, "Each One Teach One" literacy campaigns in developing countries developed literacy skills among groups of adult students in diverse communities, with the expectation that these students

would in turn share this "gift" with at least one neighbor or relative. Such campaigns have met with only modest success, however. Although the initial wave of learners may be able and personally motivated to learn to read and write or mind their own children's health, this does not necessarily translate into skills and motivation necessary to teach. Without additional booster training, monitoring, feedback, and reinforcement, using all available channels of communication and organizational support from the government sector as well as others, the quality of the communication will diminish, volunteers will drop out, and other problems will ensue.

The philosophy underlying *Motivating Health Behavior* holds that increasing effective interpersonal communication is fundamental to health promotion. Therefore, this topic is covered extensively throughout this text and is presented here only as it applies to typical social marketing areas. Instead, the present section emphasizes mass (or "impersonal") communication.

Mass Communication. Mass communication is subdivided into print and broadcast media. However, the term "mass" is somewhat misleading, as newsletters, tape recorded messages, and other forms of communication are often used to reach small numbers of individuals. Hence, the term "mini media" was coined to refer to approaches which incorporate mass media techniques to deliver messages within organizations and in other ways to smaller numbers of individuals. Generally, "print" and "broadcast media" are more descriptive of techniques in the mass media category.

The differences between **print and broadcast media** are perhaps more subtle than one would expect. Print must be proactively read or seen, whereas broadcast must be heard or seen (though print can be displayed through broadcast channels, hence adding "reading" as a broadcast mode). The second primary difference is that print generally can be read (and reread) at the reader's convenience, but broadcast stimuli must be attended to when broadcasted. Again, there are exceptions: driving past a billboard on a busy freeway offers a limited opportunity to read a particular message, whereas audio or video recordings of broadcast messages can be played back at a later time.

Other differences between print and broadcast include pricing (print costs are based on space used and are generally lower; broadcast is based on time and occasionally includes free public service announcement (PSA) slots, formats available (print generally has more), and locations available (print can be read anywhere). Finally, print is appropriate when longer attention spans are required, whereas broadcast sound bites can reach larger numbers of people for shorter periods of time. Ideally, these two as well as other channels are used to complement one another and create an optimal promotional effect.

Print Media

Print media can also be an effective component of communications or at times can "stand alone" as a health promotion tool. Among print media which emphasize behavior change are self-help books and "kits," comic books with a health theme training manual, and follow-up mailings which can serve to provide rewarding and corrective feedback to an individual attempting a self-change project. In contrast, pamphlets, brochures, flyers, and posters can help set a community agenda, but often emphasize the promotion of a specific event or the agenda once it has been set. Newsletters announcing progress and prospects of various health promotion efforts can be mailed to individuals who have demonstrated interest in the project. Indeed, all print media can be mailed through mass or targeted mailing. However, the cost of such efforts tends to be quite high, even if special mailing rates are acquired. More effective yet is to work within organizations and community groups (e.g., corporations, libraries, churches) to make use of their central locations where people can walk by and pick up various print media. Alternatively, in-house mailing systems (e.g., in paychecks, campus office mail, etc.) can also be effective in reaching large numbers of people at a relatively low cost. Some health promotion programs have even piggy-backed onto other organizations' prepaid mailing systems, such as sending health promotion literature in paycheck envelopes or in utility bills.

Terminology. Understanding the following four terms will help you become familiar with print media technology:

1. *Primary audience:* Those who are exposed to the message in its original presentation.

2. *Secondary audience:* Those who have a magazine, brochure, or other print piece "passed along" to them.
3. *Circulation:* The number of newspapers, magazines, fliers, etc., sold or otherwise distributed to the (primary) audience.
4. *Total audience:* Primary plus secondary audiences.

Formats. Formats are the varied forms of media the promotional message can take.[12] They are highly varied; program goals, resources, and experience will dictate which formats are chosen for any given effort. For example, billboards, buttons, banners, fliers, hats, posters, and even the use of the Yellow Pages may serve as excellent promotional formats for increasing awareness of a topic. Calendars, charts, grocery bag stuffers, and shelf markers serve as specific guides to subsequent behavior. The extra details afforded by the use of flip charts, newsletters, direct mail, and, occasionally, newspapers are useful for skills training. Finally, bumper stickers, t-shirts, and diplomas can serve as effective rewards for both direct and vicarious behavior change.

Clear Writing. In addition to keeping sentences and words short and comprehensible, a variety of other factors need to be considered to maximize the impact of print messages. First, the

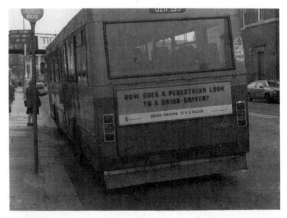

FIGURE 10–6. This clever sign in Dublin, Ireland discourages people from "drink-driving." *Photo courtesy of John Elder.*

EXHIBIT 10-1

Layout Options. Print (primarily display) layouts include the following options:*

- Conventional: an illustration covers the upper 60 percent to 70 percent of the piece, with headline, and/or copy below.
- All-type: little or no pictorial material.
- Picture-dominant (e.g., poster): illustration covers most or all of copy.
- Multi-panel (e.g., cartoon): several picture-word combinations.

Newspapers. In comparison, newspapers offer the following formats:

- Regular news coverage, with articles which may appear once, and unfortunately (in larger newspapers) in the back of the newspaper.
- Serial coverage, whereby a special article is carried for a period of days similar to that discussed above.
- Editorials and letters to the editor, which perhaps attract less attention but may be especially effective at initiating a community-involvement debate on a contentious health-related issue.
- Community calendars or columns, as discussed for television/radio.
- Paid or donated advertisements which attempt to recruit people for a certain activity or event.

*C. D. Schick & A. C. Book. (1984). *Fundamentals of Copy and Layout.* Chicago: Crain.

---

second person pronoun is usually more appropriate. Action verbs also pack more punch than passive verbs. In other words, most print should be written as though the sender were talking directly to the audience. The use of captioned photos or illustrations with careful attention to making the images relevant to the target audience adds to message impact.

Broadcast Media

Radio and television offer potentially the largest audiences of any medium, and in some cases (such as the use of radio for child survival programs in underdeveloped countries) represent the *only* means of reaching audiences in remote areas. News programs, public service announcements (PSAs), public affairs programs, and even call-in shows and straight entertainment can be used to create awareness, build skills, and provide direct and vicarious reinforcement for health promotion programs.

Health and community development have been given play in the broadcast media since the widespread use of radio began seventy years ago.

Health programming through the broadcast media should take the following factors into account:

- Comedy, drama, and music presented on television and radio are the most common forms of popular entertainment, but audiences resist being "educated" while being entertained.
- Broadcast news is a highly respected source of information and is potentially the most inexpensive method of getting the word out. However, health items—especially positive health items—are seldom adjudged "newsworthy."[13]
- Public service announcements (PSAs) represent an inexpensive means of reaching broadcast audiences, but the timing of their presentation can be less than ideal.
- Paid advertisements can be expensive, but they have a greater potential than PSAs for attracting or affecting an audience.

Public Service Announcements. Public service announcements (PSAs) are advertisement-like messages delivered free of charge by a radio or television station or paid for by a third party sponsor. They are generally ten to thirty seconds in length and can be aired at the station's discre-

EXHIBIT 10-2

RADIO REINFORCEMENT OF VILLAGE HEALTH VOLUNTEERS

The following are scripts of two radio spots used to promote motivation via vicarious reinforcement among "kader," who are Indonesian community health volunteers.*

RADIO SPOT I: JAVANESE VERSION

Intro:	(national music)
Mom I:	Well . . . Cempluk looks cheerful, healthy and lively. She's just recently recovered from diarrhea, hasn't she?
Mom II:	Thanks be to Allah, after I kept on giving her drinks and nutritious food, Cempluk seemed well.
Mom I:	Hey . . . how do you know that food and drink should not be stopped for a child who has diarrhea?
Mom II:	From the kader. That's Mother Siti who usually weighs the young kids and gives advice on health.
Mom I:	Well, that kader knows everything, doesn't she?
Mom II:	Yes, right. Since she was trained by the health center, she can give advice on how to keep children really healthy.
Mom I:	Ooohh . . . in that case, I'll go to the health post every month and do whatever she says.
Mom II:	Don't forget, Mother, if you need help or advice, you can go to her house. You don't have to wait until the monthly clinic day.
Mom I:	Okay, Mother, I'll always ask for advice from the kader.
Announcer:	Right! Kader work voluntarily, without expecting anything in return, for the future of your children, the future of your village, and the future of the nation. We thank the kader for everything they have done. Let's go to the post to keep our children healthy, really healthy.

Smash . . . fade out

*RADIO SPOT II**

Intro:	(music)
Village Chief:	Hey, Mother Kader, come in a while. Where are you going so early?
Kader:	I'm going to the health post. I have to prepare for the monthly weighing sessions and to give advice and help on other health problems for the balita in our village.
Chief:	Well, well, well . . . that's what I want to talk to you about. Please sit down, Mother Kader.
Kader:	What is it Mr. Village Chief? I'm getting nervous.
Chief:	Well, Mother Kader, after observing the activity of Mother Kader in this village, and after seeing you visit young children in their home, I feel proud. The whole community owes many thanks to you and also to all kader who make little children healthy.
Kader:	Ah . . . that's my job, Mr. Chief.
Chief:	Yes, but for that, on behalf of the people of this village, I thank you and all kader. I promise to always help the respected work of kader, whom I'll call "heroes without medals."
Kader:	Thank you, Mr. Chief.
Chief:	You're welcome and thank you, Mother Kader. May God bless you.
(music)	
Announcer:	Right! Kader work voluntarily, without expecting anything in return for the future of your children, the future of our village, and the future of our nation. We can only

EXHIBIT 10-2-Continued

	thank them and God, who will reward them. Let's go to the health post to keep our children healthy, really healthy.
Chief:	Yes, but for that, on behalf of the people of this village, I thank you and all kader. I promise to always help the respected work of kader, whom I'll call "heroes without medals."
Kader:	Thank you, Mr. Chief.
Chief:	You're welcome and thank you, Mother Kader. May God bless you.
(music)	

*Source: Thomas Reis, HEALTHCOM, Personal communication, October 1990.

tion. This often means that PSAs are broadcast at low audience times, such as late at night or early in the morning. Nevertheless, the PSA's inexpensiveness makes them a very attractive marketing format.

The bulk of production work in radio PSAs emphasizes writing for a single person's listening, whereas television PSAs must, of course, present attractive visual material as well. Given their brief period of air time, PSAs need to be carefully written. The PSA's central theme should be presented immediately and summarized at the end of the announcement. Specific behavioral actions need to be advocated, with a straightforward presentation of facts, a unifying and memorable theme (manifested in a logo, song, or slogan), and limited but effective sound and visual effects. In a brief (e.g., ten or fifteen second) PSA, little more than

---

EXHIBIT 10-3

Getting on the News. The coverage, credibility, and inexpensiveness of news programs for promoting public recognition of a project make this a compelling broadcast format. Nevertheless, getting on the news with any meaningful frequency is very difficult.

Press releases announcing upcoming or recently completed events comprise the most common form of initiating media contacts. While most broadcast stations (as well as newspapers), of course, will retain their journalistic independence, developing good working relationships with stations and reporters is a necessary aspect of preparing a marketing campaign. Also, special audience newspapers (e.g., Spanish language weeklies) and broadcast stations have a special interest in and need for news related to your program. Often, these stations and others will appreciate video tape, audio tape, or even print which they can incorporate directly into their news broadcast "other" presentation.

A major challenge, however, is finding a newsworthy event. Such events include openings of new clinics or offices, the launching of special campaigns, the presentation of prizes, gifts or awards, visits by celebrities and authorities, goal achievements, special training, seminars or program offerings, and human interest stories (which should be designed in such a way as to promote vicarious learning).*

In addition to news broadcasts, non-news programs such as talk shows can be appropriate for promoting awareness, acceptance and behavior change. Panel discussions, one-to-one interviews, testimonials, and even magazine format shows (such as "60 Minutes") all offer attractive formats for news broadcast.

*D. Bogue & T. Peigh. (1979). Formats for development of radio programming. In T. Peigh et al. (Eds.). *The use of radio in social development.* Chicago: University of Chicago Community & Family Study Center, p. 41.

reminders can be presented, whereas a thirty second or longer spot may present and repeat clear messages and behavior change prescriptions. A phone number should be read aloud and presented visually if being televised or reread if presented via radio.[14]

Advertisements are paid messages which allow the marketer to select the time and duration of the announcement rather than having that controlled by the station. They are very attractive alternatives to PSAs. Nevertheless, advertisements can be extremely expensive, especially if presented on television and during prime time.

Advertisements and PSAs can take a great variety of forms, depending on the needs of the program and the creativity and experience of the marketers. Generally, a light and humorous touch can be effective, but at times a negative appeal (e.g., through the use of sarcasm) or even a serious approach (e.g., in drug abuse prevention spots) can be appropriate.

An example of the latter is presented by the California Tobacco Control Program's rap group piece, an advertisement played in the major urban markets in the state. The video depicts a rapper showing his disgust for smoking by pulling cigarettes out of teenagers' mouths, while a funeral procession for an expired smoker marches off in the background. The refrain of the rap song is:

> "First you made us pick it — now you want us to smoke it? Get back — you must be jokin'!'',

The refrain invokes the image of enslavement to tobacco.

As deregulation by the federal government ended the enforcement of PSA programming on broadcast media, the PSA is waning as a health promotion tool. Generally, marketers prefer paid advertisements when they have the resources to develop them.

Telephone Marketing

The Pawtucket Heart Health Program (PHHP) developed an innovative approach to personal selling and interpersonal communication for health promotion.[15] Using volunteers (many of whom were retired Bell Telephone Company employees), telephone marketing was used either to promote program offerings (e.g., self-help or small group weight loss programs) or provide counsel-

ing and support to individuals already on their way to reducing their heart disease risk. Phone numbers were selected through: (a) cold calls, where Pawtucket (Rhode Island) prefixes and random digit 4-number suffixes were dialed, primarily for program promotion; (b) general program phone banks, where individuals who had participated in any general PHHP activity in the past were recontacted to determine and promote further interests; and (c) specific phone banks, where people involved in a current self-help or other low contact activity were contacted by change agents to troubleshoot or promote maintenance or generalization.

Given the technical skill required for counseling for risk reduction, the bulk of the volunteer effort went into out-call "sales" of upcoming face-to-face or self-help programs.

In a total of 97.5 person/hours, the volunteers called 1,223 households and made contact with half of those. The total number of "sales" (registration for a risk reduction program) made was 222, or 35 percent of the households contacted, requiring 5.5 calls per "sale" and just over 2 sales per volunteer hour. The advantages of this personalized approach over impersonal media make it an intriguing alternative.

Other Channels

Audio-visual (A/V) programs, in contrast, are much more labor-intensive but have a chance to generate two-way communication with an audience. These are generally slide shows, videos, films, puppet shows, or other types of presentations shown at meetings of various community organizations. The emphasis of such A/V presentations is on either building awareness of projects or educating/promoting desired behavior change.

Audio and video cassettes represent another communication channel. Many video rental stores have a "community service" section, where health and other public interest titles may be lent out free of charge to customers renting other tapes. In Karachi, Pakistan, two-thirds of housewives surveyed reported not listening to radio, but instead preferring audio cassettes.[16] These women and urban American commuters alike could be very receptive to skills training via cassette tapes.

Table 10-1 summarizes the advantages and disadvantages of these various channels of communication.

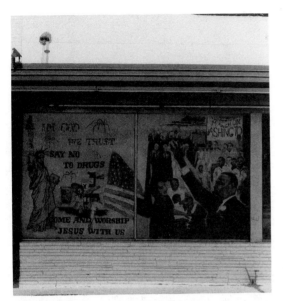

FIGURE 10–7. Consistent with a locality development model of community organization, promotional pieces need not be professionally developed to be effective. *Photo courtesy of Betsy Clapp.*

SOCIAL MARKETING RESEARCH AND PRE-TESTING

There are a variety of ways to incorporate consumer input into a social marketing campaign and otherwise enhance two-way flow of communication. Social marketing research tools especially involve those previously mentioned in the formative/qualitative research section in chapter 6.

Management Plan, Timetable, and Budget. Finally, health promoters using social marketing techniques (or any other techniques for that matter) must develop an overall management plan in terms of: (a) the identification of specific program activities; (b) which staff members and volunteers will be expected to carry out certain marketing activities; (c) when various activities and phases will take place; and (d) how much budget is needed for the various aspects of the marketing activities. Details on this are clearly beyond the scope of the present discussion. However, health promotion efforts are frequently faulted for an incomplete or inappropriate management plan.

Moreover, in this period of increasing concern about budgetary issues, methods for saving money through careful planning and creative financing should be considered.

WHERE TO GET HELP

Social marketing and communications are highly sophisticated disciplines requiring years of practice just to master a subspecialty within the technology. The health promoter can and should seek assistance from a variety of sources.

Agencies That Conduct Market Research

Radio and television stations, newspapers, advertising agencies, and other groups will have audience segmentation or other data which can expedite the pretesting or evaluation processes. Often, these agencies are willing to share these data (or their expertise in other marketing and communications areas) with nonprofit health programs. Representatives from these agencies make excellent advisory board members.

Applying Existing Materials. Thousands of posters, pamphlets, slides, PSAs and other communications pieces appropriate for your program and audience might already exist and be available at little or no expense. In the U.S., for example, the National Institutes of Health, the Centers for Disease Control, the Office of Substance Abuse Prevention, and many other federal and state agencies offer excellent materials for chronic disease prevention and control. Materials for maternal health, child survival, and family planning programs in underdeveloped countries can be obtained from the World Health Organization or its regional offices, the U.S. Agency for International Development or its contractors, Planned Parenthood International, UNICEF, and many other agencies. Materials can often be used as they are or adapted slightly to fit a program's needs.

SUMMARY

Social marketing has recently emerged as a key health promotion intervention approach. Social

TABLE 10-1

Advantages and Disadvantages of Major Channels of Communication

Channel	Purposes and Advantages	Disadvantages
Interpersonal	1. Exploits most common form of human communication and most powerful source of influence. 2. Inexpensive. 3. Involves health and other sectors in health promotion. 4. Especially effective for detailed training and reinforcement.	1. Difficult to train and motivate multipliers. 2. Difficult to monitor and manage.
Circulating Print	1. Format allows for extensive detail; good for knowledge/skill acquisition and vicarious learning. 2. Involves reader in the message. 3. News events covered by newspaper result in inexpensive, detailed promotion. 4. Magazines and pass alongs may have long life.	1. Production quality must be attended to. 2. Distribution can be logistically complicated. 3. Paid advertisements can be expensive, "newsworthy" events. Difficult to come by and contributed space is rare. 4. Reader might ignore print altogether. 5. Newspaper has short life.
Display Print	1. Can be used as points-of-purchase or otherwise where health behavior occurs. 2. Certain formats (e.g., billboards) can reach large audience. 3. Good for getting attention and promoting awareness/reinforcement.	1. Production and space rental can be expensive. 2. Not good for knowledge/skill acquisition. 3. Can be difficult to control and maintain placement.
Radio	1. Reaches large audience. 2. News items and PSAs. 3. Good for awareness/recognition reinforcement.	1. Audience attention not assured. 2. PSA timing can make it unattractive. 3. Advertisements can be expensive. 4. Difficult to develop "newsworthy" stories.
Television	1. Visual stimuli make message even more powerful; other advantages similar to those for radio.	1. Even more expensive production and air time than radio. 2. PSAs not as available as radio.
Telephone	1. Inexpensive if implemented through volunteers. 2. Especially good for initiating and maintaining behavior change programs.	1. Negative public reaction possible. 2. Takes trained change agent if behavioral counseling is required. 3. High rates for no-answers and hang-ups.

marketing and its component discipline health communication may be used to build awareness of a program, add health issues to the community's agenda, create demand for health promotion programs, or change behavior directly. The steps of health communication include planning, selecting channels, developing products and materials, pretesting and revising materials, training, implementing, monitoring and evaluating. Channels of communication include mass media and face-to-face communication. Mass communication is delivered through print or broadcast media. More recent developments in this area have emphasized audiovisual programs and telephone calls for health communication.

With this chapter we conclude the presentation of the technologies of health promotion intervention. We now are ready to examine how health promotion interventions are monitored and evaluated.

ADDITIONAL READINGS

Keep these print media within easy reach:

1. U.S. Department of Health and Human Services. *Making health communications programs work*. Washington, D.C.: National Institutes of Health Publication No. 89–1493, April 1989.
2. U.S. Department of Health and Human Services. *Pretesting in health communications*. Washington, D.C.: National Institutes of Health Publication No. 84–1493, January 1984.
3. The University of Chicago Community and Family Study Center. *The media monograph series*. Chicago: 1979. (Includes "Mass mailings for family planning," "Twenty-five communication obstacles to the success of family planning programs," "Radio and television spot announcements for family planning," "Relevant posters for family planning," "The use of radio in social development," and "Communications pretesting.")
4. Debus, M. *Handbook for excellence in focus group research*. Washington, D.C.: Academy for Educational Development, 1989.

EXERCISE

Select a health concept and divide into teams of 3–5 per team. Select a coordinator. Then, each team should develop a presentation for one com-

munication channel (e.g., television PSA, radio talk show, newspaper press release). Use videotape, audiotape, poster boards, etc., as appropriate. Content, tone, etc., should be integrated into the whole "campaign" by the coordinators. (Alternatively, have some of the groups use pre-testing and others not, and compare the results.) If appropriate, use the same topic developed in the chapter 6 exercise.

ENDNOTES

1. The authors are deeply indebted to Moshe Engelberg for his many criticisms and comments on an earlier draft of this chapter, and especially for the ideas presented in Figures 10–1 and 10–2.
2. Kotler, P. (1982). *Marketing for nonprofit organizations*. Englewood Cliffs, NJ: Prentice-Hall, p. 490.
3. In this text, *social marketing* is used as a broad, umbrella term, whereas "health communications" is used as a component of the former, roughly equivalent to Kotler's "promotion." Social marketing is more closely associated with the concept of "exchange" in the economic sense — an individual gives up a personal resource or an old habit for a new product or behavior. Communication, in turn, places greater emphasis on the dissemination of information on a large scale, connoting a one-way flow from the sender to the receiver. Social marketing uses communication techniques and adds those from behavior analysis, social psychology, economics, and other fields.
4. Weiner, L. (1987). *Media development for health promotion issues for planning*. Presented at the Community Health Promotion Conference, Kaiser Family Foundation, Menlo Park, CA.
5. U.S. Department of Health and Human Services. (1989). *Making health communications work*. Bethesda, MD: National Institutes of Health (#89–1493), p. 1.
6. Academy for Educational Development. (1983). *The HEALTHCOM project*. Washington, D.C.: Academy for Educational Development.
7. Also, see U.S. DHHS, *Making health communications work*, pp. 5–6.
8. Ibid., p. 5.
9. Bloom, P. N. & Novelli, W. D. (1981). Problems and challenges of social marketing. *Journal of Marketing, 45,* 79–88.
10. Bloom & Novelli. Problems and challenges of social marketing; Novelli, W. D. (1984). Developing marketing programs. In L. W. Frederikson, L. J. Solo-

mon, & K. A. Brehony (Eds.), *Marketing health behavior: Principles, techniques and applications.* New York: Plenum; and Kotler, P. & Zaltman, G. (1971). Social marketing: An approach to planned social change. *Journal of Marketing, 35,* 3–12.

11. Often marketers distinguish betwen "circulating print" and "display" media, with the latter depicting simple images and short messages presented on billboards, posters, etc. The present text uses "print" to describe these stimuli as well as those newsletters, brochures, and other forms of print.

12. Bogue, D. (1979). The use of radio in social devel-

opment. In T. Peigh, M. Maloney, R. Higgins & D. Bogue (Eds.), *The use of radio in social development.* Chicago: University of Chicago Community & Family Study Center, pp. 4–5.

13. U.S. DHHS, *Making health communications work,* p. 36.

14. Schwertfeger, R., Elder, J., Cooper, R., Lasater, T., & Carleton, R. (1986). The use of telemarketing in the community-wide prevention of heart disease: The Pawtucket Heart Health Program. *Journal of Community Health, 11*(3), 172–180.

15. Mirza, A. (1987). *Child health related practices in Karachi slums.* Karachi: USAID/Pakistan.

Chapter 11

Monitoring and Evaluating Health Promotion

also chp 5+6

OBJECTIVES

By the end of this chapter, the reader should be able to:

1. Define the following terms:
   - impact evaluation
   - needs/resources assessment
   - outcome evaluation
   - process evaluation
   - program evaluation
2. Identify common "pitfalls" in monitoring and evaluating health promotion programs and offer strategies for combating these problems.
3. Describe and give examples of the four categories of program evaluation data.
4. Formulate appropriate program evaluation questions in each of the following areas: organization, needs/resources assessment, priorities and goals, research, intervention, monitoring, and evaluation of impact and outcome.
5. List the major points addressed in program evaluation report.

INTRODUCTION

Much of the work of the program evaluator has already been described. The specific tasks of an evaluator depends on a variety of factors, including: (a) whether the evaluator is a member of a project team or is external to the project, (b) the source and amount of project funding (and of course, how much is budgeted for evaluation), and (c) the specific goals of the evaluation (for instance, deciding whether to continue funding versus measuring the ultimate program impact, which calls for different evaluation strategies).

Regardless of the situation, the techniques described in chapters 5 and 6 are fundamental to carrying out good program evaluation. Just as for program planning, key informant interviews, archival research, rates-under-treatment and surveys can form part of the program evaluation methodology, whereas focus groups, in-depth interviews, and observations provide additional data. Quasi-experimental or even experimental designs provide the framework for the program monitoring and evaluation.

Table 11-1 demonstrates the relationship between the various types of program "evaluation" activities and the needs and maturity of a pro-

TABLE 11–1
Critical Questions and Phasing of Program Evaluation Components

Type of Evaluation	Critical Questions	Phase
Needs/Resources Assessment	What are the actual health needs of the community? What resources are available to deal with them?	At beginning of program
Formative Research	What form should the intervention take? How can it be refined and improved?	At beginning of program and on an as-needed basis
Process Evaluation Monitoring	Is intervention being implemented as planned? With sufficient dissemination and participation?	Continuous
Impact Evaluation	Were program goals met? Were health behaviors changed?	At transition point, or end of program
Outcome Evaluation	Did the target population's health or related conditions improve?	At end of program

gram. Perhaps not typically included in evaluation, the first step is to develop and operationalize appropriate and valid program goals and objectives based on particular needs and resources. Second, specific formative or "operational" research will clarify program-related issues as they arise, e.g., will we get more bang for our buck with a marketing campaign versus a training-of-trainers approach. Third, **monitoring, or "process evaluation,"** of the program implementation and resulting dissemination and participation data (e.g., number of women who attend breast feeding classes) will tell us whether the program begins and stays off the ground (but *not* to where it's bound!). **Process evaluation is the evaluation of the implementation of a program contemporaneous with that implementation, and the attainment of short term objectives related to program inputs.** Finally, impact and outcome evaluation indicate whether behaviors and health (as defined by the community or organizational structure) were actually changed through the program efforts.

Figure 11–1 depicts the temporal relationships among these evaluation activities.[1]

A program evaluator requires general needs/resources assessment and research skills to be a well-rounded. This chapter should be useful to either an "internal" or "external" evaluator who, in addition to or instead of conducting formative research and operationalizing goals and objectives, is expected to describe the process of the program and/or evaluate its impact. Thus, this chapter extends the technology of evaluation to program monitoring and impact.

TWO AVOIDABLE MISTAKES

Brenda Williams just finished her course work for her master's degree in public health and landed her first job as a program evaluator for the health promotion office in her state's health department. Her first assignment was to conduct site visits for a variety of state-funded demonstration projects to determine which of these projects should receive two additional years of funding. She began these site visits in the community of Imperial, where a local health center was funded to promote breast feeding among women soon to give birth. As a primary part of her activities, she interviewed a variety of Imperial's key community informants, including doctors, city council representatives, and religious officials who served on the advisory

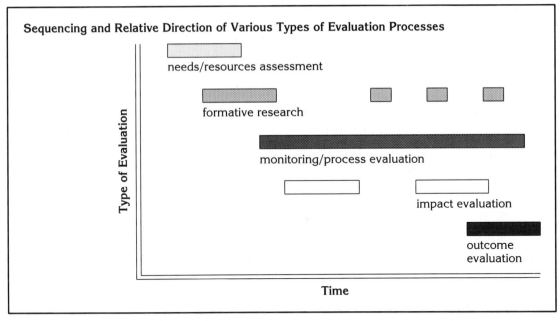

Sequencing and Relative Direction of Various Types of Evaluation Processes

needs/resources assessment

formative research

monitoring/process evaluation

impact evaluation

outcome evaluation

Type of Evaluation

Time

FIGURE 11–1.   Sequencing and relative direction of various types of evaluation processes

council for the project. Although not in the majority, several of these advisory council members had very strong objections to the way the breast-feeding project was managed. For instance, project staff were not often available to speak to civic groups upon council members' requests, which irritated these members. At other times, the staff were difficult to reach during normal working hours. These objections were sufficiently strong to have an impact on how Brenda wrote her report. In the context of limited funding for such a project and due to the relatively negative way Brenda summed up her evaluation, the state decided not to continue funding for the project. This occurred in spite of the fact that the prevalence of breast feeding among all former prenatal patients at this center increased from 21 percent to 36 percent.

Dr. Celia Gomez is the director of an Employee Assistance Program (EAP) for a large manufacturing firm. One of her recent responsibilities was to help reduce absenteeism through a reduction of drug and alcohol abuse among all employees. Her other responsibility was to prepare an outcome evaluation of the program for a point in time two years into the future. She took note of the baseline absentee rate, then launched an information, education, and communication campaign targeting drug and alcohol abuse. She also compiled a list of

community-based physicians and counselors specializing in the treatment of substance abusers, and offered a confidential referral service for employees needing individual or family treatment but did not want to use in-house health professionals. The management and union alike seemed generally satisfied with the quality and quantity of her efforts, which eventually comprised a large portion of her day-to-day activities. Finally, the two-year time period came to an end, and she peeked behind the curtain to see what outcomes she had achieved. Lo and behold, there was little to note. In the three months before the program began, January to March, 1989, the average absentee rate was 3.2 days per month per employee. In the final quarter of the program, October through December, 1991, the rate had actually increased to 3.5. She had to report this negative outcome to an unhappy executive vice-president, whose first reaction was, "we sure wasted a lot of money on this stuff."

When screening for risk factors and diseases (see chapter 6) we have to make sure our procedures are both sensitive and specific. The same rules apply to program evaluation. In the first case, Ms. Williams' evaluation was not "sensitive," in that she failed to detect that the program was effective when it was. Clearly, the project staff was having a public relations problem with some of the board members, whose personal preferences for the way things should be run were not compatible with project resources or goals. Unfortunately, this friction led to a "false negative" evaluation, which in turn caused "the baby to be thrown out with the bath water."

Conversely, Dr. Gomez' evaluative eyes were too starry, and her assessment was not "specific" to the outcome she hoped to achieve. She accepted subjective judgments of program process as valid, and allowed an ineffective (at least according to her final impact evaluation) program to continue. This "false positive" was not detected until it was too late.

Program evaluation research is as far away from the Hollywood image of Robert Oppenheimer and Madame Curie's science as Eddie Murphy's humor is from Bob Hope's. Program evaluation is applied research. While based in the scientific method, it also necessitates taking into account political pressures, subjective judgments, and the integration of seemingly incompatible data from a wide variety of sources. Moreover, it must be conducted with generally modest resources. Yet failure to evaluate health promotion programs properly can result in the premature discontinuation of good programs—as in the first case described above—or in the failure to refine or discontinue a program going nowhere. A non-sensitive evaluative judgment can result in a loss of services to needy individuals who stand to benefit from them, whereas a non-specific evaluation can result in wasting money and losing opportunities to make better use of resources. Needless to say, both can embarrass and damage the reputation of health promotion professionals and their sponsors.

What is the "right way" to evaluate health promotion programs? Not surprisingly, there is no absolutely correct approach. But within any given context, some approaches will be more valid and useful than others. Now we present the most appropriate definition of program evaluation for the domain of health promotion.

PROGRAM EVALUATION DEFINED

"Program evaluation is the systematic process of collecting and analyzing reliable and valid information at different points and processes in a pro-

gram. Its objectives are to improve effectiveness, reduce costs, and contribute to planning future actions."[2] In its emphasis on reliable, valid and systematic information, program evaluation does not differ in substance from "real" research (see chapter 6). However, through its orientation toward quality enhancement, cost-effectiveness, and planning, program evaluation may take on a much different tone than its epidemiological or clinical trial counterparts.

CATEGORIES OF PROGRAM EVALUATION DATA

The type of data collected in any program evaluation will vary substantially, depending on the goals of the program (and the type of evaluation), the time, resources and expertise available to the evaluators, and the nature of the health promotion effort itself. Ranging from the relatively informal to the scientific, these categories include **descriptive, comparative, analytic,** and **explanatory** data.

Descriptive

These data rely on words more than numbers; for example, a narrative of what happened in planning, implementing, and evaluating the program, or a lengthier version of the hypothetical cases presented above. Although such description may provide rich information about the processes and outcomes of a program and is therefore often an integral part of any program evaluation, it gives us little insight on how or why a program worked, or whether alternative approaches could have been just as effective. For such uses, we need to consider "higher" levels of data, as described below.

Comparative

Whereas descriptive data give us the "what" of program evaluation, comparisons with other programs or techniques put that "what" into a context. A novice gambler may arrive at a horse track early to watch workouts, and be understandably impressed by the grace, beauty and, of course, speed he observes as the thoroughbred,

Seven Year Itch, is taken around the track alone by his jockey. But until the races are run, he cannot determine the actual speed of this horse. The fate of his two dollar investment, of course, will depend on Seven Year Itch's speed relative to the other horses on that day and the track. However, the gambler may also want to consider a broader comparative framework by buying a racing form and studying how fast Seven Year Itch ran compared to previous efforts and against horses of similar and different caliber. With such data, our friend will make a more informed wager. However, if he were more analytical, he would probably play the stock market instead.

Analytic

When we know more about the "what" and "compared to what" of our program (as a result of descriptive and comparative data, respectively), we then turn to the who, how, and why connection. In other words, we are moving from what is typically thought of as "softer" program evaluation to the realm of time series, control group, or other forms of analytical research (see chapter 6). **Analytic data allow us to determine objectively what kinds of program inputs (people, money, other resources) using what techniques (marketing, face-to-face education, etc.) are effective with a given problem or target.** The advantages to collecting analytic data are many. With reasonable certainty or even exact statistical probability, analytical data can determine whether the program was effective, the extent to which it succeeded, and even what level of resources were required to achieve the effects. There are some disadvantages, however. The funding agency or organizational hierarchy may not be interested in sponsoring or funding this extra effort. More expertise and resources are required for the evaluator. Yet analytic data get us much closer to making appropriate decisions regarding the future of our program.

Explanatory

This category of evaluative data is an accumulation and extension of the previous three. From the first three approaches we know what our program was designed to do, how well it performed

compared to other programs, and how and why it worked. A variety of questions are still unanswered, however. Was the program differentially effective for certain people and not others or certain target behaviors and not others? Were some phases of the technology used in the program more effective than others? Are their logical reasons for the results (or lack thereof) based on previous research in this area? **This level of evaluation allows us to streamline the program to its essential components or alternatively, to project what types of target populations or problems it might be appropriate for in the future. In other words, we obtain information on how to maintain the program and how to generalize its benefits across people, behaviors, and settings.** Thus, although descriptive data begins a program evaluation, each successive level of evaluation is increasingly focused toward future decisions about the program's utility, validity, and generalizability.

Evaluation of an Exercise Program for African-Americans

Baranowski and his colleagues[3] evaluated a center-based program for promoting exercise among African-Americans in a South Texas community. In the N/RA phase of the study, extensive interviews and meetings were held with residents and key informants to design a program with optimal appeal to the African-American population. Input from these sources included opinions on the optimal location, program times, and content for the sessions.

Weekly monitoring of attendance rates showed that the initial sessions resulted in minimal participation. Therefore, additional formative research was conducted via a survey to identify reasons for these low attendance rates. This resulted in deleting the requirement that participants attend an educational session before the fitness center sessions and that they fill out daily monitoring logs.

Impact evaluation emphasized the frequency of aerobic activity as well as other psychosocial measures. **Impact evaluation is research designed to identify whether and to what extent a program contributed to accomplishing its stated goals (here, more behavioral focused than outcome evaluation.) Outcome evaluation is research designed to account for a program's accomplishments and long term effectiveness, in**

terms of health change. Outcome evaluation measures included percent body fat, and a bicycle exercise stress test for cardiovascular fitness.

Data from all four categories were collected. Descriptive data included information on the marital status, employment, income, education, and households of the participants. Monitoring of weekly attendance allowed the evaluators to make comparisons from week to week, indicating that a bomb scare, inclement weather, and a community-wide festival results in lower attendance rates, while loosening the requirements for participation brought them back up. For analytic purposes, impact and outcome data were compared to that of a control group. In spite of all their efforts, participation data and program impact were disappointing. Analytic information indicated the economic vulnerability of this population — with many changing to or from part-time employment, unemployment, or full-time work on varying shifts. The evaluators concluded that future programs must offer community-wide programs with flexible options for participation.

NON-LINEAR PROGRAM PLANNING AND EVALUATION

Formative research indicates whether a motivational procedure needs to be refined before continuing. A key member of a board of directors resigns and is replaced by someone who wants to see a different program emphasis. Our funding agency reduces our budget, then reinstates the money with an increase. Our monitoring shows that we had a 45 percent increase in attendance at screening, counseling, and referral activities after only one month.

ONPRIME presents a largely linear model of program planning, intervention and evaluation that implies a simple order to this effort, which is more or less wrapped up when we get to "E" for evaluation. Nothing could be farther from the truth. In the paragraph above, we described several events which occur frequently in any health or human service efforts.

Figure 11–2, presents the recursive nature of health promotion by showing additional decisions rather than simply proceeding to the next ONPRIME step. For example, the initial research accomplished to finalize program plans could show that we inadequately or unrealistically set program priorities. Such a finding would lead us to go back to the drawing board (and to the board of directors) to reconsider our goals and objectives. Fortunately, conducting the pre-implementation research saved us a lot of time and resources.

Careful program monitoring of the intervention process similarly leads us to learn fairly early on whether adequate progress is being made. If this is not the case, additional focus groups or other formative research can help refine the program to become more effective.

Finally, evaluation data take us into the future, or back to any point in the ONPRIME sequence. Results are presented to the program directorate and to the funding organization (if different). Successful programs may be continued, with external support gradually faded until the program becomes self-sustaining. If the program was a roaring success, the techniques used may be extended to other settings, populations, or problems. In other words, evaluation data lead us to maintenance and generalization decisions. Finally, modest results can send us back through all or part of the ONPRIME sequence: reconsidering the priorities, refining the intervention, or making the monitoring system more sensitive. (And a program that belly-flops — well, let's not go into that.)

PROGRAM EVALUATION QUESTIONNAIRES

Program evaluation is often initiated at a point where the program is well along the way or even reaching its conclusion. Even at such a relatively late date, evaluation questions should be developed to assess all points in the planning-implementation-evaluation sequence. Whether program planners used this or other models to plan their activities, ONPRIME can guide the development of specific valuative questions. The following is not an exhaustive list of questions, nor does each question need to be addressed. Unique program characteristics and problems can lead the evaluator toward extensive details and other follow-up questions in some areas, although barely touching on other topics. In any case, generic evaluation questions include:

Organization (review chapter 4)

1. Did the responsible entity exist previously? If so, what is its mission, and how does this influ-

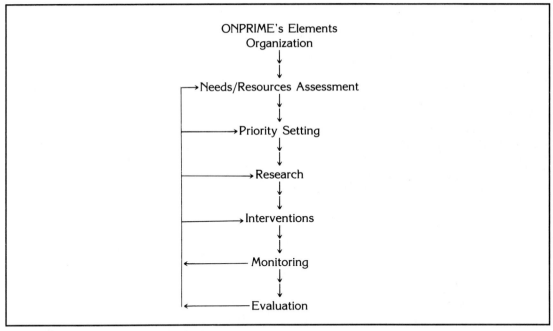

FIGURE 11–2. Recursive nature of health promotion

ence the way the program was structured and designed? If not, did the organization or coalition come together specifically to address this health issue?

2. Who are the members of the governing structure? Whom do they represent? Specifically, how well is the target population represented? In what ways do they offer resources, expertise, or access to the target population? If appointed or voluntary, what is their term of representation?

3. What is the balance of power among members of the governing board? What is their relationship to program staff? Do they hire personnel and participate in programmatic, budget, and other decisions? What is their knowledge and acceptance of program goals?

4. Who are the program staff? What is their training and experience in this type of work? In which areas are they strongest and in which are they weakest? Do they have the skills and personal characteristics appropriate for working with this target population?

5. Does the staff use a train-the-trainers approach or in other ways use community change agents to extend their impact? Why or why not? If

volunteers and/or paraprofessionals are used, how are they selected? To what tasks are they assigned? How are they trained?

Needs/Resources Assessment
(review chapter 5)

1. Who set the goals for the needs/resources assessment? What were the goals? Who designed the questions and instruments? Are these consistent with the goals?

2. How well and to what extent were resources as well as the needs of the community identified?
   a. Were data compiled from key informant interviews, archives, rates-under-treatment, and surveys/interviews (KARS)? Which sources within each of these categories were selected, which were not, and why?
   b. In what form were data from the needs/resource assessment summarized and reported? How well were qualitative and quantitative data from different sources integrated?

3. Who reviewed and "signed off on" the needs/resource assessment report?

Priorities and Goals (review chapters 5 and 7)

1. If there was a needs/resources assessment, to what extent was this used to guide program priorities? If not, on what were priorities based? Who participated in setting priorities, and why was this process selected?
2. What was the process of goal setting?
3. Are the goals operationalized? Is goal achievement readily measurable?
4. How realistic are the goals? Can they be attained within the program's time frame and budget? If there is more than one goal, are they prioritized?
5. How valid are the goals and priorities for the target population and their health and community problems?

Research (review chapter 6)

1. What formative research needs are evident, given resources and goals? What formative research was undertaken? Was it appropriate?
2. Given the research issues and the expertise of the staff, was the research design appropriate? Were results valid?
3. Were the objectives and intervention techniques appropriate for the program goals? If not, why? What improvements can be implemented?
4. Was formative research used in an appropriate and timely manner after the research had begun?
5. Did the formative research include both quantitative and qualitative aspects, as appropriate? Were results from these two approaches clearly integrated?

Intervention (review chapters 7-10)

1. Was the intervention:
   a. **accessible** to the target population? For example, are program activities offered at appropriate times and places to maximize participation?
   b. **affordable** in terms of money, time, and resources needed to make use of it?
   c. **appropriate** for the target population and its culture?
   d. **acceptable** to those for whom it was intended?
   e. **adequate** to meet the program goals in terms of type and quality of the procedure and level of effort?
2. What were the costs of the educational, motivational, marketing, organizing, and training procedures? What were the relative contributions of these components to the program impact and outcome? (See below.)
3. Were the intervention procedures "state-of-the-art"? How were they selected? Was the intervention design process participatory? What was the mix of training, education, etc.? How was this mix chosen?

Monitoring

1. Were data collected continually and systematically on:
   a. program inputs, such as resources and personnel needed to carry out the program?
   b. program processes, such as the number of people participating in various program components, the reach of various media efforts, the amount of program contributions made by the community, and the number of health-related policies changed?
2. Were data graphed or in other ways presented in a "user-friendly" way? Were such presentations made to the program staff, target population, and program governance?
3. How were the process evaluation data used? Were they used to refine the intervention and/or reinforce change agents for their efforts?

Evaluation of Impact and Outcome

1. What is the context of the program evaluation?
   a. Who requested the evaluation, and why?
   b. Are the resources adequate for the evaluation?
   c. Who is the evaluator? What potential biases does she or he bring to the evaluation, and how are these handled?
   d. How comprehensive is the evaluation plan? For example, which aspects of the ONPRIME sequence will be examined? What are the reasons for not including some components? (Obviously, this question will

probably not be included in the evaluation report, but can give the evaluator a better notion of the true context in which he or she is working, and the validity of the actual evaluation effort).

2. What is the program impact? How consistent are these with program goals? To what can the program's success or lack thereof be attributed?
3. What long-term outcomes did the program produce?
4. What are the limitations in the evaluation methodology? For example, was descriptive, comparative, analytic, and explanatory information collected and integrated?
5. What recommendations can be made with respect to (a) continuing the program, and (b) extending it to other problem areas, target populations, and settings?

TWO MISTAKES REVISITED

We now return to the two hypothetical evaluation cases presented at the beginning of this chapter. What alternative evaluation approaches and measures would have yielded more sensitive and specific information? In the first case, an outside evaluator encountered something of a political mess in terms of conflicts between certain board members. This understandably led Ms. Williams to focus on the organizational aspect of the planning and implementation sequence. However, additional information could have resulted in a report that not only avoided "axing" a generally effective program, but could also have resulted in corrective feedback to the board and staff for ameliorating the program's problems. For example, Ms. Williams could have examined why board members were chosen to serve, how they participated in setting program goals, and how well these goals were accepted and understood by the board. Through that effort she may have noted that the board members' expectations were inconsistent with the goals and objectives of the program or that staff were being inattentive to the public relations aspects of their duties, which often include keeping board members happy. In other words, the goals and objectives as written were probably incomplete.

In some ways, it appears the breast feeding project planning, implementation, and evaluation plan could have benefitted from additional formative research and more attention to the organizational aspects of the needs/resources and intervention phases. Similarly, Ms. Williams' report was not sufficiently balanced, describing difficulties in one aspect of the program, while underemphasizing some critical strengths. Had she gone beyond the descriptive level of evaluation, she would have recommended the program be continued, with additional formative research and/or staff training in consensus building to help resolve some sticky but not insurmountable problems.

As is frequently the case, Dr. Gomez evaluated a program for which she was largely responsible, which may have led her to overlook some critical elements of the evaluation. First, were the objectives (a reduction of substance abuse) consistent with the program goals (a reduction of absenteeism)? Perhaps a greater level of participation on the part of the target population in program planning may have revealed that absenteeism was more closely related to employee morale, work schedules, or other issues for which drug use *and* absenteeism are both symptoms. Clearly, more careful attention to needs assessment and formative research were warranted.

Perhaps the greatest shortcoming of this second evaluation was the lack of monitoring data, other than subjective (and probably selective) judgments on the part of certain management and union representatives. A sensitive evaluation of trends in absenteeism would have alerted Dr. Gomez that things were not going as well as hoped. Moreover, the monitoring and graphing of weekly or even daily absenteeism could have indicated what factors were related to relatively higher and lower absenteeism rates.

Additionally, a time series analytic approach could have shown that the program was actually having an effect. Instead, the first quarter of a year (when people are still adhering to New Year's resolutions?) was compared to the last quarter of a subsequent year (when higher rates of missing work could be related to the holiday season).

THE EVALUATION OF THE CALIFORNIA TOBACCO CONTROL PROGRAM: A CASE STUDY

In 1988, the voters of California were asked to vote on whether to raise the tax on a pack of cigarettes by twenty-five cents. "Proposition 99," sponsored by a coalition of voluntary health organizations and other interested agencies, stipulated that one-fourth of the money raised by this tax (estimated to yield a total of $600 million annually) would be used to conduct tobacco education and research.

The tobacco industry, alarmed at the portents of this initiative, struck back in force, spending as much as $20 million in anti-Proposition 99 media compared to the $1 million spent by the coalition from their donated funds. In spite of, or perhaps because of, the industry's campaign, Proposition 99 passed by approximately 60 percent to 40 percent. (In one ad, the industry asserted that a vote for Proposition 99 was a vote for gang violence, as the increased price would accelerate cigarette smuggling. And who would control the smuggling? Gangs, of course! The public's response was a combination of outrage and laughter, and the ad was quickly pulled). Thus, one of history's best-funded health promotion campaigns was launched, the specifics of which are presented in chapter 16.

Working with the California Department of Health Services, the Legislature then proceeded to designate specifically how Proposition 99 money was to be spent. Now transformed to "AB (for Assembly Bill) 75," the legislation designated that nearly $5 million per year of the education account would be spent on a statewide prevalence survey, media-oriented formative research, and an "independent" process evaluation.

The prevalence survey is conducted through statewide random digit telephone dialing. It measures program outcomes such as smoking and use of smokeless tobacco, including questions about the onset, maintenance, and cessation of the tobacco habit. Additional items assess anti-tobacco attitudes and behaviors, such as support for tobacco education and the willingness to protest against exposure to second-hand smoke. The survey is phased to analyze trends in statewide tobacco use which may be related to AB 75 funded efforts. The initial baseline survey overlapped somewhat with program implementation due to the necessity of getting AB 75 programs launched quickly. Subsequent survey waves are planned for every second year. Moreover, the questions in the survey are identical to or compatible with those used in many national and international smoking research efforts, allowing for comparisons between California and other regions.

A decision to earmark millions of dollars per year to statewide anti-tobacco media led to the designation of the second component of the evaluation. This component is characterized by focus groups, test marketing, and other formative research efforts, the results of which are used to refine the media campaign. Special attention is given to certain target populations about whom the least is known, such as ethnic groups (Latinos, African-Americans, Asians, and Native Americans, who make up over 40 percent of the state's population), pregnant women, and high-risk teens.

The "Independent Evaluation" looks specifically at *program processes*, especially with respect to how efficiently other "health education" (which in this case includes policy and protective) activities are implemented and the resulting program participation. Major emphases of this component are on programs developed by county health departments and schools for cessation and prevention efforts. While these organizations are encouraged to implement educational, skills-building, motivational, and marketing interventions, support is also provided for community organizing, policy innovations, and activism. Thus, the Independent Evaluation includes a variety of methods for assessing not only the number of individuals who participate in behavior change programs but also coalition building, policy development, implementation and enforcement, and activism initiated or facilitated by the local health departments. Also, an effort is made to assess the cooperation between health departments and schools, the two major institutions involved in AB 75 implementation. Finally, the initiation of policy change is measured at the state level. Since the passage of Proposition 99, the state legislature has introduced a variety of other tobacco control-related legislation, including a bill which would further increase the cigarette and smokeless tobacco tax. The level of legislative activity in this area as well as the stimulus for and outcome of these initiatives will be compared to similar bills regulating alcohol sales, as well as tobacco control legislation being initiated in neighboring states.

Various program outcomes are tracked by the Independent Evaluation, as well. First, AB 75 is expected to stimulate tobacco control efforts by health professionals and others not funded by or directly connected with this initiative. Therefore, ongoing surveys of physicians' and dentists' offices are conducted to assess their personal counseling to tobacco users as well as any non-smoking cues present in the office waiting areas. Contact is maintained with voluntary organizations (the American Lung Association, the American Cancer Society, and the American Heart Association), critical actors in the coalition which got the proposition on the ballot and passed in 1988, in order to assess additional ongoing anti-tobacco activities. The State Board of Equalization provides data on the number of packs of tobacco sold by quarter. These data allow health authorities and the Legislature to determine the role of the price increase as well as the tobacco control campaign in reducing overall consumption. Again, these "consumption" data are directly comparable to those from other states.

The initial tax increase precipitated a substantial drop in cigarette sales over one year. In the second year, purchasing gradually leveled off as the education intervention slowly geared up and consumers became acclimated to the higher price. But during the third year, purchasing again began to drop, this time probably due to intensified educational efforts and stayed at a level far below the national average. Additionally, modest but important reductions due to the educational campaign, introduced gradually beginning fifteen months after the tax increase, are finally evident.

Finally, cost effectiveness analyses are being conducted to learn which of the educational (and policy) components were most effective at reducing the prevalence of smoking. Data from both the survey and process evaluation will be used to attribute behavior change to either AB 75 programs or other events. A summary of the AB 75 program evaluation activities is presented in Table 11-2.

TABLE 11-2
California Tobacco Education Program
Evaluation Components

Evaluation Category	Measure	Description
Formative Evaluation	Reaction of target audiences and others to media	Focus group and school-based surveys
Process Evaluation	Implementation of cessation and prevention activities	Surveys of local health departments and schools
	Assessment of community organization and activism	Surveys of local health departments and schools as well as monitoring of additional legislation for tobacco control
Impact Evaluation	Prevalence and initiation of tobacco use	Statewide random digit dialing telephone survey sample of all households every 24 months
	Personal Activism	
	Amount of tobacco purchased	Telephone survey
	Generalization of activity to other settings	State Board of Equalization
	Tobacco industry counterattack	Tax Stamp (sales) data
	Cost-benefit analysis	Surveys of medical and dental offices
		Monitoring of frequency and content of ads, assessment of tobacco-related behavior change as a function of AB 75 activity, and cost of each activity.

THE EVALUATION REPORT

An evaluation is usually undertaken to provide information and insight to a supervisor, board of directors, or funding agency. The results of an evaluation should be presented in a well organized and concise fashion, with appropriate charts and summary statements. The following is a typical format for an evaluation report:

I. Summary or Abstract
II. Background for and goals of the evaluation
III. Level(s) and categories of the evaluation
   A. Reasons these were chosen
   B. Limitations
IV. Methods and instruments used
V. Results
   A. Elements of the ONPRIME sequence
   B. Charts, graphs and tables
VI. Conclusions
VII. Recommendations.

SUMMARY

Broadly defined, health promotion evaluation activities comprise needs and resources assessment, formative or qualitative research, program monitoring, and impact and outcome evaluation. Needs/resources assessment is generally conducted for program planning purposes at the beginning of an effort. Formative research is often carried out early in a program to select or develop an intervention approach, but may be needed during the course of the intervention as well in order to refine the program. Monitoring of the program implementation and responses to it should be carried out on a continuous basis once the program is underway. Impact and outcome evaluation measure the immediate and long-term effects (respectively) of the intervention.

This concludes the presentation of the basic techniques of health promotion planning, intervention, and evaluation as represented by the ONPRIME sequence. In the following section, we will explore how health promotion is conducted at four different and progressively more complex levels.

ADDITIONAL READINGS

These references will further enhance your evaluation skills:

1. L. Green & M. Kreuter. (1991). *Health promotion planning: An educational and environmental approach* (2nd ed.). Mountain View, CA: Mayfield.
2. R. Windsor, T. Baranowski, N. Clark, & G. Cutler. (1984). *Evaluation of health promotion and education programs.* Palo Alto, CA: Mayfield.

ENDNOTES

1. The authors are indebted to Dr. Dennis Foote for his conceptualization of aspects of this representation.
2. Quintero-Torres, M. & Perez-Gomez, A. (1988). *Evaluacion: Un instrumento de superacion.* Bogota, Columbia: Ministerio de Educacion Nacional, p. 16.
3. Baranowski, T., Simons-Morton, B., Hooks, P., Henske, J., Tiernan, K., Dunn, J., Burkhalter, H., Harper, J., & Palmer, J. (1990). A center-based program for exercise change among Black-American families. *Health Education Quarterly, 17,* 179–196.

Introduction to Section III: Levels of Intervention

OBJECTIVES

After reading this introduction, the reader should be able to:

1. List the four levels of intervention for health promotion and give examples of health promotion interventions for each.
2. Given a community health problem, outline a comprehensive health promotion plan linking different input levels of the community.

INTRODUCTION

The traditional focus of behavior modification has been on the behavior of individuals or that of people in small group settings. For example, mental health counselors tend to work on a one-to-one basis with individuals demonstrating various problems in personal or social functioning. Psychiatric hospitals frequently have wards where token economies are used to enhance the adaptation of the group of patients on that ward. Parent and teacher training procedures engender contingency management skills in these adults with the ultimate target being one or several children. Recently, however, it has become necessary to demonstrate a broader impact of behavior change programs by modifying behaviors of large numbers of people in churches, worksites, schools, or entire communities. Even regional and national-level behavior change programs can be developed using appropriate behavior-change technology. Therefore, change agents optimize their effectiveness by deciding on the best and most appropriate level of impact at requiring the fewest amount of resources which can be utilized to achieve optimal health outcomes. Although it may be rewarding for us to get two or three people to quit smoking for their lifetime and thereby prevent the ill effects of this habit, a larger number of individuals need to be approached to have a true public health effect. The multi-level societal structures as related to health promotion planning may be referred to as levels of impact. For present purposes, these levels will consist of "individual," "group/social network," "organizational," and "community." They may also include one higher level, namely, "national/regional."[1]

At the **individual** level, clinic-based and related activities can be used to change individual health behaviors on a one-to-one basis. These behavior change procedures involve a professional or paraprofessional helping a client set goals, develop a contingency contract, learn new skills, and/or generalize behavior change to other situations. Typical of this level are clinic-based procedures used in medical centers, behavioral medicine clinics, or hospitals. Although they may be inefficient, such procedures are appropriate when intensive "therapy" is needed (e.g., in teaching heart attack patients to quit smoking), or when such behavior change or health education efforts simply augment existing clinical services (e.g., having a hospital dietitian incorporate patient input into discharge planning in order to enhance maintenance of behavior change accomplished in the hospital). Paraprofessionals and even volunteers tend to provide some assistance in this resource-intensive behavior approach. Finally, individual level interventions sometimes provide needed information regarding how best to approach a program development effort at a higher impact-level target (see chapter 12).

Group or social networks are the next level of impact for the health promoter. Members of families, friendship groups, work groups, or neighbors can be targeted simultaneously in order to improve cost efficiency (see chapter 13). Moreover, if such groups are "naturally formed" (such as those just mentioned) and not simply a collection of strangers who show up for a clinic-based class, the potential for maintenance of behavior change may be enhanced, given that relatives and acquaintances are involved from the beginning in the behavior change process. At the group level, "early adopters" can reach out to their "later adopter" relatives or friends, thereby improving the efficiency of the behavior change efforts. For

example, a family planning program in Seoul, South Korea, used beauticians, church members, and merchants to recruit women into attending a family planning clinic. These individuals were chosen due to their fairly extensive number of acquaintances (i.e., the density of their social network) as well as the frequency with which they saw these acquaintances. Incentives were provided whereby these lay facilitators were reinforced by small cash awards for the number of attendees they recruited.[2]

The **organizational** level of intervention is the next larger and more complex level of impact of concern to health promoters. Procedures such as organizational behavior management and occupational safety and health (see chapter 14) can attract even larger numbers of individuals to attempt behavior change as part of a program in their church, school, or worksite. Indeed, approaches to intervention such as the Johnson & Johnson "Live for Life" program, the Lycoming (PA) County Health Improvement Project's interbank weight loss competition, and a variety of other efforts have had a major impact on health promotion planning in the U.S.[3]

The next impact level for our consideration is the **community** level. Communities are composites of the various individuals, families, neighborhoods, and organizations within them. Community environment also includes print and broadcast media, medical centers and health clinics, police and fire departments, and other extra-organizational institutions which allow the imaginative health promoter to develop the potential for a large effect or to support existing efforts at the individual, group, and/or organizational level. Success in community-level interventions may correlate with the degree of identity that the target population has with its community. This sense of identity may especially be present in sociologically or geographically well-defined communities. Finally, national or regional efforts are frequently beyond our purview as health promoters. However, efforts at lobbying to enact legislation such as gun control, maintaining the 55 MPH speed law, or reducing subsidies for tobacco growers are definitely of interest to those of us working in public health.

Although these levels of impact are presented separately, they should not be seen as independent of one another, but as interacting and mutually supporting processes. For example, developing political support at the community level for lobbying congressmen to support anti-tobacco legislation can be far more effective than simple individual letter writing. Developing support from a group of "early adopter" gatekeepers (e.g., managers of worksites) to give personal testimony for and otherwise indicate support of health promotion efforts, may increase the chance of such efforts being supported by a mayor and city council. The mayor and city council, in turn, could be used to help convince "later adopter" organizational gatekeepers of the advisability and benefits of participating in the health promotion effort. Small groups within churches or schools can be formed to run health education classes as well as to organize a health promotion effort for the entire organization, whereas stated earlier, individual participants and small groups may be interested in spreading the word to other individual later adopters.

We will now proceed to examine principles and examples of health promotion efforts at these four levels of intervention.

EXERCISE

Think about a community you know fairly well and a health problem it has. What health promotion strategies might you employ to address this problem, using the four-level planning scheme? Remember to link activities at different levels.

ENDNOTES

1. Abrams, D., Elder, J., Carleton, R. A., Lasater, T. M., & Artz, L. M. (1986). Social learning principles for organization health promotion: An integrated approach. In M. Cataldo & T. J. Coates (Eds.), *Health and industry: A behavioral medicine perspective.* New York: Wiley-Interscience.

2. Kwon, K. H. (1971). Use of the agent system in Seoul. *Students in Family Planning, 2*(11), 237–240.

3. Cataldo, M. F. & Coates, T. J. (Eds.). (1986). *Health and industry: A behavioral medicine perspective.* New York: Wiley-Interscience.

Chapter 12

Changing the Health Behavior of Individuals

OBJECTIVES

After reading this chapter the reader should be able to:

1. Define individual health promotion.
2. Distinguish among the philosophies of the determinists, the self-control theorists, and the social learning theorists regarding the concepts of "external" and "self" control.
3. List the main ingredients of an effective contingency contract.
4. Discuss the importance of collecting baseline data.
5. Develop solutions to improve a contingency contract that is not working.
6. Identify appropriate instances for applying negative reinforcement, response cost, punishment, modeling, and positive reinforcement.
7. Identify the role of individual health promotion in the field of public health.

INTRODUCTION

The assessment and modification of individual behavior is the foundation of motivating health behavior. Decades of laboratory and applied research in individual behavior change serves as the starting point for all current efforts of behavior change at group, organizational, and community levels. While understanding how to change individual behavior is not sufficient in itself for success at public health promotion, it is a necessary prerequisite skill. Whether you ultimately are employed as a service provider, supervisor, Peace Corps volunteer, or private health consultant earning $1,000,000 per year, one important goal will be to contribute to the behavior change of several or many individuals.

The present chapter expands on the techniques described in Section II and provides examples of how professionals from a variety of fields have approached the challenge of changing individual health behavior. Advantages and limitations of the individual change approach are then presented.

Definition of Individual-Level Interventions

Individual health promotion is the modification of health behavior and related factors through motivational procedures, skills training, communication strategies, and educational techniques delivered on a one-to-one-basis. Typically, such efforts are undertaken by professional change agents in clinical or counseling settings (e.g., physicians working with individual patients), but they can also be accomplished by lay change agents and in community settings (e.g., a mother attempting to shape healthful eating habits in her elementary school-age child). In this section, we focus on individual interventions centering around one-to-one interactions. Higher order interventions which consider individual behavior only in the larger context of the group, organizational, or community environment are discussed in the succeeding chapters.

External vs. Self-Control

A source of contention among human service professionals and behavioral scientists concerns the relative importance and scientific validity of the concepts of "external" versus "self-control." This argument parallels that in philosophy pitting proponents of determinism against those who insist on the importance or predominance of free will. In the former category, Skinner and other **determinists argue that human behavior is controlled by one's physical environment, genetic predisposition, and physiological and physical functioning.**[1] As discussed in chapter 3, Bandura, Kanfer, and other **social learning theorists** and social psychologists seek the middle ground between self-control and determinism and **maintain that while behavior is a function of environmental factors, the individual, in turn, can shape or influence the environment to his or her liking through a process called "reciprocal determinism."** Expectations regarding the potential for various consequences and confidence in one's ability to perform a behavior also help predict whether behavior will occur. Social learning theory's revision of operant psychology has proven easier to swallow for those who favor free-will explanations of behavior, which in part has contributed to the current popularity of social learning-based and self-control-based health promotion approaches.

While *Motivating Health Behavior* places a relatively greater emphasis on operant psychology's explanations of health behavior, we question the importance of the dispute among those loyal to these various models. After close examination, it is apparent that much of the argument is semantic in nature. The present chapter, for example, reviews techniques derived from Kanfer's self-control model as well as behavior modification which are often combined in intervention approaches (such as contingency contracting). These mixed-ancestry technologies often prove quite effective and are in turn advocated and embraced by followers of both camps.

CONTINGENCY CONTRACTS FOR MOTIVATING INDIVIDUALS

A contingency contract is a written contract on which a client agrees to a specific behavior change or health outcome by a given date. The contract also specifies consequences of completing (or not completing) the agreement. Contingency contracting is one of the most effective individual behavior change procedures currently employed and provides a convenient mechanism for combining two or more motivational or other procedures in one change effort. Although generally used for the specification of reinforcement criteria, it can also set the stage for practice and homework exercises needed to master new skills or educational material. Contracting allows both the consumer and the change agent to participate in the development of a behavior change procedure and makes this procedure objective, open, and effective. Contracting also provides a vehicle for supervision in clinical settings, as individual clinicians can keep copies of patient contracts in their charts for subsequent review by their supervisors. It involves the inclusion of individuals from the social support network and forces us to think in terms of both acceleration and deceleration targets. It can focus discussions for future counseling or clinical efforts, for staff behavior change, or for whatever method of change we want to consider. Therefore, contracting is considered a cornerstone for effective individual behavior change efforts.

The specific nature of a contingency contract varies from case to case. Contracts may even be verbal, with a public statement serving to "bind" the person to his or her commitment. Whenever possible, however, written contracts enhance the recall of specific contract elements and improve compliance. The first six of the following elements should be clearly written on each contingency contract, with the final three added as appropriate:[2]

1. The date the contract begins and ends (or is to be renegotiated).
2. Acceleration and (if applicable) deceleration behaviors targeted for change.
3. Amount and kind of reinforcer or other consequence to be used.
4. Schedule of consequence delivery.
5. Signatures of the consumer, change agent, and significant others.
6. Schedule for review of progress, with designation of appropriate record-keeping system.
7. Bonus clause for sustained or exceptional performance.
8. Statement of the penalties to be imposed if the specified behavior is not performed.
9. Subsequent to the initiation of behavior change, renegotiation should include clauses for generalization and long-term maintenance of behavior change.

A blank prototype form, which can easily be adapted to a variety of contracting situations, is presented in Figure 12–1. Note that stipulations for self-monitoring, goal setting, self-evaluation, and self-reinforcement — the key ingredients of Kanfer's self-control model — are included in this contracting approach.

Identifying Target Behaviors for the Contract

"Target" behaviors are the behaviors the client wants to change. Not all behaviors, however, are suitable target behaviors for contracting. A suitable target behavior must be easy to observe (at least for the consumer). It must also be a behavior that the consumer has both the skill and opportunity to perform. If the latter two conditions are not met, other procedures, such as training (chapter 9) and response facilitation (chapter 8), should be implemented prior to the contract.

Example #1

Roy Evans is a chocolate freak and couch potato, and has been one for twenty years. His favorite hobbies are "Cheers" reruns and "Jeopardy."

Behavior Change Contract for (name): _____
_____ Date:_____
Date(s) to Be Reviewed: _____
If I, (name), do the following (description of target behavior, health outcome
or both)_____
by (target date, if applicable) _____ then the following
will occur:
(description of consequence and schedule, plus bonuses or penalties
_____
_____

I also agree to keep track of the progress I am making as follows:
(description of self-monitoring procedure)
_____
_____

A copy of a self-monitoring chart is attached.

_____   _____
Signature   Witness 1

FIGURE 12–1.   The format for the contingency contract.

Behavior Change Contract for Roy Evans
June 4, 1993
Dates to be reviewed: Biweekly until December 31, 1993

I, Roy Evans, agree to lose two pounds per week by having a negative energy balance of 600 calories per day. In order to achieve this balance, I will exercise at least 20 minutes per day and consume no more than 1700 calories per day, of which no more than 200 calories will come from sweets and other junk foods. I will closely monitor my minutes of exercise, calorie consumption, and weight; and I will graph each on a daily basis (a copy of my graph is attached).

Every other week I will visit Connie Counselor at her weight loss emporium to have my weight checked and receive advice on further actions to take. Should I meet my goal weight for that two-week period, I will treat myself to a movie and a lowfat yogurt dessert at the nearby ice cream shop. If at the end of three months I have lost 20 or more pounds, I will buy myself a suit valued at $200 or more, of which Connie Counselor will pay $100 from my deposit for signing up for her program. If at the end of six months I have kept off at least 15 pounds, I will buy a new pair of shoes with the same financial arrangement. If I fail to lose weight for two consecutive two-week periods, I will not allow myself to watch "Cheers" for the next two weeks.
SIGNATURES;

_____   _____

Roy Evans   Connie Counselor, R.D.

He has several friends at work where he is liked and respected as an energetic employee. But when he hits the freeway at five o'clock, he thinks mostly about getting home to his refrigerator and remote control.

But Roy knows changes are needed. He has gained twenty pounds in the last five to six years and notices a shortness of breath when he climbs two flights of stairs. He visited with Connie, a weight loss counselor, who discussed with Roy a variety of strategies toward better energy balance. They set up the contract shown above.

The above contract is fairly typical in weight loss programs. Specific short- and long-term goals are set, with behavioral (calories and exercise) and outcome (weight) goals. Positive and negative reinforcers and the role of the change agent in administering these reinforcers are explicit. Note that the reinforcers are integrated into the theme of the change project: the loss of TV watching (sedentary behavior), low calorie yogurt, and clothes that will fit a slimmer figure. Special care must be taken, however, as stimuli associated with the ice cream shop could set off an eating binge, and failure to earn the presumably powerful reinforcer of new clothes could create counterproductive feelings of frustration.

Example #2

Jennifer Edwards is a bit of a social outcast. She has just entered graduate school in a new community and is just beginning to get to know her classmates. However, while the rest of her classmates seem to be hanging out together and interacting frequently during and outside of class, they do not include Jennifer. Her instructor assigns group projects in which her classmates give her limited and uninteresting roles.

Jennifer goes to her instructor, Dr. Dreiser, for some insight. Dr. Dreiser has observed some potentially problematic behaviors and agrees to share these observations. First, Jennifer often rolls her eyes or grimaces when a classmate makes an uninformed comment or asks a naive question. Second, Jennifer makes no attempt to participate in after-class gab sessions; instead she heads for the library or home to crack the books. While her grades are excellent, she is not benefitting from a well-rounded educational experience.

Jennifer admits she sometimes gets impatient with students less prepared or seemingly less serious than herself, but she feels this is more a function of her perfectionism than feelings of superiority. She did not realize this impatience was

---

Behavior Change Contract for Jennifer Edwards
April 5, 1992
 I, Jennifer Edwards, agree to take the following steps to improve my interpersonal relationships with my classmates:
1. Eliminate all negative facial reactions to comments made by my classmates in class.
2. Increase smiles and head nods when they make comments I find interesting or informative.
3. Try to participate in at least one post-class conversation after each class.
4. Take a one-session Dale Carnegie course to build my skills in interpersonal relations.
 Progress will be monitored by me by checking "yes" or "no" next to each of the first three items above after each class, on the attached checklist. After every two classes, I will show the checklist to my instructor for a reliability check.
 If at the end of the semester I successfully eliminate negative reactions and increase positive reactions to my classmates, and participate in one post-class conversation per week using some of the skills learned in Dale Carnegie, my husband will make all preparations for a post-semester party in our house for me and my classmates.
SIGNATURES:

_____   _____
Jennifer Edwards   Winfield Edwards

_____
Plato Dreiser, Instructor

---

apparent. Jennifer also admitted she is shy and does not know how to meet people; while she studied more than she needed to, she did not know how to pursue more sociable alternatives. She thought more about her instructor's observations and shared them with her husband. The three of them entered into the behavioral contract shown above.

The above contract specifies not only target behaviors but also a skills acquisition activity to enhance the likelihood of success in achieving contract goals. Again, a positive reinforcer consistent with the goals was chosen. No negative reinforcer or other penalty is included, with the assumption that the current state of affairs is sufficiently aversive to motivate Jennifer to change. Jennifer is on some thin ice, however, as ultimately her success is in the hands of her classmates, who could spurn her change of style (and not show up at her party!).

Example #3: A Verbal Commitment to Give Up Chewing Tobacco

Frank Pinson is the star center fielder for the Cortland High School Redlegs. Frank and others in the junior class have gone through two semesters of smoking and smokeless tobacco education, emphasizing prevention for those who have not started and cessation for those presently using the drug. Reinforced by their coach, all the other players on the team except Frank have foregone the deadly tradition of dipping snuff and chewing tobacco on the diamond.

At first his teammates ignored Frank's deviation from their healthy ways, as his bat, arm, and glove won them a lot of games and he is personally popular. But gradually they became tired of his spitting and drooling and became unsettled by the sight of a healthy friend playing Russian roulette with tobacco. They began razzing him about his habit through exaggerated imitations of his spitting between pitches. One day Coach Hutchinson sat down with him after practice and gave him a stern lecture on the dangers of the deadly weed, and asked Frank to carefully consider giving it up.

The next day at practice, Frank stepped into the batting cage to take his practice swings and announced, "O.K. you clowns, you're looking at the new Frank Pinson—no more chewing, unless it's sunflower seeds. You see me spit anything else, you can empty the cooler over my head."

"Not necessary, my man," responded Wally

Bell, who was pitching. "But tell you what — as long as you keep off that garbage, you go first in the cage every practice."

Frank is making a verbal contract with his teammates and coach to abandon his habit by publicly announcing a punishment contingency and monitoring system. Wally, in turn, suggests a positive differential reinforcement approach, whereby Frank gets the prized first turn in batting practice for not chewing. While lacking the permanence of a written contract, the public nature of such a commitment may be equally effective, negatively reinforcing compliance through avoidance of a loss of face that would occur with failure.

FACTORS TO CONSIDER IN SELF-CHANGE PROGRAMS

Whether through contingency contracting, personal unaided self-change, or other procedures, several factors should be given attention in order to maximize the possibility of success:

Target Behaviors Must Be Easy to Observe. In order to reinforce the consumer for changing behavior, it is necessary that such changes be immediately recognizable to whomever is monitoring the client's behavior. Obviously, such factors as thoughts, attitudes, and values cannot be target behaviors because they cannot be directly observed. Also, a behavior such as "coming home late" is hard to observe because the word "late" means different things to different people. A more suitable target behavior would be "coming home after 6:30 p.m." If a person other than the consumer is responsible for monitoring the consumer's behavior, the target behavior(s) must occur at times when the person can observe it.

There Must Be Frequent Opportunities for the Consumer to Perform the Target Behavior. The more often a consumer is reinforced for performing the target behavior, the more likely he or she will be to perform it in the future. Consequently, if the consumer has few opportunities to perform the target behavior, there will be few opportunities to receive reinforcers and behavior change will occur very slowly. For example, a couple that might want to eliminate arguments related to both members drinking too much at parties. However, if the couple only attends one party a month, they will rarely have the opportunity to earn reinforcers for not arguing.

The Target Behavior Must Be One the Client Has the Skill to Perform. This requirement may seem obvious and unworthy of mention, but it is not uncommon for clients to pick target behaviors they are not capable of performing. The most common example involves contracts between parents and their children. Parents frequently want their children to take on responsibilities which they are physically or intellectually incapable of carrying out.

Collecting Baseline Data Information. Once the client and change agent have identified one or more target behaviors, it is necessary to collect baseline information for each target behavior. **Baseline information refers to how often and under what conditions the client is currently performing the target behavior.** This information serves two purposes. First, it indicates whether the specified behavior is, in fact, a suitable target behavior. Occasionally, the baseline information will indicate that the specified behavior is not really a problem or that it occurs only in situations in which it cannot be accurately monitored.

Baseline information also provides data needed to evaluate the effectiveness of the contract. The feedback a client receives about his or her progress once the contract is implemented can serve as a powerful motivator. In order to collect the baseline information and monitor the client's progress, a system for observing and recording the occurrence of the target behavior must be developed (see chapter 3).

DEVELOPING A CONTRACT — PUTTING TOGETHER A PLAN

Once the target behavior(s) has been identified, a plan for changing the target behavior needs to be developed. There are four steps in developing a plan:

Step 1: Identifying Positive Reinforcers

Anything the consumer likes enough to work for can be an effective positive reinforcer. Money, food, little gifts, the opportunity to engage in favorite activities, and social recognition such as praise can be reinforcers for some people. It is important to remember, however, that a reinforcer for one person may have no appeal for another individual. It is always necessary to sit down with the client and generate a list of specific things he or she finds rewarding.

Some reinforcers are more suitable than others for use in contracting. The most effective reinforcers have the following characteristics:

- *The reinforcer can be made available each time the client performs the target behavior.* Some reinforcers, such as expensive gifts, a night on the town, etc., simply cannot be provided very often and, therefore, may not be as motivating to the client as smaller reinforcers that can be given more frequently. An exception to this rule occurs when a powerful reinforcer given infrequently is supplemented by the delivery of tokens. Tokens are discussed below.

- *The reinforcer does not become less desirable over time.* Some reinforcers can be motivating for the client initially but lose their attractiveness over time. For example, a smoker might reward himself with an ice cream cone each time he eats a meal without smoking. After a week of such rewards, however, he may lose his taste for ice cream and begin smoking during meals again.

- *The reinforcer does not seem silly.* Behaviorists have been accused of developing meaningless or patronizing reinforcement systems which may prove ineffective or can eventually backfire. Careful attention to selecting a truly desired reinforcer and a mediator who will sincerely believe it (see below) are critically important.

Denying a client access to pleasurable activities, foods, etc., typically available to him or her is a form of aversive control. For example, a woman contracts with herself to use the loss of her favorite television show as a negative reinforcer. If the woman fails to exercise, she will feel disappointed because she has to miss her show. If she does exercise, she receives nothing extra for her efforts. Aversive control of this type can be used effectively in contracting if it is used sparingly. It is

better, however, to use only positive reinforcers if at all possible. When punishers or negative reinforcers are used, it is easy for contracting to become an aversive experience for the client.

Reinforcers that punish others should not be used. A husband, for example, might want to contract with his wife to accompany him on a fishing trip once every two weeks if he baby-sits for twelve hours during the preceding two weeks. If the wife dislikes fishing trips, however, the above plan may intensify, rather than diminish, the couple's conflicts.

Social recognition and praise should be delivered each time the client earns a material reinforcer. Statements such as "good job!", "that's great!", and "thank you" are powerful reinforcers for most people. Sometimes they can be used quite effectively alone, since they can be delivered at any time and, if stated sincerely, almost never lose their potency.

Step 2: Selecting a Monitor

A monitor is the mediator responsible for observing the client's behavior and delivering reinforcers when the client appropriately performs the target behavior. An effective monitor has several important qualities:

- The monitor should have frequent opportunities to observe the client.
- The monitor should be willing to spend the time and effort needed to help develop the plan as well as observe the client and dispense the reinforcers.
- The monitor should agree with the goals of the contract and the plan for delivering reinforcers. A monitor who is unwilling to follow the contract exactly as it is written can be more harmful than helpful to the client.

It is usually best to have a person such as the client's spouse, parent, close friend, or relative act as monitor. The professional can serve as the monitor if the target behaviors are limited to those that occur during therapy (e.g., turning in homework assignments). The client can even serve as his or her own monitor. This requires a great deal of self-discipline, however, since it is easy for the client to "cheat" on the contract.

Step 3: Determining the Appropriate Steps

Contracting can produce one of two changes in a target behavior; it can either increase or decrease how often a client performs a target behavior. In most cases, the ultimate goal of contracting is either to decrease or eliminate an undesirable behavior or increase the frequency of a desirable behavior. Such goals usually represent drastic changes for the client — changes too large to be made all at once. Consequently, it is necessary to set some intermediate goals, or "steps," for the client. The general rule to follow when establishing these intermediate goals, or steps, is that the steps can seldom be too small. The worst experience a client can have as a result of contracting is to fail repeatedly to reach the specified goals. The more failures the client experiences, the more likely it is that he or she will lose interest in trying to change any behaviors. The most common method of setting up steps in a plan is to gradually increase (or decrease) the number of times the client must perform the target behavior in order to receive a reinforcer.

Clients often identify more than one target behavior they would like to include in their plan. It is usually best to work on only one behavior at a time. In addition, the behavior likely to be the easiest for the client to change should be the first behavior the client attempts to change. This is another method of building steps into a plan.

In summary, the plan should specify goals the client is sure to attain. In many cases, this involves establishing intermediate goals or steps that will eventually lead to the ultimate goal of the plan. The general rule to follow when establishing steps is that a step can never be too small.

Step 4: Establishing the Contingencies

After the goals of the contract have been established and the reinforcers selected, the rules governing how and when the reinforcer will be delivered must be established. Under ideal conditions, a reinforcer should be delivered:

1. each time the client attains one of the goals specified in the plan; and
2. immediately after the client has attained one of the goals specified in the plan.

In many clinical situations, the above rules can only be approximated. Clients might, for instance, occasionally perform the specified target behaviors when the monitor is unable to observe them. Also, some rewards, such as going to the movies, can only be delivered at certain times of the day. Tokens and social recognition (praise, etc.) often can be used to "fill in the gap" between the performance of a target behavior and the delivery of other reinforcers. It is critical, though, that the contract specify how and when rewards will be delivered. For example, a contract between a smoker and her husband might state that each day the wife smokes only one cigarette or less between 7 a.m. and 9 p.m., her husband will prepare a snack for her before she goes to bed.

It is helpful to establish contingencies that allow the client to earn more than one type of reinforcer. For instance, the plan can specify a list of reinforcers from which the client can choose each time he or she attains a specified goal. The contract can also provide large reinforcers for meeting long-term goals. In the above example, the smoker's contract with her husband could also include "going to a restaurant for dinner on Saturday night" as a reinforcer for meeting her daily goal on six of the seven preceding days.

Writing the Contract

Once the plan has been developed, it should be written down and signed by all the persons who will be involved in its implementation. Actually writing out the contract serves two useful functions. It provides everyone involved with a set of written instructions concerning what they have agreed to do. Writing out and signing the contract also underscores the commitment each individual has made to helping the consumer change his or her behavior.

The written contract should be clear, concise, and thorough. Each goal must be clearly defined.

This requires that the target behavior(s) be clearly described. The description should indicate when, where, and how often the target behavior must be performed for the client to receive reinforcement. The contingencies must also be clearly defined. This requires that the reinforcer(s) be clearly described and the time, place, and person who will deliver them be specified. The "IF (behavior occurs) . . . THEN" (consequence follows) format allows each goal and its associated reinforcer(s) to be described. The format may also include a statement defining how long the contract will be in effect and how it can be changed.

Implementing the Contract

Once the contract has been written, it is ready for implementation. It is crucial that the terms of the contract be followed exactly by both the client and the monitor. Weekly meetings of all persons involved in the contract should be held. At these meetings, the change agent needs to determine whether:

1. The monitor is accurately observing and recording the occurrence of target behaviors and is delivering the reinforcement in the manner specified in the contract.
2. The client is attaining the goals specified in the contract.

The monitor's recordings of the client's behavior are the major, and often the only, source of information as to the client's progress. Consequently, it is critical for the professional to praise the monitor's efforts.

It is the rare contract that works perfectly the first time. The change agent can expect some problem to develop requiring a revision of the contract. Table 12–1 outlines various potential problems and possible solutions.

OTHER METHODS FOR CHANGING INDIVIDUAL BEHAVIOR

Stimulus Control

In some situations few, if any, opportunities to reinforce behavior are available. Such is often the case in public health promotion where we have minimal face-to-face contact with the majority of

individuals we serve. Even clinicians, however, see their clients infrequently and cannot be sure reinforcement procedures can be used reliably.

Stimulus control (discussed briefly in chapters 3 and 8) refers to the alteration of antecedent conditions that develop the potential for a behavior to be reinforced. In other words, we are modifying the "A-B" link, with the hope that a naturally occurring "B-C" link will subsequently support healthier behavior. Much of dieting, for instance, involves the stimulus control of appropriate eating and noneating, as dieters are taught to reorganize their environment (e.g., by not having as many fattening foods present or visible, by having weight loss charts highly visible on a refrigerator door). Although such prompting is an important component of stimulus control, smoking cessation techniques generally involve some form of fading as well. Initially, the smoker smokes in the presence of a large variety of stimuli. Gradually, he or she is instructed to smoke only in "Situation X" and not in "Situation Y," while the list of "Ys" gets larger and larger.

Recommendations for the appropriate use of stimulus control include the following:

1. First, identify by observation the actual functional links between antecedents and target behaviors to be accelerated.
2. Identify cues for inappropriate behavior.
3. Remove cues for inappropriate behavior.
4. Make cues for appropriate behavior more conspicuous. For example, if signs prompting

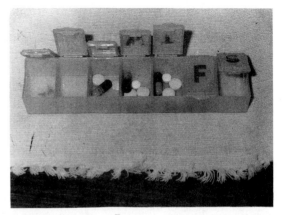

FIGURE 12–2. Stimulus control procedures provide cues for appropriate behaviors such as accurate self-medication

TABLE 12–1
Troubleshooting the Contract

If the client is not meeting the goals specified in the contract, check the following problems:

Problem	Suggested Solutions
1. Do all the involved parties understand the goals, reinforcers, and contingencies specified in the contract?	Re-explain and, if necessary, rewrite the contract so that all parties understand it.
2. Are all the involved parties in agreement with the goals and plans?	Renegotiate any part of the contract on which there is disagreement.
3. Is the system being used to monitor the target behaviors providing the necessary information?	Revise the system if it is inadequate. Provide the monitor with more training in the use of the system. Reinforce the monitor more often for his or her efforts.
4. Is the client receiving reinforcers specified in the contract?	Modify the contingencies if they are impractical. Re-emphasize to all parties the importance of delivering reinforcers in exactly the manner described.
5. Does the client feel he or she is being reinforced sufficiently for his or her efforts?	Break the plan down into smaller steps or in some other way change the contingencies to provide for more reinforcement. If punishers are being used, decrease the frequency with which they are being delivered. Determine whether the client is receiving some form of secondary gains from maintaining the old behavior.
6. Is there a potential for long-term change?	Add reinforcers for long-term goals.

the use of safety equipment in a worksite are effective in prompting the wearing of protective eyewear, make them larger, more colorful, and in places where people are likely to see them.

5. Do not "overwork" a stimulus control procedure. For example, change the placement and artwork on signs and posters frequently.

6. Arrange for stimulus control procedures that can be generalized to natural environments or environments outside the actual intervention, should this be necessary.

An Example of Stimulus Control and Reinforcement for Healthier Snacking.   Stark and her colleagues worked with eight children, ages three to eight, in teaching them how to choose relatively healthy snacks.[3] During "nutrition training," stickers were used to reinforce appropriate snack choices. The children were shown pictures of available foods and asked which ones they would pick for snacks. After selecting one of the pictures, the child received feedback on its appropriateness in the presence of the other children. The feedback included the use of the colors red and green, such as calling potato chips red foods and saying they were not as good as green foods and then mentioning a fresh vegetable that was a green food. The children were given a second opportunity to choose from the pictures if they made a mistake on the first opportunity. They received praise following green food choices. In the subsequent phase, children were given the opportunity to pick actual foods and were immediately praised if they chose a green food. They were also given a sticker as a reinforcer. Although red foods were allowed, the trainer essentially said or did nothing when they selected them. Then, the children were taught to say phrases such as, "I picked a good snack, didn't I?" The child then received praise for correct selection and a sticker for making the spontaneous statements. The children were also instructed to make the statements at home as well. The trainer stayed in touch with the parents to determine whether they were using these procedures at home and gave them feedback and extra training as needed.

A second study used the same procedures except for training the children to make statements. These two studies showed that children at this age

could be easily taught to discriminate between healthy and nonhealthy snacks in that with the "cuing statements" this skill acquisition generalized to the home setting. However, without the cuing statements, generalization failed to occur to the same extent. Also, the effects diminished over time, indicating the need for booster sessions.

PROCEDURES FOR CHANGING INDIVIDUAL HEALTH BEHAVIOR: EXAMPLES

In this section, we describe a few of the hundreds of examples in the health promotion literature on the modification of individual behavior. These examples are organized according to general categories of behavior change procedures. However, most used several motivational procedures concurrently.

Contingency Management for Infant Nutrition

While mothers in the Philippines were found to have adequate levels of knowledge about infant nutrition, especially with respect to breast feeding, inadequate numbers were acting on this knowledge.[4] Therefore, a group of health promotion researchers attempted to establish a reinforcement system for appropriate feeding behaviors by mothers and weight gained by infants. Specifically, mothers were encouraged to continue breast feeding, supplement breast milk with appropriate nutritional complements, obtain weight gain in their infants, plant green leafy vegetables for home consumption, and visit the health center at least once a month.

At each visit to the center, the mothers were given health coupons for successful accomplishment of each of the five steps. At the end of every three-month period, lotteries were held whereby numbers corresponding to some of the coupons were drawn for prizes of sacks of rice or corn. Later, however, some mothers complained that through this random process some mothers who had very few coupons were winning prizes while others with many coupons won nothing. Thereafter, a trading stamp system was substituted whereby certain numbers of health coupons could be substituted for T-shirts, sugar, or soap.

In a second village, mothers were reinforced for treating malnutrition appropriately and/or keeping their child within the normal band of growth. The reinforcer used was a Kodacolor print of the mother and child which was available one month following the time it was taken. This added an additional incentive to appear for the next month's appointment. The results indicated that while the two reinforcement conditions were equally effective, both were substantially more effective than a "usual care" control in preventing moderate malnutrition. The authors concluded that the long-term natural reinforcement of seeing a baby grow adequately through appropriate feeding may not be sufficiently powerful to override difficulties in breast feeding, childhood infections which cause feeding complications, and other natural barriers or punishers which occur on a frequent basis. They advocated the use of some form of external reinforcement when these types of complications are present.

The Relationship of Consequences and Chronic Pain

Chronic pain, such as chronic back pain, may be caused by a variety of factors including repetitious work, inappropriate stress on relatively weaker muscles, continual vibration, and other factors. However, subsequent "pain behaviors" may not be directly related to these causes.[5] For instance, positive consequences for the expression of pain include pain medication, the attention of others, and avoidance of work. Punishment of "healthy behavior" can occur simultaneously, such as when a relative or friend criticizes the patient for trying to engage in some activity and then does the activity him or herself. Therefore, strategies for changing pain behaviors emphasize both the reduction of pain behaviors and the acceleration of healthy behaviors. Techniques include teaching the members of the social support system to extinguish pain behaviors while reinforcing health-related activities. Medication is given on a fixed-time schedule rather than contingent on the expression of pain. Exercise is included as a differential reinforcement target. Rest and attention are also used as reinforcers.

Reinforcing Long-Term Behavior Change

Contingency contracts may be used for maintenance of behavior change as well as for the initial behavior change itself. Kramer and his colleagues worked with 72 women and 67 men between 130 percent and 150 percent of their ideal body weight.[6] Each of these individuals had to deposit $195 for subsequent incentives. One hundred and twenty dollars of this amount was used for the actual maintenance of weight loss. Participants forfeited $10 for each of ten follow-up discussion sessions they missed, and their total refund was withheld if they weighed more than pre-treatment weight. This financial incentive approach was not significantly different in terms of success in comparison to a standard skills training approach. Also, there was a large dropout rate for those in the financial incentive condition. However, this condition yielded the most promising results in terms of the total number of successful participants.

A Unique Approach to Weight Control. A good example of the use of the negative reinforcement (as well as stimulus control) of dieting behaviors is provided by a study in which individuals attempting to lose weight kept clear plastic bags filled with pork fat (which presumably was of an unappetizing or even disgusting visual quality) in the refrigerator. These individuals were then instructed to remove the bag equivalent to the amount of weight they lost contingent upon the actual loss of that weight.[7]

Feedback as a Consequence. Feedback may not only serve the same function as accelerating or decelerating consequences but also provides information about the target response. A form of feedback commonly used in behavioral treatment settings is biofeedback. **Biofeedback is providing physiological data to clients in order for them to monitor and change a physical or physiological condition.** Raynaud's disease is characterized by attacks of poor circulation to the hands or feet. These attacks are generally precipitated by a cold or emotional distress. Biofeedback for treating Raynaud's disease involves giving thermal feedback from the middle finger of the dominant hand. Such feedback allows the client to monitor the temperature of his or her fingers and use relaxation and other techniques to increase blood flow and thereby raise body temperature.[8]

Stimulus Control, Contingency Management, and Combined Procedures for Enhancing Participation in Treatment

Treatment compliance is of critical importance for effective clinic-based interventions and is a frequent target for health behavior change efforts. Conversely, noncompliance can usually be linked to behavioral causes, as well.

At times simple antecedent interventions such as prompts and advice can be sufficient to produce at least short-term, yet important, behavioral compliance. For instance, obstetric recommendations call for twenty-two to twenty-seven pounds of weight gain during pregnancy. Gaining less than this amount, or certainly gaining less than sixteen pounds, greatly increases the likelihood of adverse pregnancy outcomes. One study found that simple physician advice to gain at least twenty-two pounds resulted in substantial compliance with this advice. This advice may be especially effective for high-risk groups such as very young or less educated pregnant women.[9]

Physicians and other health care providers can be very important agents of promoting other types of behavior change in patients as well. It is estimated that persistent advice from physicians could yield smoking cessation in one out of every ten smokers, which would add substantially to cessation rates. As physician interventions become more intensive and their attempts become more frequent, cessation rates go up. Their effectiveness can also be augmented by self-help materials, cessation kits, nicotine gum, and other auxiliary interventions. However, physicians and their assistants often do not provide anti-smoking advice as they apparently feel unsuccessful in getting smokers to quit. We suggest physicians consider a 10 percent cessation rate as being very successful rather than something to be discouraged.[10]

Other studies have examined specifically what physicians can do to enhance compliance with recommendations such as smoking cessation. In one study, tape recordings of patient and doctor interactions were monitored to explore approaches for remediating noncompliance among patients. Tactics used by the physicians were generally as follows: medical threat, exchange of opinions in an indulgent atmosphere, authoritarian tactics (e.g., stressing the doctor's superior position and professional knowledge), medical information (i.e., giving the patient information concerning the treatment and the rationale for the regimen), withdrawal (reducing the physician's involvement in the case), trying to determine causes of noncompliance, and altering the regimen with which the patient had not complied.

While clinicians take the lead in clinic-based procedures, self-control processes further enhance their effectiveness. For example, self-monitoring is an important ingredient in clinic-based interventions. Whereas extensive self-monitoring can be effective in complementing or directly producing behavior change, self-monitoring assignments must be carefully tailored to the individual and must involve a minimal degree of difficulty and intrusiveness. For instance, Pierce and his colleagues found daily self-monitoring of blood pressure among hypertensive patients to be relatively ineffective.[11] Such an extensive self-monitoring assignment resulted in a large dropout rate among individuals assigned to this task, and many of the people asked to monitor their blood pressure did so only once or twice.

Participation and compliance problems may limit the effectiveness of screening efforts. For example, as we are as yet unable to prevent colon cancer, current colorectal cancer control efforts focus on the early detection of this problem. The testing of the stool for the presence of blood is one of the most common techniques used for colorectal cancer screening. However, participation in colorectal cancer screening is often quite low. Blalock and her colleagues identified two behaviors inhibited by various barriers to be overcome for individuals to participate in blood screening.[12] First, the agreement to participate must be obtained. Second, compliance with actual appointments and screening procedures must occur after the agreement to participate has been obtained. Barriers or punishers to obtain an agreement include embarrassment, distaste, worry, discomfort, inconvenience, problems with diet, and objections to the procedures. Similarly, embarrassment and worry were found to be the most significant predictors of noncompliance. Fecal occult blood screening efforts therefore must focus on methods to eliminate these punishers and reduce these barriers before full agreement and participation can be expected.

Compliance with prescribed drug treatment and general clinical assignments is often disappointingly low. Compliance drops off quickly soon after the treatment is initiated. Shelton and Levy[13] and Kulik and Carlino[14] propose approaching the compliance problem with the following strategies:

1. Ensure treatment assignments are presented with sufficient yet not overly technical detail.
2. Give skill training for medication use.
3. Reward compliance verbally or materially, if needed.
4. Begin with easy assignments and proceed to more difficult ones.
5. Give the patient take-home calendars, stickers, and other antecedent cues to prompt compliance.
6. Anticipate, minimize, and by all means address the negative effects of compliance.
7. Closely monitor compliance as frequently and with as many people as possible (e.g., by having a receptionist, nurse, and/or family member check on whether compliance is occurring).
8. Have the patient make an oral and written promise or commitment to comply with the treatment regimen. This should be witnessed by family or other members of the support network.

As noted in the final recommendation, sometimes a simple verbal commitment to engage in a behavior provides sufficient negative reinforcement for future compliance with that commitment. For instance, Kulik and Carlino[15] found that simply having physicians ask mothers, "Will you promise to give all the doses?" and getting their affirmative response was sufficient for them to comply with full treatment recommendations for their children suffering from otitis media (inner ear infection). These mothers complied significantly more than mothers who did not make such a commitment. Giving mothers a choice among types of antibiotics rather than simply telling them which type of antibiotic to use, in contrast, made no difference on ultimate compliance.

Altering both antecedents and prompts are more typical of applied interventions for increasing compliance than is using one of these components alone. For example, Friman and his colleagues demonstrated the effectiveness of a combination of mailed and telephone reminders (within five days and twenty-four hours, respectively) and reduced response requirement and increased compliance with appointments at a pediatric clinic.[16] The reduced response time in this case was the mailing of a parking pass needed to park in the clinic rather than having the parent come into the clinic after parking and going back to her or his car to put the permit in the car. This combined treatment package substantially increased the percentage of appointments kept in five different pediatric clinics.

Training

A final set of examples demonstrates how stimulus control, practice, and the use of consequences can be applied separately or as components of a "package" to help individuals acquire and refine various behavioral skills.

To decrease the potential for infant injury, for example, Matthews and her colleagues worked with one adult and three adolescent mothers of one-year-old infants in their homes.[17] The mothers were taught appropriate child proofing and given feedback on their efforts once attempts were made to make the home environment safer. Throughout the remainder of the intervention, each of the four mothers was given ongoing feedback on the safety of the home. "Time out"[18] in a playpen was also taught for unavoidable dangers. Essentially, mothers who needed to take an action to prevent a potential problem (e.g., child playing with a plug and an outlet) were taught to say "no," pick the child up, and put him or her in a playpen with soft toys until the child was quiet for five to ten seconds. The procedure was first modeled by the trainer, then the mother actually role-played putting the infant in time out and was given feedback on the accuracy and appropriateness of her technique. The total instruction time for each mother varied between one and two hours. The percentages of intervals in which the children were engaged in dangerous behavior were recorded in both baseline and intervention periods. These percentages were reduced dramatically for each of the four infants, and these reductions were maintained at a seven-month follow-up. (One child actually engaged in dangerous behaviors in 80 percent of the intervals recorded in one baseline observation session. This was reduced to nearly zero during the intervention period.) Mothers also reported a generalization of the management strategies to antisocial behavior as well (e.g., hitting, biting).

Periodontal disease is a major cause of tooth loss in adults over the age of thirty-five. The prevention of periodontal disease is largely dependent on the behavior of the individual, especially flossing. In a study by Dahlquist and Gil, a therapist used prompts, self-monitoring, plaque detection, and reinforcement for plaque reduction, as well as corrective feedback to improve flossing skills of four seven- to eleven-year-old children.[19] Parents were then trained to continue the reinforcement and feedback procedures to enhance the maintenance of flossing in their children. Three of the four subjects maintained low levels of plaque compared to baseline over the course of a four-month follow-up.

Modeling and vicarious reinforcement can be used to train "coping skills" such as those involved in anticipating and dealing with hospitalization for surgery. In one study, parents of children hospitalized for surgery were taught deep muscle relaxation and then learned how to prepare for stress, confront and handle a stressor, cope with their feelings of stress, and reinforce themselves for successful coping.[20] They viewed a videotape of the use of these skills by a parent and their children. The videotape first depicted puppets in a hospital setting. The text for this part of the tape was as follows:[21]

1. Preparing for Stress
   —(Nurse Puppet): "I will be bringing the medicine you need to take before your operation."
   —(Parent Puppet): "It's time for your medicine, honey. How can you get ready to have the medication?"
   —(Child Puppet): "Oh yeah—I know what I'll do. I'll make a plan to help me."
2. Confronting and Handling Stress
   —(Nurse Puppet): "It's time for your medication."
   —(Child Puppet): "I'll take a deep breath and relax. My plan is to close my eyes, hold still,

and think about the fun we had at my last birthday party or playing with my friends."
   —(Parent Puppet): "It's OK, I'm right here."
3. Coping with Feelings at Critical Moments
   —(Child Puppet): "I know it will be over real soon—it hurts but I'll be fine real soon. I'm thinking real hard about the fun I had before, and about _____ ."
4. Rewarding Things to Say
   —(Nurse Puppet): "That was great! You handled that well."
   —(Parent Puppet): "You really did!"
   —(Child Puppet): "Boy, I know just what to do whenever I feel afraid."

As can be seen, the puppets model preparation for an event, behavior during the event, and reinforcement afterwards. This technique was superior to other techniques which involved only the provision of information or anxiety reduction. Effectiveness was apparent in terms of the number of child behavior problems experienced by children, including physical problems without a known cause, sleeping difficulties, and acting-out.

Patients (especially in pediatric settings) must sometimes receive training to ensure they have the skills to comply with prescriptions. For instance, Blount and his colleagues used modeling and shaping to teach six- to fourteen-year-old children to swallow pills and capsules.[22] These children were initially shown a grab bag full of gift wrapped prizes and told they would have to swallow a training pill twice consecutively to get a prize. These prizes had been specifically tailored to the children based on interviews with the parents. Next, the therapist modeled placing a pill on the back of his tongue, keeping the tongue flat, taking water into the mouth, tilting the head back slightly and swallowing. The child then attempted to imitate this sequence. The therapist provided corrective feedback when the child was unsuccessful and praised the child when successful. When the child had swallowed correctly twice in a row, he or she was allowed to choose a prize and unwrap it. The therapist and patient repeated this sequence with five gradations of larger and larger pills or capsules. Not only was substantial success noted over baseline levels of ability to swallow pills, but the success was maintained over a three-month follow-up period.

In the past two decades, much of health promotion research in industrialized countries has emphasized the role of training and other techniques for the prevention of heart disease. Lovibond, et al., for example, worked with twenty-five Australian subjects in an eight-week behavioral treatment program.[23] They emphasized weight, blood pressure, and aerobic fitness in their group-based intervention, which consisted of the following procedures:

1. Regular assessment and feedback of coronary risk-factor status and overall risk. Participants received information on how their risk compared to others of their age and what their chances were of having a heart attack or other disease outcome within the next five years.

2. A detailed health education program on heart disease and risk factors. This component consisted of written material, lectures, and video material presented didactically to give the subjects a better understanding of heart disease risk factors.

3. Instructions in the development, maintenance, and modification of risk-related behaviors. Subjects were given specific information on behavior change principles in order to establish the general framework for their specific behavior change approaches.

4. Behavioral assessment. Patients and professionals cooperated in determining the frequency of various risk-related behaviors and the environmental conditions related to these behaviors.

5. Establishment of realistic short- and long-term goals. Specific behavior change (e.g., calorie reduction) and outcome (e.g., weight loss) goals were established on both a short- and long-term basis. This way, the participants knew generally where they were going (e.g., toward ideal body weight) and how they were going to get there on a week-by-week basis (e.g., through the loss of one and a half pounds per week). This approach essentially involved the use of shaping procedures, with the participant being fully aware of both the short- and long-term criteria.

6. Detailed information tailored to the individual's needs. With respect to the previously discussed goals, each participant was given information specifically on how to go about attaining these.

7. Training in a variety of self-management procedures aimed at facilitating self-control over dietary, stress, exercise, and drug behavior patterns. These procedures include self-monitoring of behaviors and environmental antecedents and consequences, stimulus control procedures aimed at narrowing and eliminating the range of stimuli listing undesirable behaviors, contingency management procedures aimed at strengthening desirable behaviors and weakening undesirable ones, and supervision by the therapist in the implementation of these procedures.

8. Objective measurement and regular feedback of changes in subject's coronary risk-factor status, overall risk, and projected risk. Participants were given specific physiological measures which were compared and contrasted with the daily self-monitoring they were collecting. These measures included the treadmill test, blood pressure measurement, and occasional serum cholesterol measurement.

This intensive intervention was compared to one which was relatively minimal. The group receiving this intensive behavioral intervention showed substantially more favorable blood pressure, weight, and aerobic capacity profiles at the end of treatment, maintenance, and four-year follow-up phases.

The use of behavioral training techniques to educate and motivate individuals in behavioral health skills has increasingly expanded both in areas of application and technology. For example, the "Learn Not To Burn" curriculum addresses the reaction skills of primary school students to fire.[24] The curriculum emphasizes fire safety behavior change identifying twenty-five behavioral objectives in the following categories: protection (when a fire occurs), prevention (before the fire occurs), and generalization to others. It involves the school, home, and community and integrates fire safety into existing subject areas. Included in the curriculum is an effort to increase awareness and understanding of fire safety and burn prevention, including the "drop and roll" method, the fact that clothing burns and does not protect, the survival behavior of crawling under the smoke, the necessity to develop an escape plan and to avoid excess rushing, and focusing on low-income groups and others at high risk for home fires. Also, general first aid knowledge is imparted. Curriculum and community-backed programs emphasizing these and similar approaches in the past have resulted in substantial savings of life and injury in communities as diverse as Memphis, Tennessee, and Rochester, New York.

Kirschenbaum and his colleagues noted that nearly all patients treated in hemodialysis units rely on trained staff to direct their treatment.[25] They therefore speculated that the enhancement of self-directed care by hemodialysis patients could save millions of health dollars while patients may derive emotional benefits from directing their own treatment. They began working toward this goal by first developing a behavioral observation system for defining and measuring self-directed treatment of hemodialysis. This behavioral checklist identified specific behaviors as those involved in preparation, checking vital signs, machine setup, treatment monitoring and cleanup. The nurse simply observed the patient going through the process of self-hemodialysis and checked whether or not the patient successfully completed each of the required steps.

After the baseline assessment, each patient was introduced to the rationale for the intervention. The nurse explained what the patient could gain from participating and talked about the benefits the patient could receive by taking care of his or her own treatment. Second, decision-making strategies were reviewed and a behavioral contract was established. This behavioral contract allowed the patient and staff to negotiate most of the key components of the treatment procedure and clarified expectations and consequences with respect to compliance with the procedures. Next, patients were taught why and how to self-monitor using the checklist described above, and finally, weekly meetings with the nurses were established to further promote and maintain patient problem-solving abilities and self-care effectiveness. Four elderly patients were exposed to this intervention by four different nurses. Three of the four experienced substantial improvements in their ability to conduct self-directed hemodialysis.

Although typical educational training approaches involve little if any opportunity for feedback and shaping to occur, variations of the Personalized System of Instruction (see chapter 7) have shown us what dramatic differences the use of shaping procedures can make in assisting students to acquire health or other academic knowledge. Recently, such educational shaping procedures have been applied to health promotion activities as well. For instance, Levenson and

Morrow used interactive video lessons on smokeless tobacco to orient young college students to the problems associated with smokeless tobacco and develop their knowledge and skills accordingly.[26] With the use of the interactive video, students saw segments of the video which were stopped with questions then being posed on a computer screen to ascertain the student's understanding of that segment. When incorrect answers were given by the student, the computer either repeated the question series, gave corrective feedback, or allowed the student to review the video segment that he or she did not totally understand. A control group simply saw the entire set of video segments and then responded to questions at the end without feedback. The interactive video group demonstrated the most accurate and comprehensive recall of the smokeless tobacco subject matter.

LIMITATIONS OF THE INDIVIDUAL APPROACH

As can be seen, individual behavior changes are the cornerstone of behavioral health promotion. Mastery of individual change techniques can be a valuable part of the armanentarium of the health promoter. Moreover, consumers' problems can at times be so complex as to require the intensive individual attention of a professional or other change agent.

On the other hand, the individual approach is severely limited for parallel reasons. Although it has been demonstrated that "clinically significant" change can be achieved at various times (i.e., an individual client's problems can be alleviated), others question whether such intensive professional efforts can indeed prove cost-effective. Relatedly, the public health significance of individual interventions can be seriously questioned. For example, if we work intensively with five severely overweight people on a one-to-one basis, we may get two or three of them to lose enough weight to improve their health substantially. However, let's assume each of these individuals was seen in a clinic for two hours per week over a period of four months to get them to lose the weight. In other words, ten hours a week of work (5 clients x 2 hours per week) were required to significantly improve the health of three people. At this rate, one professional could improve the health of thirty-six of these weight loss consumers per year on an individual basis with moderate to good rates of success. One could argue that this was a year's work well invested and, indeed, fairly successful. In general, however, such individual efforts will have little effect on public health.

SUMMARY

Individual-level health promotion extends the technologies of motivation and training to the clinic and community settings where one-to-one health promotion is appropriate. The contingency contract, formalizing commitments to change behavior, is a good vehicle for promoting individual change. Given its inherent inefficiency, however, the individual approach is of marginal relevance for public health. This limitation is less true of group and higher-level efforts.

ADDITIONAL READINGS

For those individuals seeking more help in this area, see:

F. Kanfer & A. Goldstein (Eds.). (1986). *Helping people change.* New York: Pergamon Press.

EXERCISE

1. A self-change activity: Using appropriate targeting and behavioral assessment techniques, you should set goals, select strategies, choose a monitoring system, develop a contingency contract, select an evaluation system, and graph your relevant data on a frequent basis.
2. In groups of three, take turns role-playing a change agent and one member of a couple (marital, friendship, etc.) coming to you for help in getting one of them to change a health behavior. Draft an appropriate contingency contract and present it to the class.

ENDNOTES

1. Self-control theorists, as well as Judeo-Christian philosophy, Anglo-Saxon legal tradition, etc., in contrast, assert that behavior is largely under the control of the person's thoughts and choices, with the environment playing a secondary role to this self-control.
2. The student should review the content of chapters 3 and 8 in order to master this section fully.
3. Stark, L. J., Collins, F. J., Osnes, R. G., & Stokes, T. (1986). Using healthy reinforcement and cuing to increase healthy snack food choices. *Journal of Applied Behavior Analysis, 19,* 367–377.
4. Fernandez, T. L., Estrera, N. O., Barba, C. V. C., Guthrie, H. A., & Guthrie, G. M. (1983). Reinforcing mothers for improving infants' diets with local available food. *Philippine Journal of Nutrition, 36,* 39–48.
5. Fordyce, W. E. (1976). *Behavioral methods for chronic pain and illness.* St. Louis: Mosby.
6. Kramer, F. M., Jeffery, R. W., Snell, M. K., & Forster, J. L. (1986). Maintenance of successful weight loss over one year: Effects of financial contracts for weight and maintenance or participation in skills training. *Behavior Therapy, 17,* 295–301.
7. Penick, S. B., Filion, R., Fox, S., & Stunkard, A. J. (1971). Behavior modification in the treatment of obesity. *Psychosomatic Medicine, 33,* 49–55.
8. Jobe, J., Sampson, J., Roberts, D., & Kelly, J. (1986). Comparison of behavioral treatments for Raynaud's disease. *Journal of Behavioral Medicine, 9*(1), 89–96.
9. Taffel, S. M. & Keppel, K. G. (1986). Advice about weight gain during pregnancy and actual weight gain. *American Journal of Public Health, 76*(12), 1396–1399.
10. Ockene, J. K. (1987). Physician-delivered interventions for smoking cessation: Strategies for increasing effectiveness. *Preventive Medicine, 16,* 723–737.
11. Pierce, J. P., Watson, D. S., Knights, S., Gliddon, T., Williams, S., & Watson, R. (1984). A controlled trial of health education in the physician's office. *Preventive Medicine, 13,* 185–194.
12. Blalock, S. J., DeVellis, B. M., & Sandler, R. S. (1987). Participation in fecal occult blood screening: A critical review. *Preventive Medicine, 16,* 9–18.
13. Shelton, J. & Levy, R. (1981). *Behavioral assignments and treatment compliance.* Champaign, IL: Research Press.
14. Kulik, J. & Carlino, P. (1987). The effect of verbal commitment and treatment choice on medication compliance in a pediatric setting. *Journal of Behavioral Medicine, 10*(4), 367–376.
15. Ibid.
16. Friman, P. C., Finney, J. W., Rapoff, M. A., & Christophersen, E. R. (1985). Improving pediatric

appointment keeping with reminders and reduced response requirement. *Journal of Applied Behavior Analysis, 18,* 315–321.

17. Matthews, J. R., Firman, P. C., Barone, V. J., Ross, L. V., & Christophersen, E. R. (1987). Decreasing dangerous infant behaviors through parent instruction. *Journal of Applied Behavior Analysis, 20,* 165–169.

18. An applied form of extinction where the child is removed from all potential environmental enforcers.

19. Dahlquist, L. M. & Gil, K. M. (1986). Using parents to maintain improved dental flossing skills in children. *Journal of Applied Behavior Analysis, 19,* 255–260.

20. Zastowny, T. R., Kirschenbaum, D. S., & Meng, A. L. (1986). Coping skills training for children: Effects on distress before, during, and after hospitalization for surgery. *Health Psychology, 5,* 231–247.

21. Ibid., 237–238.

22. Blount, R. L., Dahlquist, L. M., Baer, R. A., & Wuori, D. (1984). A brief, effective method for teaching children to swallow pills. *Journal of Applied Behavior Analysis, 17,* 260–270.

Medication is commonly prescribed in a liquid form. However, liquid medication yields less compliance than does medication in pill form, and not surprisingly, the error in the amount of medication consumed is considerably greater when patients are prescribed liquid as opposed to pill medication.

23. Lovibond, S., Birrell, P., & Langeluddecke, P. (1986). Changing coronary heart disease risk factor-status: The effects of three behavioral programs. *Journal of Behavioral Medicine, 9,* 415–438.

24. Donovan, M. K. (1987). Do nurses know and teach burn prevention and safety in practice? *Issues in Comprehensive Pediatric Nursing, 10,* 13–32.

25. Kirschenbaum, D. S., Sherman, J., & Penrod, J. D. (1987). Promoting self-directed hemodialysis: Measurement and cognitive-behavioral intervention. *Health Psychology, 6*(5), 373–385.

26. Levenson, P. M. & Morrow, J. R. (1987). Learner characteristics associated with responses to film and interactive lessons on smokeless tobacco. *Preventive Medicine, 16,* 52–62.

Chapter 13

Modifying the Health Behavior of Groups

OBJECTIVES

After reading this chapter, the reader should be able to:

1. Define group-level health promotion interventions.
2. Describe the importance of social networks in achieving successful group behavior change programs.
3. Give examples of each of the following methods that can be used for group health promotion: skills training, competition and cooperation, setting individual and group goals concurrently, using social support, enlisting a group member as the behavior change agent, and modeling.
4. Describe a situationally-based "social skills" conceptual scheme and give examples of social skills in the four types of situations.
5. Describe guidelines for videotape modeling programs.
6. Discuss the advantages and limitations of group health promotion interventions.

BACKGROUND

At the next level of intervention we consider working with multiple individuals simultaneously in groups. Why is group health promotion important? Considerations of both efficiency and effectiveness are relevant to this discussion. Clearly, working with twenty individuals in a weight loss group or worksite safety training class is more efficient than attempting to carry out these efforts on a one-to-one basis. Moreover, individuals are afforded many opportunities to learn from the success and failures of their co-members who can serve as live "coping models." Yet more important, perhaps, is the recognition that all of us are gregarious by nature. We are participants in our "social networks" which, among other things, are major sources of influence on health.

Social Networks and Health

An understanding of social network parameters can enhance the "diffusion" (i.e., generalization to others) and maintenance of health behavior change. Studies of social network structures and their influence on health behaviors from medical sociology, social psychology, and anthropology

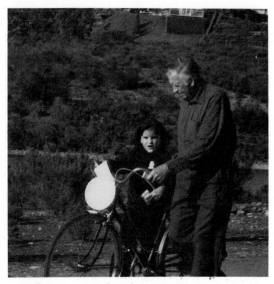

FIGURE 13–1. Through modeling and social support, interest and skills in physical activity is transmitted from grandparent to grandchild. *Photo courtesy of Betsy Clapp.*

have shown how these factors (such as frequency, degree of mutual acquaintance, supportiveness, or range of contacts between members) can moderate health care use, the transmission of health-related attitudes, and health-enhancing behaviors.[1] Social network factors have also been shown to have a direct influence on health status.[2] The technology for facilitating group health changes in social network structures and the feasibility of doing this on a large scale has therefore been advocated for clinical, worksite, and public health promotion.[3]

DEFINITION OF GROUP-LEVEL INTERVENTIONS

Group-level interventions are those which emphasize the interpersonal process, which is a material part of everyone's daily interactions with friends, relatives, and others as a part of the health promotion effort. Thus, such interventions may actually seek to modify this process directly through emphasizing interpersonal acceleration and deceleration of target behaviors, which in turn, generally lead to more adaptive functioning. For example, spouses may be taught to be less

critical of the other's excesses (e.g., alcohol and calorie consumption) and alternatively how to be more complimentary of behaviors incompatible with these problems (e.g., exercising). Second, group interventions may simply be used to target behaviors or outcomes of entire groups, thereby indirectly affecting the interpersonal process. For example, a teacher may decide to treat her entire class of seventh graders to a pizza party at the end of the semester if the entire group is not smoking. Assuming this reinforcer is of sufficient magnitude and that students were convinced that the carbon-monoxide breath test she was going to use was valid, beneficial peer pressure would hopefully develop whereby students discouraged smoking among one another, at least until the time of the party.

Group interventions are often conducted among friends or family members, but may be considered for virtually any collection of individuals. It should be noted, however, that not all interventions in group settings are "group interventions." For instance, a medication compliance group in which a clinician goes around a room asking her patients one-by-one whether they are having problems with their prescriptions would constitute a series of individual interventions, assuming that intragroup interactions were not encouraged. Failure to promote such group interaction, in turn, generally represents a missed opportunity for maximizing the potential for behavior change.

METHODS FOR GROUP HEALTH PROMOTION

Many of the techniques described for individual behavior change are equivalent to those used for groups, especially to the extent that individual acceleration, deceleration, and maintenance goals can be achieved in the group setting. However, groups can be perceived as both the environment for the individual change and an entity which itself can be changed through the efforts of various individuals within the group. Thus, reciprocal influences between individuals can act in such a way as to promote or discourage adaptive or maladaptive behavior. Such influences between individuals and their families and groups of friends can be especially powerful.[4]

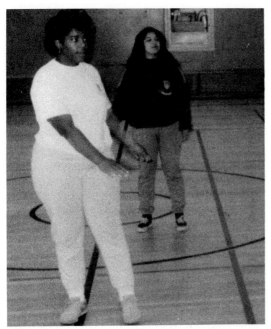

FIGURE 13–2. Exercise and other health behaviors may be more enjoyable (and more likely to be maintained) when done in groups of friends or neighbors. *Photo courtesy of Tere Aparicio.*

Social Skills Training

Gambrill studied the concept of **"interpersonal"** or **"social skills,"** those behaviors which persons engage in while interacting with members of their social network (or, on occasion, with casual acquaintances or strangers).[5] These behaviors can be categorized as "proactive" or "reactive," and occur in situations which are "pleasant" or "unpleasant." The following summarizes this conceptual scheme:

	BEHAVIOR	
	Proactive	Reactive
Pleasant		
Unpleasant		

(row labels on left margin: S I T U A T I O N)

A variety of general social skills can be applied in the "pleasant/proactive" category. For example, individuals may want to focus on how to give and solicit social support from important people in their lives. Teaching them to give compliments to others who have made health behavior changes or to request support from others in an effort to make behavior change may be important. For example, a man may say to his fiancee, "I really admire the way you've started swimming and doing other exercises this past year. I, too, want to make a change in my life. Would you help me lose weight by helping me choose restaurants with low-calorie options when we go out to eat?" This is an example of a statement which combines both giving and requesting support.

Most of us are reasonably good at reacting naturally to pleasant situations. However, at times people may negate compliments and other forms of support they receive, thereby making it less likely that they will continue to receive this support in the future. Adults who make fun of children's efforts to perform health-related homework (which includes getting the parent to be healthier) would also be an example of a failure to respond to a positive, health-promoting situation.

Frequently we find ourselves (or our clients) in the role of having to be assertive in rather unpleasant situations. It is relatively easy for health promoters to teach children how to request their parents to put on their safety belts while driving. Indeed, parents may not be the least bit negative about such a request and may even feel kindly disposed to the child making it. It is somewhat more difficult, however, to get a friend who has been drinking too much to turn the keys to his car over to you so you can drive home. A delicate combination of tactfulness and assertiveness is required in this type of situation. Finally, sitting in a no smoking section in a restaurant when someone at the next table lights up may call for a yet more assertive response. Again, it is important for people to not feel inhibited from responding assertively in such a situation, assuming they are acting within their own personal rights to do so.

The concept of responding to negative peer pressure is discussed in detail in chapters 16 and 20. However, it should be noted that this is perhaps a prime example of social skills which apply to the "unpleasant/reactive" category. Pressure exerted by friends and siblings to smoke, take drugs, or drink alcohol is perhaps the single leading factor in determining whether a child or adolescent will begin these unhealthy habits. Adults, however, can also be notoriously negative. Individuals working on making lifestyle changes in diet, exercise, or even smoking cessation must at times learn to respond to criticism from (supposed) friends and relatives for doing so. One author (JE), for instance, noted that while conducting worksite smoking cessation classes, individuals would leave the smoking cessation group only to be accosted by fellow workers who would offer them cigarettes and then light one up themselves in front of those trying to quit. Such inappropriate teasing must be ignored or at least responded to appropriately if the person's change efforts are to be successful. In other cases, men who use condoms may be berated by their friends for doing so. Mothers in developing countries seeking to leave the home for a day to have their children vaccinated or take a variety of other health protective measures must be prepared for the potential criticism from their mates who, in turn, inadvertently place barriers in the way of full health for their children. Health campaigns seeking to promote activities such as immunizations must take this negative situation into account and help prepare both parents for appropriate responses.

Competition and Cooperation

A responsible and skilled trainer is careful to promote the cooperation and mutual supportiveness of various group members attempting behavior change. Indeed, such cooperation can actually be reinforced directly by setting group goals and having groups go through the self-directed behavior change process in a parallel fashion to that described for individuals. When groups set their own goals, monitor their own data, and receive reinforcement only when group goals are met, members cooperate with one another to achieve the health promotion goals for everyone. Should the group members clearly desire the given outcome, it is possible that excessive pressure will be placed on one another to make sure the group goal is being met. Thus, it is the group leader's responsibility to ensure that such pressure is never more than mildly negative and does not lead to the attrition of one or more participants who feel

they cannot keep up the pace. A group member who prefers to walk and occasionally jog in an exercise group (and who is left behind or otherwise ignored for being slower) is more likely to drop out of that group than someone who is accompanied by a fellow group member who, although capable of running, is much more interested in everyone achieving a moderate level of success.

Competition can also provide a variety of potential benefits and problems. Classrooms competing with one another, in terms of the proportion of students with clean teeth every day, can generate a spirit of enthusiasm with respect to a competition whereby the classroom with the highest percentage of students with verified clean teeth wins a prize. However, suppose all classrooms made significant progress toward the goal of adequate dental hygiene throughout the course of the intervention. There is a danger that classrooms which did not receive the prize for best level of performance would feel punished for their efforts rather than motivated to try harder in the future. Therefore, the spirit of competition which contributes to cooperation can also lead to the feeling of being a "loser," and actually punish future attempts at health promotive behavior in the class. The health promoter should consider carefully whether such a danger exists in a group-based reinforcement program.

An Example of Competition

Competition can be applied to a variety of health issues and population ages. For instance, Swain and his colleagues developed a toothbrushing competition game whereby groups of students in two classes (first and second grade) in a public school were reinforced for adequate oral hygiene through winning prizes.[15] The effects of this competition showed dramatic increases in oral hygiene among all the students as measured by a disclosing tablet. Results were maintained nine months following the intervention.

Recent innovations in modeling include the use of videotape models. Clients can be shown videotapes of individuals or groups engaging in appropriate behavior and then prompted to imitate this appropriate behavior.

Integrate Individual and Group Goals

Self-help groups, health education classes, and a variety of other types of groups include individuals of varying needs and aspirations. Therefore, the person coordinating group activities should be careful to respond to these individuals' needs and not attempt to impose uniformity where it should not exist. The challenge to the health promoter working with groups is to take into account each individual's unique needs and goals and to address these adequately while getting individuals to contribute to overall group progress as well. Therefore, not everyone should be expected to contribute equally to "numbers of pounds lost" or similar group goals. One example of individual and group goals being concurrently considered would be for each individual to work on his or her own goals while groups are reinforced for percentage of individuals achieving goals. This not only engenders appropriate cooperation but also allows modeling of appropriate health behaviors and generalization from one skill area to another to take place among group members.

Social Support

For years, smoking cessation researchers have speculated about the importance of social support for quitting smoking, yet have been somewhat vague as to the specific mechanisms of social support which may assist the person trying to quit. In a study by Venters and his colleagues, the smoking behavior of the social contacts of smokers, former smokers, and people who never smoked were studied.[6] It was found that while the smokers (not surprisingly) had the largest proportion of other smokers as social contacts, ex-smokers resembled "never smokers" in having relatively few social contacts who smoked. The authors suggested that individuals trying to quit smoking should attempt to enlarge their number of nonsmoking social contacts which, in turn, should help them prevent relapse.

At times existing social support can be targeted for modification, but at other times "artificial" social support must be generated to ensure accomplishment of health promotion goals. In British Columbia, a group of health promoters developed a "breast feeding consultation" system whereby new mothers were assigned a breast-feeding consultant by the community's only hospital.[7] During these consultation visits at the mother's home, the visiting nurses inquired about any problems with breast feeding and offered advice on ways to increase the milk supply and address other problems. At their home visits, the consultant spent as much as two hours talking with the mothers about the condition of her breast, the baby's feeding habits, and other general problems. This consultant also observed the mother breast feeding and gave feedback on the breast feeding performance (e.g., positioning of the baby). She also provided instructions on latching, nipple care, hand expressing, and general lifestyle factors important to breast feeding (e.g., diet, rest, and family relationships). At the end of these home visits, each mother was given a card with a telephone answering service number for contact regarding any problems. Subsequent to this two-hour visit, the consultant made weekly phone calls to the mother with additional phone calls and home visits as necessary. Although the added effectiveness of this procedure was relatively modest, it provides a good example of how training and social supportiveness can be established in clinical settings and then extended to natural settings.

The health professional interested in engineering social support must be very careful to tailor the specific mechanism of social support to the health promotion problem being addressed. For example, Brownell and his colleagues studied weight loss among obese adolescents assigned to one of three groups: mother and adolescent together, mother and adolescent worked with separately, and adolescent alone.[8] They found that the superior approach was to work with both the mother and the adolescent separately. In this treatment condition, mothers and adolescents received social support for dealing with the sensitive aspects of their therapy from people having similar problems (i.e., other mothers with obese adolescents and other obese children). Apparently, working with mothers and children together on a jointly shared problem was too sensitive an issue to achieve maximal success.

While emphasizing the adaptive potential of peer groups, we must keep in mind that the "support" received from a peer group may often turn into peer pressure which, in turn, negatively reinforces maladaptive or destructive behavior. For instance, Kanin found that sexually aggressive male college students (i.e., those who had attempted rape) reported a relatively large amount of pressure from their peers in the form of stress to "score" with a female.[9] Those who reported less emphasis from their peers regarding this process were less aggressive sexually, as well.

The Family as the Target Group

In spite of the long-standing evidence that a child's car safety seat provides far greater protection for a young child riding in a car than no car seat or just a safety belt, parents were initially reluctant to use such car seats.[10] Perhaps this was due to the fact that children making a transition from no safety seat to a car safety seat expressed their displeasure in such a way as to make the car ride for everyone extremely unpleasant. Subsequently, however, it has been noted that children who "grew up" in child safety seats were actually better behaved during automobile trips than children who did not ride in child safety seats. Such indirect reinforcement of safety seat use increased the likelihood that parents would use such safety devices over and over again, as the natural and immediate reinforcer of improved child behavior supplanted the long-term and less concrete reinforcer of child protection.

Often health promotion combines family and other interventions to maximize treatment effectiveness. One example of this is in the design of curriculum for pre-school and school-age children suffering from asthma.[11] Six one-hour classes were conducted for either parents only or the child and parent together. These classes focused on breathing control skills (controlled intake and prolonged exhalation), body relaxation skills, bronchial hygiene and airway clearance skills, physical conditioning, and additional miscellaneous topics. The families in both skill training and control conditions kept records of the frequency and severity of asthma episodes. The skills training groups showed a relative decrease in the number of episodes but no change in severity of the episodes. The results suggest that skills training can be effective in reducing episodes and increasing skills, but record-keeping alone may be sufficient to orient the parents to the problem.

The Group Member as the Change Agent

Although many of us are accustomed to thinking of ourselves and other professionals as having the optimal skills necessary for facilitating health behavior change, recent efforts have emphasized the abilities of lay leaders in conducting their own groups. For example, Lando found lay facilitators to be as effective as highly trained facilitators in

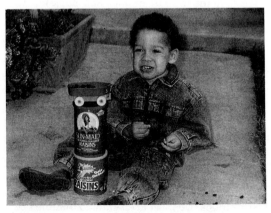
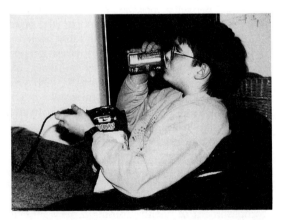

FIGURE 13–3. Nutritional habits—both good and bad—are learned at early ages, making the family an important health promotion target. *Photo "A" courtesy of Craig Molgaard, Photo "B" courtesy of Bill Powell.*

getting individuals to quit smoking.[12] These lay facilitators managed to get group participants to quit at a 40 percent abstinence level at twelve months, strongly verifying their ability to work in this area.

Peterson and her colleagues demonstrated that volunteers can be as effective (if not more) than professionals in accomplishing weight loss among participants of a weight loss clinic at a worksite.[13] These researchers used a "double endorsement" system to pick volunteers from among the group members to lead the weight loss group. This double endorsement system consisted of having the participants use a modified secret ballot to nominate a fellow participant in the group ("other-endorsement") to lead the group. Those who received the most endorsements *and* desired to lead the group ("self-endorsement") were recruited as change agents. This group did as well as a comparison group consisting of factory workers whose class was led by weight loss professionals.

Innovations in Group-Based Training

Gilchrist and Schinke described a group-based intervention model for developing sexual and contraceptive responsibility among adolescents.[14] Their general intervention outline consists of four steps, including provision of accurate information about human reproduction and sexuality; having the adolescents apply this information to themselves; having the adolescents acquire "affective, cognitive, and behavioral skills"; and having adolescents practice applying the information and skills to everyday situations. Group leaders used a variety of examples, role play and (as appropriate) humor to give the rationale and overview of the program. They then discussed future situations involving sexual behavior with the adolescents and demonstrated sexual and contraceptive self-management strategies. One of the strategies included "self-instruction" whereby the adolescents practiced repeating to themselves what to do in various sexually-related situations so that they would be able to think through the appropriate response when the situations actually occurred in the real world (see chapter 20). Generally, self-instruction began with the adolescents repeating the phrases out loud, eventually switching to a whisper and then to a subvocal repetition. This "shaping" procedure maximized the opportunity

for generalization of the skills to the actual situation. Gilchrist and Schinke taught such statements as "keep calm," "Stop! I need to think this all the way through," and self-reinforcement such as "I did great!" Role-play vignettes were developed to depict typical dating situations. Finally, contingency contracting was used to reinforce students for homework, such as discussing sexual abstinence with same-sex friends, obtaining contraceptive information from a vendor who sold contraceptives, or discussing birth control with parents or dating partners.

THE IMPORTANCE OF GROUP HEALTH PROMOTION

A variety of factors contribute to the potential effectiveness of group as compared to individually-based health promotion, especially from a public health perspective. First, maladaptive behavior and risk factors tend to "run in packs." If a child is using drugs, an adult is consuming excessive fat, or a young mother is not breast feeding, it can be assumed that the peers or relatives of these people are having similar health-related problems. Therefore, an identification of a person's appropriate social network and support group for concurrent interventions may extend the effectiveness of the intervention or health.

Additionally, of course, individuals have a greater opportunity to learn from the accomplishments and mistakes of their peers if they are attempting behavior change in group situations. They in turn can participate in teaching other members with methods shown to be effective in the two studies cited previously. In essence, training individuals to be health promoters can be much more effective if accomplished in a group situation. The generalization of behavior change from one behavior to another (e.g., from dieting to exercise), or from one person to another, as well as from the classroom or training situation to the "natural" situation, can be increased substantially through group-based health promotion.

LIMITATIONS OF GROUP-BASED HEALTH PROMOTION

Occasionally, working with a group, especially if a naturally-formed one (e.g., family), can backfire. Group participants who are not completely sold on the behavior change program may develop resentment toward it and sabotage the efforts of friends or relatives sincerely dedicated to the behavior change program. Group leaders must be carefully attuned to these potential pitfalls and be ready to deal with them. Although more cost-effective than individual approaches, group health promotion is not likely to result in true public health change. Programs for individual and group change should be developed only in the context of broader organizational, community, and policy interventions.

SUMMARY

The social network is the single most important feature of the environment in which individual health behavior occurs. Social skills training, competition and cooperation, and engineering social support are group-level interventions which take advantage of an individual's existing social network or change it in order to reinforce healthy behavior and promote its generalization to others.

EXERCISES

Take turns working in groups of five to ten people and pretend you are all participants in a smoking prevention, weight loss, or other group health program. Each individual in the group can take on certain roles, e.g., leader, recalcitrant participant, saboteur, person who tries to do too much, and exemplary role model. If possible, videotape the session, focusing on the group leader and his or her strengths and weaknesses in leading the group and responding to each individual's needs as well as the group's needs.

ENDNOTES

1. McKinley, J. (1976). Social network influences on morbid episodes and the career of help seeking. In L. Eisenbert & A. Kleinman (Eds.), *The relevance of social science for medicine* (Boston: D. Reidel, 1980); and Cobb, S. (1976).
2. Berkman, L. F. & Syme, L. (1979). Social networks, host resistance and mortality: A nine year follow-up of Alameda County residents. *American Journal of Epidemiology, 109,* 186–204.
3. Abrams, D. B., Elder, J. P., Carleton, R. A., Lasater, T. M., & Artz, L. M. (1986). Social learning principles for organizational health promotion: An integrated approach. In M. Cataldo & T. Coates (Eds.), *Health & Industry, A Behavioral Medicine Perspective.* New York: Wiley.
4. Ibid.
5. Gambrill, E. (1978). *Behavior modification.* San Francisco: Jossey-Bass.
6. Venters, M. H., Solberg, L. I., Kottke, T. E., Brekke, M., Pechacek, T. F., & Grimm, R. H. (1987). Smoking patterns among social contacts of smokers, ex-smokers, and never smokers: The doctors helping smokers study. *Preventive Medicine, 16,* 626–635.
7. Lynch, S. A., Koch, A. M., Hislop, T. G., & Coldman, A. J. (1986). Evaluating the effect of a breast-feeding consultant on the duration of breast-feeding. *Canadian Journal of Public Health, 77,* 190–195.
8. Brownell, K. D., Kelman, J. H., & Stunkard, A. J. (1983). Treatment of obese children with and without their mothers: Changing in weight and blood pressures. *Pediatrics, 71,* 515–523.
9. Kanin, E. (1967). Reference groups and sex conduct norm violations. *Sociological Quarterly, 8,* 495–504.
10. Christophersen, E. R. (1977). Children's behavior during automobile rides: Do car seats make a difference? *Pediatrics, 60,* 69–74.
11. Whitman, N., West, D., Brough, F. K., & Welch, M. (1985). A study of a self-care rehabilitation program in pediatric asthma. *Health Education Quarterly, 12,* 333–342.
12. Lando, H. A. (1987). Lay facilitators as effective smoking cessation counselors. *Addictive Behaviors, 12,* 69–72.
13. Peterson, G., Abrams, D. B., Elder, J. P., & Beaudin, P. A. (1985). Professional versus self-help weight loss at the worksite: The challenge of making a public impact. *Behavior Therapy, 16,* 213–222.
14. Gilchrist, L. & Schinke, S. (1986). Increasing sexual and contraceptive responsibility. In A. Stiffman & R. Feldman (Eds.), *Advances in adolescent mental health* (Vol. 2). Greenwich, CT: JAI Press.
15. Swain, J. J., Allard, G. B., & Holborn, S. W. (1982). The good toothbrushing game: A school-based dental hygiene program for increasing the toothbrushing effectiveness of children. *Journal of Applied Behavior Analysis, 15,* 171–176.

Chapter 14

Organizational Health Promotion

OBJECTIVES

By the end of this chapter the reader should be able to:

1. Define the following terms:
   - organizational interventions
   - Organizational Behavior Management (OBM)
   - PIP (performance improvement potential)
2. Compare two distinct types of organizational interventions.
3. Compare the ONPRIME model with the Pawtucket Heart Health organizational-level intervention model.
4. Categorize various organizational-based incentives in terms of types of behavior-consequence relationships.

INTRODUCTION

We now turn to a content area of health promotion that is one of the most popular and intensively studied today. Organizational health promotion is currently being advocated as one of the most effective and efficient approaches to changing the behavior of large numbers of people. The focus of organizational health promotion has been on any variety of health promotion efforts at the worksite. This emphasis accounts for as much as 80 percent of the literature in organizational health promotion. However, we are expanding the scope of the discussion of organizational health promotion to include two other aspects. First, we discuss members of any of a variety of non-worksite organizations and their potential for health promotion opportunities. For instance, members of various places of worship or other organizations with "voluntary affiliation" should be interested in seeing the health of their fellow members improve as well as their own.

From a different perspective, organizational health promotion can include the mobilization of employees to serve consumers better through health-related efforts. We also consider organizational behavior management (OBM) procedures which can be applied in health service organizations or agencies to maximize the effectiveness and productivity of health workers, volunteers, and other change agents. Indeed, many of these techniques overlap considerably with those directly promoting employee health.

DEFINITION OF ORGANIZATIONAL LEVEL INTERVENTIONS

Organizational interventions emphasize individual (and group) behavior in the context of membership or participation in an organization; e.g., an employee of a worksite or a member of a union, a member of a religious organization or club, or similar entity. (Organizations are smaller than communities, but generally larger than a group of relatives, friends, or colleagues.) Changes in the organizational environment may be undertaken separately or concurrently to affect the behavior of individuals and groups within the organization or the entire membership at once. Policy changes (e.g., prohibiting smoking), endorsements, and encouragement by gatekeepers (e.g., a pastor reading the names of participants in a church-sponsored exercise club), and organization-based feedback (e.g., monthly posting of lost time injuries at the employees' entrance to a mine) are typical of organizational interventions.

Organizational interventions may include the modification of health professionals' behavior for purposes of better serving the clientele or target population of a health clinic or agency. Incentives to improve the quality or quantity of service provided, other health agency management policies, and in-service training are examples of OBM procedures included in this category. Thus, organizational health promotion considers the entire organizational environment as an opportune target for change while concurrently considering efforts at the individual and group levels.

THE PROCESS OF ORGANIZATIONAL HEALTH PROMOTION

How do we access the members of organizations? How are "gatekeepers" best approached, and what health promotion roles should they play? How do we determine what health services to provide and where should we start? The focus of the ONPRIME model can be narrowed for an organizational context: organizing, needs assessment, priority-setting, and other procedures are carried out (with necessary modifications) just as they are in a community setting. One model similar to ONPRIME for addressing organizational health issues, developed by the Pawtucket Heart Health Program (PHHP),[1] was used to contact worksites, unions, churches, clubs, schools, and service organizations. Specific PHHP approaches to promoting health included individual and group behavior and OBM techniques.

The PHHP promotion effort begins with an assessment of the various organizations in the community. This general assessment examines such factors as what types of activities an organization is currently involved in, who the "gatekeepers" are in the organization, and whether these individuals are likely supporters of a health promotion effort. Second, the gatekeeper is contacted and the health program is explained to him or her. If the gatekeeper agrees that the health promotion activity would be valuable for the members of the organization, a general promotion consisting of social marketing efforts using in-house media is conducted, with members given general information about their health promotion options. Subsequently, an assessment of specific areas of health enhancement in which the members are interested is undertaken, as well as ideas regarding who among the members might be interested in forming a task force for coordinating and evaluating the health promotion program in that organization. This task force participates in setting goals for health behavior change, selecting various behavior change activities, and proposing environmental changes. Environmental changes might consist of any of a variety of strategies, including the installation of showers for those interested in exercising, increasing healthy food options at the worksite cafeteria, and changing the physical environment of the organization to facilitate healthy behavior or inhibit unhealthy behavior. Subsequently, the task force, as well as the professional health promoters, undertake an evaluation of the initial efforts and provide feedback to the members and gatekeeper regarding progress achieved. At this point, the task force may elect to continue present efforts or generalize the efforts to other individuals or areas of needs. This general approach was used by the PHHP to improve the heart health of members of worksites and religious congregations in Pawtucket, Rhode Island.

ORGANIZATIONAL BEHAVIOR MANAGEMENT (OBM)

Public health promotion involves more than changing the health-related behaviors of individuals or small groups of patients, clients, or other consumers. In order to have a public health impact which will ultimately result in large scale changes in health practices, behavioral scientists working in the health area need to think on much larger scales than typically represented in the behavior modification literature. The behavioral health promoter must therefore be familiar with two powerful techniques which could potentially alter the behavior of large numbers of individuals rather than one or two at a time. **Organizational Behavior Management (OBM) is one such set of techniques designed for changing the behavior of change agents, as well as employees. The change agents are typically employees or professional staff in the health care or health promotion setting (e.g., medical clinic, health department office, nonprofit health promotion agency). However, these techniques also apply to managing and supervising volunteers, students, or other individuals who may be seeking to prevent disease and promote health among other people.**

By "pyramiding" our efforts, we have the potential to reach far larger numbers of individuals, as represented in Figure 14–1.

Problems

A South American country recently embarked on a nationwide vaccination campaign with the goal of inoculating all "under fives" in the country against measles, tetanus, polio, and diphtheria. In spite of the provision of free vaccinations for individuals unable to afford them, attendance at the clinics providing the vaccinations was very low. Consultants were brought in to observe the vaccination process in various clinics and saw a variety of problems, including the fact that mestizo staff members frequently patronized, ignored, or at times even verbally abused their primarily Indian clientele. These consultants ultimately recommended that a certificate be developed to rein-

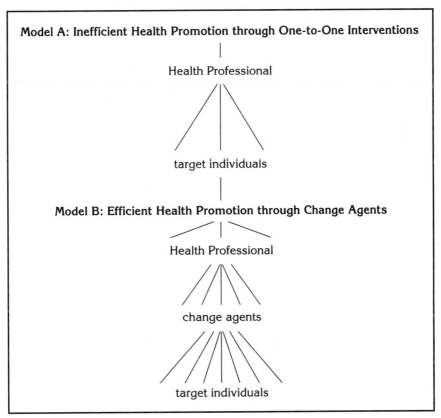

FIGURE 14–1. Inefficient and efficient models for large scale health promotion

force mothers for attendance at these clinics with the potential backup reinforcement system of a lottery whereby food, small transistor radios, or other reinforcers could be used to increase attendance.

A community in the U.S. received a federal grant for a community-wide heart disease prevention program. The stipulations of the grant were that the group of hospital workers receiving it would have to evaluate systematically the prevalence of risk factors in the community, and the incidence and prevalence of heart disease at baseline, and then again five years later. As the staff began to plan their intervention process, they frequently encountered disagreement among each other with respect to which direction to take to demonstrate a statistically significant improvement in heart disease incidence and prevalence. Several false starts preceded an eventual agreement on a plan, which was implemented some ten months behind schedule.

Both of the above cases are real-life examples of problems encountered in health promotion activities. Both contain mistakes by well-intentioned people. Are such mistakes avoidable? What can the public health professional do to contribute to the planning of programs such as the two mentioned above? For now, let's consider some dimensions of organizational behavior management, which represent the extension of behavior change principles to planning, managing, and evaluating the performance of change agents.

Before considering the application of OBM to health promotion, it's instructive to consider a few of its dimensions.

1. Systems Analysis.

Systems analysis is the study of an organization's activities in order to define its goals and purposes and to discover the operations and procedures for accomplishing these goals and purposes most efficiently.[2] Implicitly, systems analysis studies the behavior of two or more people with a common "purpose." Systems analysis, therefore, considers the input, process, and output of an organization. Inputs include capital, staff, clients/consumers, and other entities defining wholistically the structure and boundaries of the organization. The process is the conversion of these inputs into new behaviors (e.g., pain management technique in a behavioral medicine clinic, a class on automobile safety, and a

driver's education program at a public high school). Outputs are actual health changes.

2. Behavioral Leadership.

Previous models of organizational leadership emphasized the traits or characteristics of the leader and, in some cases, define those leadership traits most suited to a particular organization. In contrast, an OBM perspective emphasizes the specific functions of leaders or supervisors, including: (a) their use of educational objectives and task analysis as well as training or shaping techniques (chapter 9) to meet the needs of employees; (b) their use of reinforcement, emphasizing in this case results (or outcome) rather than process (or behaviors); (c) reinforcing groups of workers rather than reinforcing individuals, assuming the individuals in the group can contribute adequately to the group goals; and (d) using a "behavior analytic" approach to hiring and job placement, which involves developing criteria for optimal skill levels and assessing the skills of the applicant or employee with respect to these criteria. Professional credentials such as academic degrees or number of years experience would not necessarily be emphasized in such a hiring/placement scheme. In other words, OBM professionals are more interested in what individuals can do than in who they are.

In summary, OBM is the application of behavior change principles to organizational management.

3. Measuring and Improving Performance.

Gilbert discussed behavioral procedures for improving employee performance in terms of a particular numerical index termed the **"potential for improving performance," or "PIP."**[3] The PIP is simply the ratio of the performance of a typical or target worker to that of the best worker, or **"exemplar."** For example, the exemplar in a well-baby clinic may be able to average an 80 percent monthly return rate among the mothers she works with. The "typical" worker is able to achieve only a 40 percent return rate. Therefore, this worker's PIP is $80 \div 40$, or 2. Gilbert emphasized the need to focus on the potential for improvement and avoid punitive measures which may simply lead to a variety of undesirable side effects. He also noted several qualifications and recommendations including:

- The larger the PIP, the easier it is to improve performance. Therefore, we should not worry about workers who are at an initially low baseline, but simply whether their progress is satisfactory toward a level of performance similar to that of the exemplar.

- We should also note that the attainment by others of the criteria set by the exemplar may not be practical.
- More complex jobs will result in higher PIPs.

The use of the PIP is certainly not without implementation problems in OBM, but it does at least allow us to make several decisions to improve staff performance. Specifically, using the PIP or a similar system, we can come to some decisions regarding (1) what are we doing, why, and how well?; (2) whose performance is in greatest need of improvement?; and (3) why is the performance of the typical worker or an atypically poor worker less than that of the exemplar? Inadequate performance may be a function of (a) inadequate information, (b) a lack of good job models or inadequate past job analysis, (c) inadequate training opportunities, and/or (d) inadequate feedback and reinforcement procedures. Gilbert's PIP model therefore requires the application of appropriate behavioral assessment and intervention strategies for effective management.

Summary of OBM

In summary, OBM procedures are a more complex version of individual behavior change approaches discussed earlier (e.g., chapter 8). They involve (1) selecting a level of job performance or results as a goal; (2) breaking down the goal into steps or levels that can be met sequentially over a period of time; (3) selecting appropriate reinforcers for attaining goals or sub-goals; and (4) reinforcing and maintaining behavioral improvements or deriving and implementing alternative approaches to goal attainment.

Although OBM procedures are directly applicable to changing staff performance, they apply to general health promotion activities in other sectors, as well. Contacting gatekeepers, working on both individual and group programs within an overall organizational context, and making the organizational environment generally conducive to health behavior change are applicable both to staff performance and to individual health change efforts. Mastery of OBM techniques generally allows the health promoter to be more effective, either as a management consultant or as one trying to set up programs at worksites, places of worship, schools, or any number of organizational settings.

EXAMPLES OF IMPROVING STAFF PERFORMANCE

Modifying the Behavior of Health Service Staff

Elder and his colleagues conducted a series of studies designed to improve the performance of clinic workers in a comprehensive community mental health center in rural Appalachia.[4] A variety of problems with existing performance was noted, including inadequate and unreliable charting, the use of questionable or outdated treatment procedures, and reliance on a handful of workers to "carry the load" for the entire clinic. Given the staff's unreliable charting and that baseline data from charts are a prerequisite to determining appropriate intervention and evaluation procedures, it was decided to develop an OBM approach to improve the charting before attempting other interventions. First, systematic and simplified charting procedures were developed with specific steps prescribed for appropriate admissions statements, treatment plans, progress notes, and discharge plans. Staff were taught the information to include and not include in each document. Teams of four staff and a supervisor per team reviewed compliance with these procedures on a team-by-team basis, whereas the clinic director reviewed the progress of the entire team with its supervisor. These reviews were conducted on a weekly basis. Compliance with the appropriate charting procedures improved from 60 percent compliance at baseline to over 90 percent immediately after the intervention and six months later.

The data from this study demonstrated that these staff could be trained to chart reliably but still used clinical intervention procedures which were deemed inadequate, outmoded, or inappropriate. The management's major concern involved the heavy emphasis or dependence of the staff on psychiatric referral for treating "anxious" or "depressed" outpatients rather than using appropriate and current behavior therapy techniques for such treatment. Therefore, the staff were given intensive training on deep muscle relaxation and self-control procedures for anxiety and depression management and were asked to see each client for at least four sessions before referring for psychiatric evaluation.[5] During the intervention phase, staff were required by their supervisors to attend the four treatment sessions and develop a new treatment plan if they desired to make a referral for psychiatric consultation. Subsequently, this combined skills training and response cost procedure reduced referrals to psychiatrists and medications by approximately 30 percent.

CPR Training

Staff training is frequently used by behaviorally-oriented managers to enhance the skills of health workers. However, such training must be designed and implemented carefully. Despite widely available training, it has been questioned whether certified emergency medical technicians have mastered essential CPR skills. Previous studies suggest a need for more extensive practice, during and after training. Seaman and his colleagues compared a standard training approach to CPR with a behavioral training approach.[6] In the standard training, the instructor modeled the steps of CPR using a mannequin, after which trainees practiced on the mannequin and then received feedback from the instructor. In the behavioral training condition, the trainer continued to work with the trainees who had received standard training and offered feedback regarding each specific step of the CPR with respect to whether or not the trainee had performed it correctly (e.g., opened patient's airway, established breathlessness, ventilated patient, established pulse, activated EMS system). The trainer also used charts to present feedback publicly to each trainee. Trainees who received this additional behavioral training and feedback performed more effectively over the short- and long-term than those who received only the standard package.

Promoting Health Among Members of Organizations

Enhancing Worker Safety. Organizational Behavior Management can also be used to influence the health of individual workers in large industries where occupational safety and health is a major management priority. For instance, Ritschel and colleagues used an organizational behavioral approach to reduce accidents in a chemical plant.[7] "Protective poker" involved the use of incentives given to individual workers as a consequence of not having an injury serious enough to require the use of sick days. Using a modified lottery procedure (whereby cards were won for each period of noninjury, and a poker hand could eventually be developed to compete with other workers), ten workers and one supervisor per month were chosen as winners. Although this program had some weaknesses, eventually both the frequency and severity of injuries decreased.

A token economy using trading stamps as tokens was instituted at two dangerous open pit mines in Wyoming and Arizona.[8] Miners earned stamps for injury-free work time, for being in injury-free work groups, for not being involved in equipment-damaging incidents, for making safety recommendations, and for emitting specific behaviors that could prevent injury or accident. They also lost stamps if they were injured or others in their group were injured, caused equipment damage, or did not report accidents or injuries. This intervention resulted in large reductions in days lost from work due to injuries and the costs of accidents and injuries. And these improvements were maintained for more than ten years. Additionally, the union at one of the mines requested that the token economy system be written into the company-union contract. Improvements occurred in spite of the fact that workers had previously received intensive safety training during baseline years. The authors did note that this training could have been important as a precondition for the subsequent success of the intervention.

Economic Incentives. Warner and Murt described "economic mechanisms" such as taxes, insurance premiums, income incentives, and other incentives that employers and others have used to alter behavioral and environmental factors related to health at the worksite and elsewhere.[9] They classified health-related incentives as being direct or indirect. Direct incentives include "income enhancement or reduction" or "price changes." Indirect incentives include "changes in other opportunity costs" and "regulatory policies." Indirect incentives also include such things as provision of exercise facilities, time off, preferred parking, and reduction of barriers to health promotion. Incentives can be offered on a one-time-only or periodic basis. The motivation for providing incentives may vary among intervention agents. For instance, employers promoting smoking cessation clearly want to reduce employees' smoking behavior directly, whereas insurance companies reducing premiums for nonsmokers are seeking to market their policies more effectively. In contrast, increasing the cigarette excise tax is seldom, if ever, intended to discourage smoking, but instead generally to raise tax dollars.

A major incentive for employers to promote health promotion is to reduce costs for health benefits and increase productivity through reduction in sick time and inefficiency on the job. Employers generally have not been able to manipulate health benefits directly as this would have a severely deleterious effect on employee morale. Therefore, health promotion activities are undertaken to reduce expenses related to health care, disability and other insurance, worker compensation, absenteeism, and employee turnover. Warner and Murt concluded that prevention of alcoholism, cessation of smoking, and hypertension control, and exercise will generally have a positive economic benefit. However, most studies have not thoroughly evaluated the cost effectiveness of health promotion at the worksite. Prolongation of life through such successful health promotion efforts may actually tax the ability of some companies to provide pensions to their former employees. In any case, most health promotion programs are attractive to the employee and therefore important to employers.

Income incentives are used whereby employees are rewarded or punished for defined health actions. Incentives generally involve cash or in-kind income including vacations or consumer goods. They may be awarded to the individual or group and may be given in one lump sum or over a period of time. Whereas the use of positive reinforcement is more typical, certain employers such as fire departments have begun to refuse to employ smokers or others at high risk for illness based on the potential dangerousness of the work involved. Cash is a common incentive used to promote worksite smoking cessation. Employees at the Speedcol Corporation, for instance, received an extra $7.00 per week if they did not smoke on the job. After one month of this program, the percentage of employees smoking on the job fell from 67 percent to 43 percent, and four years later the percentage fell as low as 13 percent.[10] This ongoing periodic bonus was shown to be more effective than the one-time lump sum bonuses provided by other corporations.

Cash incentives have since been applied to exercise and weight control programs. Jeffery, Wing, and Stunkard compared the effectiveness of a $30.00, $150.00, and $300.00 bonus in motivating weight loss.[11] Although the larger bonuses resulted in more weight loss at post-treatment, differences were nonexistent one year following this intervention as all groups relapsed toward being overweight.

In 1977, the Mobil Oil Corporation developed a program whereby an annual bonus was paid to groups using employer-provided medical services below a certain target level. These bonuses averaged $55.00 for each employee belonging to one of the groups reinforced.[12] Blue Shield of California has developed the "health incentive plan" where employees are reinforced for keeping their medical expenses below $200 to $500. An employee can draw upon whatever money has not been spent by the end of a year.

Most of these programs have been used to change the behavior of individuals. Much still needs to be explored regarding the use of group contingencies to create peer pressure for changing group behavior. Two types of incentives can actually contribute to ill health or ill health behavior at the worksite.[13] First, disability insurance and early retirement provisions for disability may increase the likelihood of people making claims on this insurance. Second, certain employers (e.g., military, construction) pay higher wages for higher risk jobs. In a sense, this may be reinforcing people for risking their health.

Insurance and tax policies provide incentives for beneficial behavior change through altering prices of various practices or behaviors. For instance, the "risk rating of premiums" is a well-established practice in the insurance industry, whereby life insurance and other forms of insurance are priced based on characteristics of the person being insured (e.g., smoking status, medical history). Although such premiums may be insufficient to motivate people to quit, they do seem to be popular among nonsmokers and provide a useful marketing tool for companies. Also, more and more companies are reducing their insurance premiums for drivers of cars with passive safety belts and/or air bags.

Taxation can be used directly or indirectly to motivate health behavior. For instance, it is estimated that a 10 percent increase in the price of cigarettes would decrease total cigarette consumption by 4 percent.[14] Moreover, this same increase would result in a 14 percent reduction in the number of cigarettes for adolescents who smoke. Such excise taxes would at least offset some of the cost of health damaging behavior. In contrast, Wikler talks about "positive price incentives" which could subsidize relatively healthy or nutritious items (e.g., exercise equipment, fresh fruits and vegetables) or health programs (e.g., hot school lunches, free immunizations).[15]

Incentives for the employer also include a variety of categories of behavior-consequence relationships. For instance, Chadwick proposed that insurance companies offer preferred rates or premium reductions to worksites with relatively healthy indices on aggregate variables (e.g., percentage of workers who smoke, percentage of workers overweight, etc.).[16] Alternatively, insurance companies could reinforce employers for having health promotion programs such as aerobic exercise programs. Employers are currently receiving reinforcement for providing health insurance. Others have encouraged the taxing of waste created by factories, as this in turn harms an economy or health of the community surrounding the factory.[17]

Some have noted that the U.S. Government could save a substantial amount of tax revenues as well as reduce alcohol consumption by eliminating alcohol-related business entertainment as allowable deductible business expense. Mosher showed that this type of deduction has exceeded $8 billion, nearly 12 percent of the total amount expended on alcohol in this country.[18] He also argued that current policy encourages drinking and contributes to potential drinking problems. Occupational safety promoters, on the other hand, have few economic inducements available to promote compliance with laws. Whereas the potential to levy fines for employers ignoring occupational safety regulations, inspections from the U.S. Occupational Safety and Health Association (OSHA) result in few actual reports of violations with small fines per violation.[19] In other words, the cost of noncompliance is much less than the cost of compliance. Indirectly, however, regulations such as restricting employees' smoking in a worksite can result in extra barriers for employees who smoke and therefore potentially limit their smoking.

In using incentives to reduce undesirable health-related practices, we are often faced with the problem of not knowing exactly how to avoid antagonizing individuals who are already at healthy levels on this practice. One possible solution is provided by Rosen and Lichtenstein, who reported the results of a smoking control program at a small (thirty-one employee) ambulance company.[20] Employees were given a small financial bonus for every month they did not smoke on the job, regardless of whether or not they were initially smokers. Twelve of the sixteen employees who were smokers elected to participate in the program. This was not accompanied by any other smoking cessation program. At a one-year follow up, a third of the smokers were still reporting abstinence during the working period.

Appropriately implemented policy changes can be effective at promoting health promotion. The Group Health Cooperative of Puget Sound, Washington, for example, implemented a smoking prohibition policy for staff and patients in its thirty-five facilities.[21] This policy was implemented gradually in three stages over one year and was developed with the cooperation of smokers and nonsmokers. Results of an evaluation indicated that the vast majority of the employees approved of the decision to go smoke-free, and the overall rate of smoking decreased. Many staff also believed their work performance and that of their co-workers improved. The developers of this policy recommend that such policies be introduced gradually with provisions made to offer opportunities for those who disagree with the policies to express their disagreement.

Worksite Competitions. An example of the use of competitions at worksite settings were provided by Klesges and his colleagues in a competition among several banks in Fargo, North Dakota.[22] A standard smoking cessation clinic was offered to five different banks. Additionally, at a kickoff press conference the chief executive officers of four of these banks challenged one another to come up with the greatest reductions in percentage of smoking employees. Organization-wide prizes included $100 to the bank with the highest participation rate, $150 to the bank with the greatest success in reducing carbon monoxide (a trace element of smoking) among participants, and a $250 prize to the bank with the greatest reductions at a six-month follow-up. Also, a grand prize for the bank with the highest cessation rate included a catered meal served to all employees of the winning bank by the executives of the three losing banks. Individual prizes augmented the organizationally-based incentives. A comparison condition was held in the fifth bank where the clinic itself was offered. Results of the competition showed a mean 16 percent cessation rate for all smokers in the four competition banks compared to only a 7 percent reduction in smokers at the clinic-only bank.

Group competition has also been used success-fully to motivate individual weight loss. A study of the effects of weight loss competition was conducted to determine which type of competition in a worksite setting would be most effective.[23] This study compared competitions between teams versus one among individuals. The majority of the participants were blue-collar factory workers in a light manufacturing firm. For the inter-team competition, employees were randomly assigned to one of three teams with equal numbers of men and women. At an introductory meeting, participants' heights and weights were measured and a weight-loss goal was set for each individual, based on the midpoint of his or her ideal body weight. The maximum goal for each participant was twenty pounds over twelve weeks. To enter the program, each participant contributed $5.00 which was matched by the factory management. To increase program commitment, participants were weighed weekly in the cafeteria during their lunch hour. These employees were thereby able to see their teammates as well as opponents being weighed. Also, a poster with a large weight-loss thermometer, similar to that used by the United Way in providing feedback and reinforcement for annual contributions, was posted in the workplace that displayed each team's progress toward their overall cumulative goal on a weekly basis only. Team feedback was given rather than individual feedback in order to foster the team's spirit. At each weekly weigh in, participants received a one-page sheet of weight-loss instructions based

on behavioral principles, including stimulus control, self-monitoring, behavior change, and social support. It is noteworthy, however, that no formal program was conducted, nor were any professional weight-loss staff used in the competitions.

In the comparison condition, employees were recruited in the same manner and also contributed $5.00 to a pool matched by the management. However, the competition was carried out between individuals rather than teams. Participants who reached their goal weight received a full share of the winnings, and those who reached between 75 percent and 95 percent of their goal weight received a half share of the winnings. In other words, the fewer participants reaching goal or partial goal weight, the more money available to divide among those who reached their goal. Therefore, the only incentive was for competition, with no incentive for cooperation. As in the team-competition condition, participants were not aware of the weight change of the other participants. Although both types of competitions produced substantial weight loss and reasonably low attrition rates, the inter-team competitions did much better with regard to these two variables than did the individual competition. These results suggested that competition can be an effective means of attracting participants and promoting health promotion goals as well as maintaining participant interest in a weight loss program. However, team support in the context of competition was the critical contributor to the success of this group.

Recruitment of participants is, of course, at least as important as the actual effectiveness of worksite health promotion programs, at least if a broad-scale impact is desired. Interpersonal communication can be very effective in recruitment, whether using face-to-face or telephone methods. One study examined 119 smokers who stated on a questionnaire that they would be interested or very interested in quitting smoking.[24] Some members of this group were sent letters by the director of the quit smoking program and invited to the program, whereas other individuals received a phone call from a health educator inviting them to participate. None of the former group responded to the invitation, but 16 percent of those receiving a phone call did participate. Although neither of these results is very encouraging, they do underscore the importance of following through with interpersonal recruitment after an initial commitment to change health behavior is made.

LIMITATIONS OF ORGANIZATIONAL HEALTH PROMOTION

Organizational Health Promotion clearly offers us a myriad of opportunities for public health behavior change in worksites, churches, schools, and other settings. Working through the behavior of health service providers can be especially effective in rapidly multiplying the effectiveness of our change, whether these providers are professionals, paraprofessionals, or volunteers.

A variety of limitations are associated with organizational behavioral approaches to health promotion, however. One of these limitations involves determining who makes the decision on what behaviors will be changed in this type of intervention. In factories, for instance, are the particular behaviors targeted of special interest to the employees or are they simply chosen by management as a way to promote their public relations or to appease certain worker demands? In staff behavior change efforts, who decides how hard the staff should be working? To what extent do staff have a right to participate in goal-setting, and how is their input balanced against that of their supervisors? Who, in turn, monitors the supervisors' behavior to ensure they are being as effective as possible?

A final issue related to behavioral health promotion is reflected by the unevenness of the reviews of the examples presented in this chapter. The vast majority of organizational health promotion efforts have been conducted at worksites. This is probably due to the fact that many worksites can afford to pay for worker health promotion activities whereas churches, schools, and other public or nonprofit private organizations cannot. Does this mean we should not attempt to accomplish health promotion in these alternative sites? Perhaps more research is needed, both to determine the potential effectiveness of health promotion in alternative (i.e., non-worksite) organizational settings as well as to explore alternative methods of financing such efforts. Only through this type of approach can we ensure that not only workers but also dependent populations, homemakers, and others who are not easily reached

through worksite interventions can have equal access to health promotion programs.

SUMMARY

Organizational-level health promotion is conducted with individuals or groups in the context of their membership or participation in organizations such as worksites, churches, and schools. They also include modifying the behavior of health professionals or other change agents to provide better service to clients. Public health promotion in organizational settings may include each of the ON-PRIME steps, only within the organizational environment. Nevertheless, the full public health potential of a health promotion program can only be realized through community-level interventions, discussed in the next chapter.

ADDITIONAL READING

M. Cataldo & T. Coates (Eds.). (1986). *Health and industry*. New York: Wiley.

EXERCISES

1. Refer back to the vaccination campaign and heart health examples at the beginning of the chapter. How might OBM have improved these efforts?

2. While physicians during the Cold War felt that patient education on nuclear war and its medical and social consequences was important, very few actually provided education to their patients on this subject. It appeared that physicians were afraid of hurting the doctor-patient relationship by bringing up such anxiety-provoking issues. This natural punisher served to diminish a potentially socially important response.[25] What types of OBM procedures might be used to diminish these barriers? Which of these interventions are realistic?

3. Infections are a major problem for infants and toddlers in day-care or preschool settings. Among recommendations for preventing the onset or spread of infections in these settings are the following:[26]
   a. As often as possible, children should wash

their hands after blowing or wiping their nose. Nasal drip should be washed off the children and their toys.

b. Windows should be opened daily to dilute respired air with fresh air. Filters in central air conditioning or heater units should be changed frequently.

c. All surfaces touched during diapering should be washed twice daily, including the changing table, sink, faucets, soap dispenser, etc.

d. A regular diaper changing procedure should be used instead of the finger check approach.

e. Soiled diapers, washcloths, and tissues should be placed in a plastic-lined receptacle with a step opening lid.

f. Soiled clothing should be handled as little as possible and should be sent home in a plastic bag.

g. The changing surface should be covered with a paper towel provided on a roller at each change table. Of course, this paper should be changed after each toddler has been changed.

h. Infants, children, and adults all should wash their hands before handling any food items.

i. Staff should not be discouraged from taking an appropriate number of sick days.

Design an OBM intervention to promote compliance with some or all of these procedures.

ENDNOTES

1. Elder, J., McGraw, S., Abrams, D., Ferreira, A., Lasater, T., Longpre, N., Peterson, G., Schwertfeger, R., & Carleton, R. (1986). Organizational and community approaches to community-wide prevention of heart disease: The first two years of the Pawtucket Heart Health Program. *Preventive Medicine, 15,* 107–117.

2. Krapfl, J. & Gasparotto, G. (1982). Behavioral systems analysis. In L. Frederiksen (Ed.), *Handbook of organizational behavior management.* New York: Wiley.

3. Gilbert, T. F. (1978). *Human competence.* New York: McGraw-Hill.

4. Lovett, S., Bosmajiam, P., Frederiksen, L., & Elder, J. (1983). Monitoring professional service delivery: An organizational level intervention. *Behavior Therapy, 14,* 170–177; and Elder, J., Sundstrom, P., Brezinski, W., Calpin, J., Boggs, S., & Waldeck, J. (1983). An organizational behavioral approach to quality assurance in a community mental health center. *Journal of Organizational Behavior Management, 5*(3), 4, 19–35.

5. It should be noted that not only were psychiatric evaluations expensive, but also over 75 percent of all individuals being evaluated were eventually given psychotropic medications by the psychiatrist. This rate was deemed inappropriately high, given behavioral treatment alternatives available as well as problems inherent in prescription of tranquilizers, anti-depressants, and related drugs.

6. Seaman, J. E., Greene, B. F., & Watson-Perczel, M. (1986). A behavioral system for assessing and training cardiopulmonary resuscitation skills among emergency medical technicians. *Journal of Applied Behavior Analysis, 19,* 125–135.

7. Ritschel, E., Merman, R., Hall, R., Sigler, J., & Hopkins, B. (1976). *Personal safety program: A behavioral approach to industry safety.* Unpublished manuscript. In L. Frederiksen (Ed.), *Handbook of organizational behavior management.* New York: Wiley, 1982.

8. Fox, D. K., Hopkins, B. L., & Anger, W. K. (1987). The long-term effects of a token economy on safety performance in open pit mining. *Journal of Applied Behavior Analysis, 20,* 215–224.

9. Warner, K. E. & Murt, M. A. (1985). Economic incentives and health behavior. In J. Rosen & L. Solomon (Eds.), *Prevention in health psychology.* Hanover, NH: University Press of New England.

10. Ibid.

11. Jeffery, R. W., Wing, R. R., & Stunkard, A. J. (1976). Behavioral treatment of obesity: The state of the art. *Behavior Therapy, 9,* 189–199.

12. Fielding, J. (1979). Preventive medicine and the bottom line. *Journal of Occupational Medicine, 21,* 79–88.

13. Warner & Murt, Economic incentives and health behavior.

14. Lewit, E. M. & Coate, D. (1982). The potential for using excise taxes to reduce smoking. *Journal of Health Economics, 1,* 121–145.

15. Wikler, D. (1978). Coercive measures in health promotion: Can they be justified? *Health Education Monographs, 6,* 223–241.

16. Chadwick, J. (1982). Cost-effectiveness of health promotion at the worksite? In R. S. Parkinson & Associates (Ed.), *Managing health promotion in the workplace* (pp. 288–299). Palo Alto, CA: Mayfield.

17. Kneese, A. & Schultze, C. E. (1975). *Pollution, prices, and public policy*. Washington: Brookings Institution.

18. Mosher, J. F. (1983). Tax-deductible alcohol: An issue of public health policy and prevention strategy. *Journal of Health Politics, Policy, and Law, 7*, 855–887; and Mosher, J. F. (1982). Federal tax law and public health policy: The case of alcohol related tax expenditures. *Journal of Public Health Policy, 3*, 260–263.

19. Viscusi, W. K. (1983). *Risk by choice*. Cambridge, MA: Harvard University Press.

20. Rosen, G. M. & Lichtenstein, E. (1977). An employee incentive program to reduce cigarette smoking. *Journal of Consulting Psychology, 45*, 957.

21. Rosenstock, I. M., Stergachis, A., & Heaney, C. (1986). Evaluation of smoking prohibition policy in a health maintenance organization. *American Journal of Public Health, 76*, 1014–1015.

22. Klesges, R. C., Vassey, V. M., & Glasgow, R. E. (1986). A worksite smoking modification competition: Potential for public health impact. *American Journal of Public Health, 76*, 198–199.

23. Cohen, R. Y., Stunkard, A. J., & Felix, M. R. J. (1987). Comparison of three worksite weight loss competitions. *Journal of Behavior Medicine, 10*, 467–480.

24. Lowe, J., Windsor, R., & Post, K. L. (1987). Effectiveness of impersonal versus interpersonal methods to recruit employees into a worksite quit smoking program. *Addictive Behaviors, 12*, 281–284.

25. Cohen, D. A. (1987). Physicians' attitudes toward patient education on nuclear war. *Preventive Medicine, 16*, 837–842.

26. Keenan, K. & Holm, B. J. (1985). *Problems and prevention of infection for infants and toddlers in group care*. La Mesa, CA: Child Care Health Project.

Chapter 15

Community-Level Health Promotion

OBJECTIVES

By the end of this chapter, the reader should be able to:

1. Define "community-level intervention."
2. Describe
   a. Six guidelines for designing and implementing community interventions.
   b. Advantages and limitations of community-level work.
3. Critique examples of community-level programs according to six guidelines or criteria.

BACKGROUND

Behaviorists view the "community" as part of the environmental factors of interest in understanding and changing behavior, whereas social learning theorists emphasize the reciprocal nature of the interaction between person and environment. Just as individuals, groups, and organizations may show varying degrees of "self-control" (see previous sections), communities, too, may be guided through a variety of "community regulating" mechanisms.[1] The ultimate challenge for health promotion to become a *public* health technology lies in whether we can have an impact at the community level while simultaneously affecting change at the three subordinate levels: among individuals, groups, and organizations. Community-wide application of the four health promotion strategies underpinned with effective community organization will help us meet this challenge.

Definitions of Community-Level Interventions

Community-level interventions involve changes in the community's social and/or physical environment in such ways as to promote individual, group, and/or organizational health. These relatively remote interventions can have a direct influence on health or indirectly support more immediate interventions occurring concurrently at other levels. For example, a menu marking program in a popular restaurant may lead to the selection of relatively lower sodium and lower fat items by clientele eating there. Alternatively, it could be part of a larger multi-level intervention whereby

237

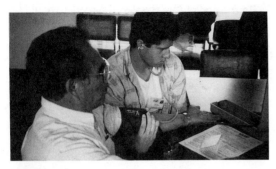
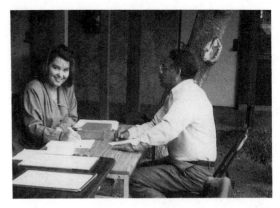

FIGURE 15-1.   As part of the community-level health promotion program of a primary care clinic, health educators provide counseling to a man who has just had his blood pressure and cholesterol checked. *Photos courtesy of Betsy Clapp.*

hypertensive patients in a community clinic, members of a running club, and participants in a church-sponsored cooking class are encouraged to select this restaurant and others citing the menu marking system. Community-level interventions typically involve working with key individuals and agencies whose status or function brings them into contact with large segments of the population (e.g., politicians, heads of inter-organizational committees, fire fighters and police, chambers of commerce). They may target cultural (e.g., the African-American "community" in Pittsburgh) or political (e.g., "Allegheny County") entities.

GUIDELINES FOR COMMUNITY HEALTH PROMOTION

Techniques

Attention to several specific guidelines and principles related to the development of community health promotion programs presented below can lead to a more favorable end result.[2] Although these techniques are represented throughout the ONPRIME (and especially the STEM) process (and expanded on in detail in the other chapters of this text), a brief summary is presented below, followed by examples of various community-level interventions.

1. Case-Control Assessment.   The case-control logic, a key element of epidemiology and public health research, is also crucial to planning effective community (and other) interventions. No one knows better how to deal with a community's problems than people in that community (or communities like it) themselves. The health professional must rein in the natural urge to prescribe a solution and instead find out (a) how this community addressed similar or other problems in the past; (b) what did and did not work and why; and (c) what other communities of similar size, geography, and socio-demographic characteristics have done in the past. Although this is only part of the needs and resources assessment (chapter 5), it will help us promote long-term community ownership of the program while avoiding stumbling around needlessly in search of something that works.

2. Community Compatibility.   Behavior change interventions must be compatible with existing community norms. Programs should be couched in local terms and language as much as possible. Professionals should be careful to adhere to specific local customs in implementing a given behavior change technique. The dissemination of behavior change through modeling and marketing should emphasize program adoption by local personalities rather than strangers.

An emphasis on the use of positive reinforcement will further serve to enhance the acceptability of behavioral procedures. Opportunities for the use of positive reinforcement should be the first consideration (see chapter 8). As much as possible, program goals should be phrased in terms of increases in target responses and outcomes (i.e.,

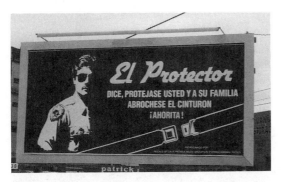

FIGURE 15–2. Whether it is social marketing or direct behavior change, community intervention approaches should always be compatible with the culture and language of the target population. *Photo courtesy of Betsy Clapp.*

"acceleration targets"). Determinations of appropriate reinforcers for such targets can then be made. When policies or other procedures use potentially unpleasant consequences, the health professional should solicit participation by those actually targeted by the program. The use of public commitments or monetary deposits may help people avoid losing "face" (or money) without engendering resentment toward the program.

3. Feedback, Shaping, and Fading. The effects of any intervention or behavioral procedure must be readily apparent to a community before widespread adoption of the procedure will take place. Through vicarious learning and other procedures, the early successes of the intervention must be continually fed back to the community in an easily understandable form. For instance, a simple chart on the evening news depicting a reduction in a "city's weight" (i.e., the cumulative weight loss in the various weight reduction programs) or in the number of smokers who have quit would provide the entire community information on how well it is doing and positive reinforcement for pro-health gains. Similarly, a target population should be gradually shaped toward a criterion through programs which initially offer minimally burdensome participation opportunities.

Fading offers the health professional the opportunity to reduce gradually his or her involvement in the community intervention and optimize the potential for long-term success. While professional involvement may initially be very intensive, indigenous change agents who rely on community resources should gradually come to the forefront.

4. Multi-Level Interventions. Procedures should be concurrently applicable to as many of the four levels of intervention as possible. A population can be taught ways in which each individual can contribute to an overall health goal by himself; as a member of a family; as a member of a church, school, or other organization; and as a member of the community at large. The technology of behavior change can be shared with all so that each may serve as his/her own change agent as well as a co-participant in larger scale applications. Mediators of health enhancement as well as the ultimate target population can be motivated by positive feedback and reinforcement.

5. The Interface between Scientific Evidence and Public Perceptions. Population-based efforts to prevent atherosclerotic coronary heart disease and stroke require a sequence of events. Credible scientific evidence for a causal role of a factor (e.g., smoking and heart disease) and the relative importance among factors must first be established. Then, the efficacy of changing such a

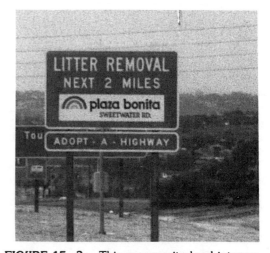

FIGURE 15–3. This community level intervention combines vicarious and direct positive reinforcement for promoting litter control. *Photo courtesy of Betsy Clapp.*

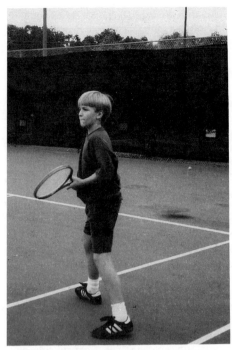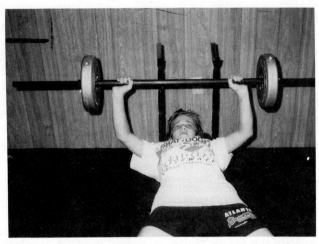

FIGURE 15-4. The field of health promotion often has to struggle to correct public misconceptions about health. Although weight-lifting and tennis may improve fitness through developing body tone and quickness, they may be less likely than other activities to improve cardiovascular health. *Photos courtesy of Tom Schmid.*

factor (e.g., lowering cholesterol levels to lower the number of heart attacks) should be established by clinical trials.

Although much remains to be learned, the scientific evidence for several risk factors and for the efficacy of change for coronary and cerebral vascular disease is well established. The public perceptions of relative importance and of change efficacy, however, differ in some key regards. These public perceptions should be recognized and addressed in any major health education effort, including applications of behavior modification described previously.

An example of the occasional difficulty in arriving at this interface between scientific knowledge and public perceptions is demonstrated in Table 15-1, which presents apparent rank orders of diverse risk factors for heart disease. As shown, the rank orders differ depending upon the importance of change.

For example, public preparedness to lose weight, manage stress, and gain the pleasures of regular exercise often lead to programs that em-

phasize these elements in initial activities. Later, addressing the important risk factors from a scientific perspective (changes in fat intake/cholesterol level, blood pressure control, and smoking) is advocated. An ongoing and active dialogue between health professionals on the one hand and representatives of the target population on the other, as well as the use of appropriate techniques, yields a balance between scientific information and public concerns. Equally important, however, is that scientists are able to listen to a community whose citizens may not equate standard of living to cholesterol change.

Finally, the populace must either initiate actions to improve its health or be persuaded that the specific risk factor(s) is of importance to them. Further, an agreement must be reached that the specific risk factor change is feasible as well as important. Health education efforts to influence individual, group, and population-wide behaviors need to transmit new knowledge, attitudes, and risk (reduction) related behaviors as the scientific evidence evolves.

6. Affordable Costs Related to "Acceptability."   Material, equipment, medical, and logistical procedures should be developed within the context of "appropriate technology" (i.e., within the technical, cultural, and economic realities of the target population). Behavioral technologies also should be sufficiently inexpensive to minimize restriction to public participation. For example, the use of lotteries with inexpensive reinforcers awarded on a periodic basis is preferable to reinforcing every person who meets a criterion with relatively more expensive reinforcers.

Volunteers, paraprofessionals, and other facilitators may be recruited and trained for various types of program operation. Existing agencies and programs which offer low-cost health promotion alternatives should be joined. When possible, screening and specific behavior change services should be provided free of cost or very inexpensively to consumers. At a minimum, healthier alternatives should be no more expensive than the behaviors they are meant to replace. For example, a "menu marking" effort for promoting healthy food choices in restaurants should also highlight items which cost no more than the greasier and saltier selections.

EXAMPLES OF COMMUNITY-LEVEL INTERVENTIONS

The Rockford Trash Man

In Rockford, Illinois, a special city-appointed "trash man" randomly selects addresses to inspect whether residents have sorted aluminum and paper from the rest of their garbage. If the lucky resident is chosen and has indeed piled "pure trash" separate from his or her bottles, cans, and newspapers, she or he will receive a weekly cash prize of $1,000. The prize increases $1,000 each week for every week it is not claimed. This has resulted in a doubling of the number of Rockford residents who have separated their trash as part of the city's campaign to promote recycling.

This environmental protection effort is very simple and straightforward, and yet has the potential for making an important and cost-effective impact. Most community health issues are somewhat more complicated, yet have solutions which may begin with simple steps such as the above. For example, incentives, feedback, and prompts have been used successfully to change electrical

TABLE 15–1
Scientific Knowledge and Importance of Public Perceptions of Cardiovascular Disease Risk Factors

Cardiovascular Disease Risk Factors	Scientific Evidence of Importance	Public Perception of Importance	Public Perception of Ease of Changes
Elevated Cholesterol	1	6	6
Smoking	2	4	5
High Blood Pressure	3	5	4
Obesity	4	2	2
Sedentariness	5	3	3
Stress	6	1	1

Note: Rank orders from 1 = top rank to 6 = bottom rank.
Adapted from J. Elder, M. Hovell, J. Lasater, B. Wells, & R. Carleton. (1985). Applications of behavior modification to community health education: The case of heart disease prevention. *Health Education Quarterly, 12,* 167.

energy consumption.[3] Transportation energy consumption was reduced through offering prizes for driving-mileage reductions[4] and through media-delivered feedback on the amount of gasoline consumed in a southwestern town.[5] Instructional technologies have been used to increase skills in community canvassing,[6] peer teaching,[7] and interracial communication.[8] The HEALTHCOM Project has blended social marketing and motivational strategies for dramatic increases in immunization rates and oral rehydration in underdeveloped countries. Increasingly, community change agents at all levels have emphasized the importance of behavior change techniques in promoting health and the quality of life.

Community Heart Disease Prevention

The best known community-level health promotion efforts in Western countries have focused on heart disease prevention. For example, the North Karelia Project in Finland provided a broad range of risk factor intervention services to their community.[9] Interventions were conducted at individual, group, organizational, and community levels. Individual and group interventions included semi-annual stop-smoking programs, instructional efforts to teach housewives how to reduce salt and dietary cholesterol in their food, and the enrollment of lay volunteers to provide health advice to members of their natural support networks. Community-level strategies included direct interventions with food producers and distributors, manipulation of economic incentives (e.g., a discount for low-fat milk), and a media campaign. Together, these efforts resulted in a reduction in heart disease morbidity and mortality in the target region. The Stanford Heart Disease Prevention Program used mass media campaigns, counseling for individuals at high risk, and other techniques in attempting to reduce heart disease in this pioneering American project.[10] The program was based on a combination of principles derived from macro-level communications theory and social learning theory, with special emphasis on print and broadcast media. The Minnesota Heart Health Program subsequently combined cardiovascular disease risk factor screening and counseling, smoking cessation contests, mass media, and other interventions to reduce heart disease risk in three Minnesota communities.[11]

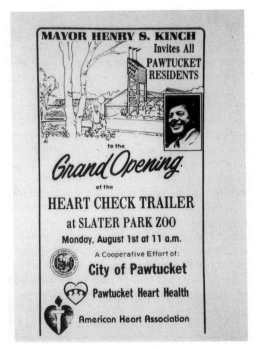

FIGURE 15–5. This newspaper ad announcing a forthcoming heart disease risk screening, counseling, and referral activity appeared in a Pawtucket newspaper. Issued by the mayor's office without prior knowledge of the Pawtucket Heart Health Program, it indicated the beginning of a sense of community ownership of the program. *Photo courtesy of Pawtucket HHP.*

The Pawtucket Heart Health Program (PHHP) initially approached the intervention city through local organizations and volunteer change agents to accomplish risk-factor behavior change in the population.[12] After eleven months, PHHP complemented its programs in organizations with activities open to all city residents, in order to accelerate participation by the target population. Seven months into this phase, it was decided that community activities should be the major focus of the intervention approach in order to assure a level of participation adequate to make a measurable impact. The PHHP smoking cessation efforts illustrate community-based behavior change programming.

As the initial emphasis of PHHP was on the development of risk factor programs within specific churches, worksites, and other organizations in the community, these organizations' members were offered smoking cessation clinics.[13] At the end of nine months of programming, however, only one organization had elected to begin a stop-smoking program. Given the community smoking prevalence of over 40 percent, it was decided that larger-scale interventions were required. Therefore, a communitywide campaign was mounted to recruit as many participants as possible into the "Up-in-Smoke" cessation program. A lottery was added to this program, with the reward contingency based on program attendance rather than cessation per se. Initially, 103 participants, including residents of neighboring communities, enrolled in three Up-in-Smoke lottery groups. At a three-month follow-up, only eleven smokers (7 percent) from the Up-in-Smoke lottery reported that they were not smoking (10 percent of those actually contacted).

For a variety of reasons, the "Quit and Win" approach was later adopted by the PHHP as the primary smoking intervention. Rather than reinforcing attendance, Quit and Win participants were rewarded for quitting through whatever method they chose. One month after the end of the contest, 20 percent of those contacted reported not smoking. The percentage of quitters for the Up-in-Smoke program increased, while the Quit and Win rate decreased over longer periods of follow-up. These and other data were compared with those of participants of a screening program conducted concurrently. Lotteries in general and face-to-face recruitment in large crowds (especially at the local "Octoberfest") were shown to be effective recruiting methods for large-scale smoking cessation programs.

Later, the PHHP conducted a two-month cholesterol education campaign called "Know Your Cholesterol."[14] During this campaign a series of screening, counseling, and referral events (SCORE) were held in the community, which included the then newly developed finger stick serum cholesterol measurement. People with high cholesterol were given immediate prescriptive dietary feedback and encouraged to obtain a second test in a doctor's office. At a two-month follow-up, over half of the one thousand participants who had high cholesterol had lowered their blood cholesterol by an average of 30 mm/dl.

A program developed in New Zealand called Waistline used behavioral, social, and community support to achieve weight loss in peer-led groups.[15] Waistline was one of the health promotion projects based in "community houses" in New Zealand, small neighborhood centers where citizens meet to determine their own health and social needs and work on them. Over 80 of these community houses in both rural and urban settings are currently in operation in New Zealand. The Waistline program developed as a result of the expressed needs of individuals in a variety of these houses. Components of the Waistline program include contracting, goal setting, self-monitoring, and actual behavior change reinforced by group support. Leaders are graduates of the program who are given some training and backup and receive a small payment for their group leadership efforts. The courses are advertised through local newspapers, often in columns which require no financial outlay. After depositing a $5.00 fee as part of the weight loss contract, individuals meet for eleven weekly sessions. Each session starts with a weigh-in and a review of the weekly summary forms. Topics for each of the sessions are as follows:

1. *Diet:* This is an outline of the primary dietary recommendations of the Waistline program, including a 1,000 calories a day consumption for women and 1,500 for men through the course of the weight loss effort.
2. *Diet Review:* Here, nutritional principles, record-keeping, calorie counting procedures, and meal planning are discussed.
3. *Exercise:* Principles of aerobic exercise and establishment of initial exercise goals are reviewed.
4. *Exercise Review:* The recording of exercising, the preference of aerobic versus calisthenic exercises, and other issues are reviewed.
5. *Planning Your Day:* Participants plan a day-by-day approach to eating and exercising.
6. *Keeping Positive 1:* Participants talk about coping with discouragement and high-risk times like holidays.
7. *Family for Better or Worse:* Participants discuss how families help or hinder ways to generate support and minimize problems with family members while losing weight.
8. *Dealing with Others:* Again, the social environment is discussed, this time targeting friends, workmates, and other nonfamily ac-

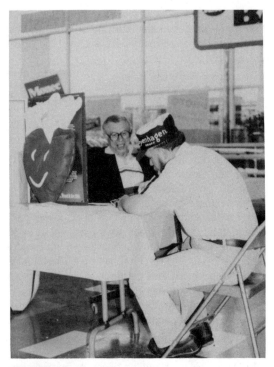

FIGURE 15–6. This retired dentist working with the Pawtucket Heart Health Program was one of many volunteers who assisted in blood pressure checks and other screening, counseling, and referral activities in grocery stores and elsewhere. *Photo courtesy of John Elder.*

quaintances with whom one interacts with frequently.

9. *Dinners and Parties:* Individuals plan in advance for high-risk situations.
10. *Keeping Positive 2:* Participants look ahead toward plateaus and consider weight control as a life-long process.
11. *Evaluation:* Participants are weighed in at the end of the last session and get their contract money returned if they have reached their goal. A party is held (with low-calorie food and some wine) and discussions of weight maintenance or further weight loss activities occur. An "after" Polaroid photo is taken of each participant for comparison with one taken before the initial weigh-in.

The Waistline program has several noteworthy advantages. First, the cost to the participant was only about $13.00 plus behavioral contract loss if applicable. This is approximately 20 percent of the cost of the Weight Watchers program in the United States. This lower cost is due to the fact that Waistline is a noncommercial enterprise run by its participants and lay leaders.

Second, while emphasizing group methods, Waistline identifies with its local community. The low attrition rate of 12 percent is remarkable and demonstrates that group leaders and group members were able to provide potential dropouts a substantial amount of support to keep them sufficiently encouraged to continue with the program.

Third, the Waistline program was integrated with other health promotion efforts occurring at these community houses. Specifically, dietary recommendations from Waistline focused not only on reduction of calories but also on reduction of dietary fat, increase in fiber, reduction of dietary sodium, and reduction of the use of additives in carcinogenic substances.

Fourth, Waistline uses a community "strength-building" philosophy which provides local people with a program they desire in which they can organize and lead in any way they want. Professional assistance is available but not imposed. Relatedly, this program has potential for widespread dissemination, given its low cost and reliance on community resources. Over the period of a year, the Waistline program resulted in an average weight loss of more than twelve pounds per participant, with nearly ten pounds lost per participant at a twelve-month follow-up.

An exemplar of community-based multiple risk-factor reduction programs for heart disease prevention is the County Health Improvement Program (CHIP) of Lycoming County Pennsylvania, which involved the mobilization of an entire community to improve its health.[16] This program focused specifically on cardiovascular disease in a north central rural Pennsylvania county of 118,000 individuals. It combined resources and efforts of the Pennsylvania Department of Health, Pennsylvania State University, and a social marketing firm. While similar to the Stanford Heart Disease Prevention Program and other community heart health programs, CHIP's budget was relatively modest compared to these federally funded efforts. As a result, community participation in program development with an almost total reliance on existing resources was of utmost importance in the CHIP effort.

Like the other heart health programs, CHIP targeted smoking, elevated serum cholesterol, hypertension, physical inactivity, obesity, and coronary-prone behavior for reductions in the intervention community. The CHIP program began with a meeting of the state's Secretary of Health, who was favorably impressed with the results of the previously mentioned North Karelia Project in Finland as well as various other projects in the United States, specifically in Pennsylvania. Although some external funding was received, the field staff never numbered more than four persons.

One of the first program planning and evaluation activities was the development of a community resource inventory. This inventory identified any institution which had at least 100 members and conceivably could be mobilized for health promotion purposes. A total of 157 different institutions of this nature were identified in Lycoming County, representing the following categories:

1. Health organizations.
2. Government offices (federal, state, and county).
3. Social service organizations.
4. Civic, service, and fraternal organizations.
5. Business and industry.
6. Unions.
7. Schools and colleges.
8. Religious organizations.
9. Professional and trade organizations.

This resource inventory identified key agencies to undertake the intervention and allowed researchers access to community data for determining the level of health promotion activities.

Five basic principles of community organization were followed in CHIP: community analysis, an integration of professional and local planning, consensus building, application of existing community resources, and the use of a community change agent. The community analysis consisted of activities such as developing a resource inventory and a baseline risk factor survey. Joint professional and local planning included a search for opinion leaders in the development of a steering committee which included the director of planning for the local hospital, newspaper editor, president of the local college, a bank president, an industry personnel manager, a Junior League member, a general manager of an industry, a bank vice-president, and others. Consensus building exercises resulted in group agreements and compromises. Existing community resources included the use of facilities and media at low or no cost. Media campaigns were both diffused and focused, with the former including efforts to reach large numbers of people in a relatively superficial manner, whereas the latter reached relatively smaller numbers of people with the hope of achieving more profound extensive change.

Media channels included newspaper, radio, TV, worksites, the health sector, schools, and various voluntary organizations. A television program introduced the program to the community in order to: (a) establish credibility, (b) increase knowledge about heart disease risk reduction, (c) alter health attitudes and behaviors in desired directions, and (d) provide information about specific CHIP activities.[17] Although mass media initially played a dominant role with respect to the first two objectives, it eventually focused more on providing information about specific activities and then assumed a subordinate role.

Worksite intervention became a major hallmark of the CHIP program, and involved the following fourteen steps:

1. Introduction of the program to top management through a letter and personal presentation.
2. Announcement of the program to the employees through company newsletters or personal letters sent to employees' homes.
3. Recruitment and organization of the corporate heart health committee, including both labor and management.
4. In-house communication planning using company newsletters and the later developments of a CHIP newsletter.
5. Perception and risk factor surveys measuring both interest and needs of the employees.
6. Formation of an intervention and evaluation subcommittee for each of the five risk factors.
7. Exploration of community risk factor reduction programs to determine existing resources that could be adapted and at what cost.
8. Community review and program selection by the risk-factor subcommittees and the overall health community (e.g., local doctors, nurses, etc.).

9. Development of a program proposal as a blueprint for future development.
10. Discussion of the proposal with management in order to enhance communication and obtain management support in the form of release time, financial assistance, and at least partial payment for various programs.
11. Promotional programs and recruitment of employees for each program.
12. Scheduling programs (based on the employee survey).
13. Program implementation.
14. Peer evaluation and feedback.

Programs ultimately selected were generally those in which (a) employees expressed interest, (b) were already available in the community, and (c) were easy to implement at the worksite. Two major strengths of the CHIP worksite program were in its inexpensiveness and feelings of ownership and empowerment it generated among employees. Additionally, worksite weight loss competitions, whereby various worksites challenged one another to lose the greatest total amount of weight, generated a substantial amount of enthusiasm among the various employees throughout the community.

In the CHIP program, health promotion through the health sector emphasized the involvement of physicians. Although physicians were initially reluctant to support the CHIP program, they gradually came to accept it and in some cases actively supported it. This activity was especially evidenced in their participation in the "go get squeezed" hypertension control effort, whereby individual physicians were given assistance in monitoring compliance with antihypertensive treatment. Other physicians also attempted to enhance their clinic-based smoking control efforts.

Due to limitations in resources, the CHIP program activated community schools later. However, school interventions occurred with little delay once activation occurred, as the school gatekeepers already knew a substantial amount about the CHIP program. Smoking prevention and weight control programs comprised the bulk of the school-based interventions.

Finally, voluntary organizations such as the American Heart Association and American Lung Association were used to enhance communication for increasing knowledge about heart disease risk, motivate people to participate in special events

sponsored by these organizations, expand the networking that occurred among the "voluntaries," and provide personal and material resources. While many of these volunteer organizations were active in the CHIP process, their membership turnover and perhaps preset agenda led them to be less instrumental in the overall CHIP system than had initially been anticipated.

Safety Promotion

Often, the relatively straightforward implementation of barriers for promoting health comes through the passage of legislation. For instance, the Poison Prevention Packaging Act of 1970 mandated child resistant safety caps for medication bottles. This resulted in a dramatic reduction in both aspirin ingestion overdoses among children as well as decreased mortality due to inappropriate medication ingestion by children.[18]

Although passive barriers and restraints can promote vehicular safety, drunken and other unsafe driving may require an active intervention on specific deceleration and acceleration targets (see chapters 18 and 19). For example, during the Thanksgiving holiday week of 1987, the San Diego police used a form of differential reinforcement to decrease irresponsible driving during this period. Whenever they saw a driver going out of his or her way to be courteous or safe (e.g., by stopping for a pedestrian, letting a car in from a merge ramp, maintaining safe distances for speed and driving conditions) and were able to do so, they pulled the car over and presented the surprised driver with a certificate for a free turkey at participating supermarkets. Unfortunately, the stress, anxiety, and inconvenience from being pulled over by a police officer made this program unpopular among numerous drivers. An alternative approach would be for police officers to record the license numbers of prize winners and then contact the vehicle owners later for prize delivery.[19]

Controlling excessive alcohol consumption (and subsequent drunken driving) need not emphasize punishment procedures. For example, unsupervised bars at parties allowing free access to liquor can lead to excessive consumption, as can the serving of liquor on trays by waiters or waitresses. In contrast, the use of bartenders or jiggers which limit the amount of liquor poured into each drink can serve to reduce the alcohol content of mixed drinks. Also, hosts and hostesses who make it clear beforehand that free chauffeur services or bedrooms are available for individuals too impaired to drive can eliminate the risk of injury or death from excessive alcohol consumption (see chapter 18). The discontinuation of serving alcohol an hour before the end of a party can also give individuals time to sober up, as well as providing coffee and other impairment-reducing beverages and foods.[20]

Promoting Healthier Dining-Out

Health promoters can either teach consumers to generalize their healthy behaviors from training to natural settings or directly intervene in the natural setting. Good examples of the latter are "point-of-purchase" interventions for promoting healthy nutrition. Stimulus control procedures can provide an effective method for influencing food choices at retail food outlets. For instance, Dubbert and her colleagues posted caloric information on various food items at cafeterias.[21] This labeling increased the probability that low calorie vegetables and salads would be selected, but not necessarily entrees. The authors concluded that preferences for meat and other entrees are probably more firmly established in a person's behavioral repertoire and are therefore more resistant to such minimal interventions. On an encouraging note, they pointed out that overall volume of food purchases (and implicitly profits) did not change due to their intervention. This could serve as a potential promotional concept for restaurant or cafeteria managers who might be concerned about the effects of health promotion efforts on overall profit.

A variety of factors should be considered when attempting to influence the selection of foods in restaurants and other points of food purchase. Colby and his colleagues at the Pawtucket Heart Health Program (PHHP) tested the effectiveness of three different messages: one promoting healthy foods, one promoting health as well as flavor, and a third nonspecific message as a control stimulus.[22] The results indicated that patrons of the restaurant selected healthy specials when the promotion emphasized flavor. For example, messages such as "tender chunks of light tuna tossed gently with fresh lemon juice and dressing team

up with a plump red tomato for a low-calorie, low-cholesterol choice" were preferred to health messages such as "for a low-calorie, low-cholesterol choice . . . tuna-stuffed tomato with a fresh garden salad."

Using the results of these findings, the PHHP subsequently developed a "Four Heart System" with each heart representing one of the following four aspects of a menu item: flavor, low fat, low cholesterol, and low sodium. Four small hearts were placed next to items on menus at a large number of restaurants to promote these specific items. Variations of this system were developed for supermarkets, as well. Participating food retailers, in turn, were given free promotion by the PHHP as a method of reinforcement. Also, they were provided the necessary paraphernalia including brochures, table tents, posters, and other materials explaining the menu-highlighting program. The emphasis was on minimizing barriers to participation by not requiring chefs to modify menu items but instead emphasizing existing items which were relatively healthy. Subsequently, restaurants developed their own innovations and variations, including incentive coupons for purchasing four heart meals and flyers prompting reduced use of condiments to maintain the low-fat, low-sodium content of a four heart meal. Finally, one of the pioneering restaurants in the four heart system conducted a heart healthy cooking demonstration.

Governments can also get involved in making restaurants healthier places to patronize. The Allentown (Pennsylvania) Bureau of Health sought to increase (a) the number of food service establishments with designated nonsmoking dining areas, (b) personnel trained in CPR and antichoking techniques, and (c) the employment of a certified food service manager to minimize problems with noncompliance with food sanitation codes.[23] When implementing interventions, food service establishments received an annual rebate of $25.00 to $75.00 on their licenses and operational fees. In spite of this small amount of monetary reinforcement, the number of food service establishments with designated smoking areas increased from fifteen to eighty-eight in the first ten months of the program. The number of establishments with certified employees for CPR and antichoking techniques increased from three to sixty-one, and those who employed a certified food service manager increased from fourteen to forty-three. Moreover, the incentive program attracted the attention of the print and broadcast media, and thus received broad-based political and public support.

Community Interventions for Child Survival

As shown in chapter 2, the mortality profile is much different in developing countries than in industrialized ones, with young children being the highest risk group in developing countries. Yet community interventions follow parallel principles and blueprints. In the winter of 1983–84, a large-scale, intensive immunization program was conducted in Delhi, India.[24] This program involved intensive community recruitment to optimize community participation. The emphasis was on using personnel for face-to-face communication with mothers in order to acquaint them with the program and convince them of its necessity. Also, posters portraying information about the diseases to be prevented with the immunizations and schedules of the immunizations were distributed, as immunization cards were prepared for all eligible children. Immunizations were provided at centers for preschool children to be easily within walking distance of all potential participants. Puppet shows with representations of children dying because of the parents' refusal to have them immunized and other shows where puppets represented five vaccine-preventable diseases also contributed to transferring information about the immunization program through school children to their parents.

In order to evaluate the impact of this intensive immunization program, researchers interviewed mothers who (a) had their children immunized before or during the program, (b) had their children partially immunized during the program, or (c) did not have their children immunized. Through a variety of questions regarding various barriers and punishers inhibiting immunization as well as reinforcers for immunization, the researchers recommended the following:

1. The initial focus of a communications campaign on immunization should be on conveying one simple message: children might die without appropriate immunization.
2. Shortly after the introduction of this basic message, mothers need to be informed about

where and when their children can be immunized.
3. Women who bring their children in for vaccination should be given further information about immunization (especially about follow-up).
4. Just after each immunization, the mothers have to be reminded that children need to receive all required doses or they are still susceptible to the diseases.
5. Interpersonal as well as other forms of communication can be effective forms of motivation. All forms of communication should be used simultaneously so mothers can receive multiple exposures to messages.
6. Communication should also target fathers, paternal grandmothers (an important source of familial power in the Hindu society), and older children (as targeted through the puppet shows).

Hubley discussed five general behavior change targets for increasing sanitation in the residential areas of developing countries, including motivation, construction, correct use, maintenance, and hygiene and health.[25] "Motivation" concerns overcoming an individual's reluctance to use shared latrines, as they dislike the notion of a common community use of this type of facility, they dislike the smell or flies, and are fearful of contact with other people's feces. Construction involves getting people to choose among various options for latrines and to participate in the building of them. Correct use means that security (especially for children) must be safeguarded and, if necessary, a method for noting when the latrine is in use should be developed. Maintenance involves minimizing the smell and dirt associated with latrines, checking the fly screens, and occasional repairs. Hygiene and health involves having hand-washing facilities near the latrine and ensuring that they are used appropriately. More general hygiene would involve personal cleanliness, food protection, and clean storage of drinking water. Finally, drinking water should be removed from a container with clean cups rather than allowing one's hands to touch the drinking water source.

LIMITATIONS OF COMMUNITY HEALTH PROMOTION

Clearly, interventions which simultaneously target the community environment as well as organizations, groups, and individuals, tend to influence the public's health far more than interventions targeting only one of these levels. Interventions which include large-scale involvement of the community are especially effective in promoting and maintaining public health.

Community-level interventions do have certain limitations. First, they can take more time to develop and implement than do organizational or individual interventions. A wider variety of key individuals and other actors needs to be included in the planning process which, of course, takes time and extra effort. Moreover, these individuals and the organizations they represent may have different and, at times, contradictory points of view as to which direction should be pursued. The community's residents may also disagree with public health "experts" as to what the community needs for its public health. For example, heart disease prevention is probably not a high priority concern in a community with a high crime rate or a high unemployment index. Priorities are usually set by people with excellent scientific credentials, and these priorities in turn determine which types of programs are funded for tax-supported grants. A grant coming from a federal agency, for example, can only address that agency's priorities and generally would not be sufficiently flexible to meet community needs which are not totally compatible with the grant's objectives. Such factors limit the potential for real community ownership of public health promotion efforts.

SUMMARY

Community-level interventions emphasize physical and social environmental changes which support health changes at subordinate levels. Guidelines for conducting community interventions include the use of case-control assessment, compatibility with existing norms, the use of feedback and fading, concurrent multilevel interventions, resolving differences between scientific evidence and public perceptions, and minimizing costs.

This concludes the presentation of the fundamental principles and techniques of public health promotion. Multilevel applications of ONPRIME to specific health issues are presented in subsequent chapters.

EXERCISE

Locate a detailed description of a community-level health promotion program which includes at least some evaluation data. Critique the program from the perspective presented in this chapter.

ENDNOTES

1. Meyers, A. W., Craighead, W. E., & Meyers, H. H. (1974). A behavioral-preventive approach to community mental health. *American Journal of Community Psychology, 2,* 75–85.
2. Elder, J., Hovell, M., Lasater, J., Wells, B., & Carleton, R. (1985). Applications of behavior modification to community health education: The case of heart disease prevention. *Health Education Quarterly, 12,* 151–168.
3. Palmer, M. H., Lloyd, M. E., & Lloyd, K. E. (1977). An experimental analysis of electricity conservation procedures. *Journal of Applied Behavior Analysis, 10,* 665–671.
4. Foxx, R. M. & Hake, D. F. (1977). Gasoline conservation: A procedure for measuring and reducing the driving of college students. *Journal of Applied Behavior Analysis, 10,* 61–74.
5. Rothstein, R. (1980). Television feedback used to modify gasoline consumption. *Behavior Therapy, 11,* 683–688.
6. Fawcett, S. B., Miller, H. H., & Braukmann, C. J. (1977). An evaluation of a training package for community canvassing behaviors. *Journal of Applied Behavior Analysis, 10,* 501–509.
7. Matthews, R. W. & Fawcett, S. B. (1979). Community-based Information system: An analysis of an agency referral program. *Journal of Community Psychology, 7,* 281–289.
8. Ivey, A. E. (1978). *Microcounseling innovations, interviewing, counseling, psychotherapy and psychoeducation* (2nd ed.). Springfield, IL: Charles C Thomas.
9. Puska, P., Tuomilehto, J., Salonen, J., et al. (1981). *Community control of cardiovascular diseases.* Copenhagen: World Health Organization.
10. Farquhar, J., Maccoby, N., Wood, P., Alexander, J., et al. (June, 1977). Community education for cardiovascular health. *Lancet,* 1192–1195.
11. Blackburn, H., Luepker, R., Kline, F., Bracht, N., Carlow, R., Jacobs, D., Mittlemark, M., Stouffer, L., & Taylor, H. (1985). The Minnesota Heart Health Program: A Research and Demonstration Project in Cardiovascular Disease Prevention. In J. Matarazzo, S. Weiss, J. Herd, N. Miller, & S. Weiss (Eds.), *Behavioral health: A handbook of health en-*

hancement and disease prevention (pp. 1171–1178). New York: Wiley.

12. Elder, J., McGraw, S., Abrams, D., Ferreira, A., Lasater, T., Longpre, N., Peterson, G., Schwertfeger, R., & Carleton, R. (1986). Organizational and community approaches to community-wide prevention of heart disease: The first two years of the Pawtucket Heart Health Program. *Preventive Medicine, 15,* 107–117.

13. Elder, J., McGraw, S., Rodrigues, A., Lasater, T., Ferreira, A., Kendall, L., Peterson, G., & Carleton, R. (1987). Evaluation of two community-wide smoking cessation contests. *Preventive Medicine, 16,* 221–234.

14. Lefebvre, R. C., Peterson, G. S., McGraw, S. A., Lasater, T. M., Sennett, L., Kendall, L., & Carleton, R. A. (1986). Community intervention to lower blood cholesterol: The "know your cholesterol" campaign in Pawtucket, Rhode Island. *Health Education Quarterly, 13,* 117–129.

15. Raeburn, J. M., & Atkinson, J. M. (1986). A low-cost community approach to weight control: Initial results from an evaluated trial. *Preventive Medicine, 15,* 391–402.

16. Stunkard, A. J., Felix, M. R. J., & Cohen, R. Y. (1985). Mobilizing a community to promote health: The Pennsylvania County Health Improvement Program (CHIP). In J. Rosen & L. Solomon (Eds.), *Prevention in health psychology.* Hanover, NH: University Press of New England.

17. Ibid.

18. Clarke, E. R. & Walton, W. W. (1979). Effective safety packaging on Aspirin ingestion by children. *Pediatrics, 63,* 687–693.

19. Rudd, R. & Geller, E. S. (1985). A university-based incentive program to increase safety belt use: Toward cost-effective institutionalization. *Journal of Applied Behavior Analysis, 18,* 214–226.

20. Geller, E. S. & Russ, N. W. (1986, February). *Drunk driving prevention: Knowing when to say when.* Paper presented at the SAE International Conference and Exposition, Detroit.

21. Dubbert, P. M., Johnson, W. G., Schlundt, D. G., & Montague, N. W. (1984). The influence of caloric information on cafeteria food choices. *Journal of Applied Behavior Analysis, 17,* 85–92.

22. Colby, J. J., Elder, J. P., Peterson, G., Knisley, P. M., & Carleton, R. (1987). Promoting a selection of healthy food through menu item description in a family-style restaurant. *American Journal of Preventive Medicine, 3,* 171–177.

23. Gurian, G. L. (1987). Promoting the community's health through a food service establishment incentive program. *American Journal of Preventive Medicine, 3*(1), 42–44.

24. Luther, S. (1984). *Immunizing more children: Towards greater community participation.* UNICEF: Regional Office for South Central Asia, New Delhi, India.

25. Hubley, J. (1987). Communication and health education planning for sanitation programmes. *Waterlines, 5,* 2–5.

Section IV:

Applications

Chapter 16

Taking on Tobacco

OBJECTIVES

By the end of this chapter, the reader should be able to:

1. Define the following terms:
   - market defense
   - market offense
   - market creation
2. Apply the ONPRIME model to the problem of tobacco use.
3. Generalize from strategies for tobacco control to those of addictive substances in general and other "illness industry" products.
4. State and justify a personal position regarding the ethics of aggressive anti-tobacco interventions.
5. Describe disadvantages of promoting smoking cessation from a public health perspective.
6. Describe major elements of effective prevention, media, policy, and activism approaches.

INTRODUCTION

And as for the vanities committed in this filthie custome, is it not both great vanitie and uncleanenesse, that at the table, a place of respect, of cleanenesse, of modestie, men should not be ashamed, to sit tossing of *Tobacco* pipes, and puffing of the smoke of *Tobacco* one to another, making the filthie smoke and stinke thereof, to exhale athwart the dishes, and infect the aire, when very often, men that abhorre it are at their repast? Surely smoke becomes a kitchin far better then a Dining chamber, and yet it makes a kitchen also oftentimes in the inward parts of men, soiling and infecting them, with an unctuous and oily kind of Soote as hath bene found in some great *Tobacco* takers, that after their death were opened.

—King James I of England
A Counterblaste to Tobacco
1604

In July, 1989, a researcher/anti-tobacco activist was busily taping the nationally telecast New Jersey Meadowlands Grand Prix auto race. This researcher was not interested in which cars were crossing the finish line, but instead wanted to find out the extent of advertising of tobacco—specifically, Marlboro—on this program. You may be thinking, "Wait a minute—advertising tobacco on television is illegal—this must be a mistake." It is true that the direct advertisement of cigarettes with fifteen or thirty second spots has been illegal for two decades. Cigarettes can no longer be sold like soap or cereal. But can the tobacco industry find a way around this law?

In the 93-minute broadcast of this race, a small raceway Marlboro ad was shown 4,998 times, and a large billboard advertising cigarettes was exposed to the TV viewing public 519 times. Cars with the Marlboro logo passed by the cameras 249 times. Jumpsuits, jackets and caps, trophies and other awards, and even television screen graphics all displayed the Marlboro insignia for a total of nearly **6,000** distinct exposures, or approximately one exposure per second. The Marlboro logo was visible for nearly 50 percent of the total viewing time.[1] And we thought we were getting the upper hand with the tobacco industry?

The scientific community had linked tobacco with deadly diseases at least three decades ago.[2] In the U.S., one of the world's major tobacco producing countries, this mutual acknowledgement led to the now landmark *1964 Surgeon General's Report*[3] about the dangers of tobacco and a warning to the public that their smoking habit was killing them. The decade following the release of this report witnessed a proliferation of smoking cessation programs for the increasing number of people (mostly upper class white males) who wanted to quit. At the same time, a small but growing outcry against the marketing of tobacco ensued, resulting in mass media anti-tobacco campaigns funded by private donations.

As with many other scientific and social developments against the tobacco-using practices of Americans, however, the tobacco industry successfully countered each anti-tobacco action with a variety of counter-control strategies. At the political level, they worked with friendly legislators from tobacco states and elsewhere to introduce mildly-worded legislation to limit tobacco advertising somewhat, with the agreement that anti-tobacco ads would also be limited. (As we can see

from the above example, it has proven to be easy to work around even these modest limitations.) At the marketing level, they introduced a variety of lower tar/lower nicotine implicitly "safe" cigarettes, suggesting that while perhaps the previous brands were a little harmful, the new products were not.

If we are to do anything about controlling the tobacco industry, we must come to grips with the sinister brilliance that goes into planning, implementing, and sustaining their marketing efforts. Robert Miles classified these strategies as market defense, market offense, and market creation.[4] Defensive strategies characterize the tobacco industry's tenacious grip on its turf, no matter the cost in human lives. **Market defense is the stand an organization or company makes to protect and advance their product and its legitimacy.** All tobacco companies cooperate in fighting tobacco control legislation and civil lawsuits which seek damages for permanent disabilities or deaths caused by smoking. The tobacco industry is represented almost everywhere, from the hallways of the U.S. Senate to small town meetings, whenever tobacco control statutes are being discussed. Industry representatives and their "front" organizations make campaign and civic contributions to help persuade lawmakers to vote on their side or at least abstain. For example, all but 8 of the 120 members of California's lawmakers have received campaign contributions from tobacco interests.[5] Phillip Morris has even gone so far as to "sponsor" the bicentennial of the U.S. Bill of Rights, with the not-so-subtle implication that tobacco is the "American Way," and killing oneself and others with this mass-scale drug addiction is not only a right, but a sociocultural mandate.

"Market Offense" refers to typical brand marketing that one sees in magazines and on billboards. This is the only one of these three strategies in which the different tobacco companies compete among themselves. Here we see very slick ads adorning our billboards and magazines, the marketing of new products for select subgroups of smokers, the use of discount coupons included with each cigarette pack, and a variety of other more traditional forms of advertising. At least ostensibly, the companies are competing for existing smokers' brand loyalties. Yet even this claim seems doubtful. The figures shown in the many Virginia Slims, Newport, and Winston ads depict healthy, young, and upper-income

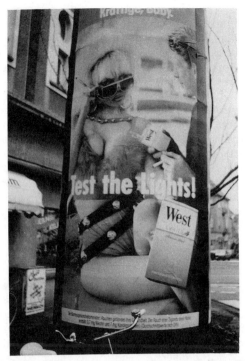

FIGURE 16–1. In Germany, as well as in the U.S., tobacco companies use sexual and other imagery to promote their deadly product. *Photo courtesy of John Elder.*

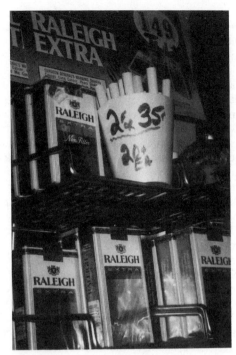

FIGURE 16–2. The sale of individual cigarettes, although illegal in most states, makes them more affordable for adolescents and harder to pass up for the individual smoker trying to quit. *Photo courtesy of Project T.R.U.S.T.*

smokers, hardly typical of this group. And how many people over twelve years of age really relate to the infamous "Smooth Character" cartoon representing Camel?

Market creation is the promotion of a product to a new market, such as minorities, a new state, or a new country. The "creation" of new markets receives the tobacco industry's greatest attention these days. In order to survive well into the next century, the industry is promoting two types of "generalization"—other products and other potential tobacco markets. For example, R. J. Reynolds owns Nabisco Company and supports all their food products.

In the market creation category, the industry has made concerted efforts to target minority groups in the U.S. (The Camel "smooth character" is readily recognized as *el tipo suave* in Latino communities.) Also, the industry has been one of America's most successful in marketing its product abroad, especially in underdeveloped countries. Tobacco traditionally has been included

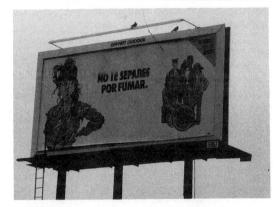

FIGURE 16–3. A part of their "Right Decisions—Right Now" campaign purportedly to combat smoking among youth, R.J.R. Nabisco produced this Spanish language billboard. However, the message ("Don't stand apart to smoke") seems to suggest instead that teens should not feel that they can't smoke among their non-smoking friends. *Photo courtesy of Betsy Clapp.*

in "Food for Peace" and other aid programs, where the federal government buys surplus agricultural products and donates them to the starving peoples of the world (apparently, smoking will help control hunger pangs). Not satisfied with this bilateral humanitarian approach, the industry has "barnstormed" through Africa, Asia, and Latin America, where fewer advertising regulations and lower or no sales taxes make it easy to introduce new products.[6] In countries where people can expect to barely reach the age of fifty-five, smoking may soon become the #1 killer. Meanwhile, America sends money, arms, and troops to cocaine-producing countries to destroy drugs that cause less damage than those which we sell.

These skillful defensive, offensive, and creative strategies masked societal anti-tobacco efforts, leaving cessation as the prominent tobacco control approach until the mid 1970s. Nevertheless, Americans grudgingly and gradually began giving up the habit, either through successfully quitting or by getting lung cancer, emphysema, or smoking related heart disease. Yet the struggle continues. Let's examine the state-of-the-art in tobacco control with reference to the ONPRIME model, while not losing sight of the industry's perspective. Recall from chapter 1 that ONPRIME is an acronym for Organizing, Needs/resources, assessment, Priority setting, Research, Interventions, Monitoring, and Evaluation. How do we counter their market defense, offense, and creative strategies?

ORGANIZING AGAINST TOBACCO

Early attempts at tobacco control emphasized educating the public to the health risks involved in its use and encouraging smokers to quit. The annual Great American Smoke Out (adopted by many other countries, such as "No Smoking Day" in the U.K.) is an example of this rather basic, upbeat message: "Let's all quit for a day and prove to ourselves that we can quit permanently." Later, cessation and prevention programs gradually came to include more advanced **skills training** and **motivational** strategies, while community programs such as the Stanford Heart Disease Prevention Project promoted these efforts through **social marketing.** Yet few of these approaches addressed the freedom enjoyed by the tobacco industry to continue to exploit the public. This

license to push drugs legally, both domestically and abroad, finds its historical parallel in the Opium Wars a century ago, when the imperial force of Great Britain compelled the Chinese to buy opium (and even demanded Hong Kong as a concession for their initial refusal).

The 1980s witnessed the development of a somewhat less conservative approach to tobacco control, partly in recognition of the fact that while smoking rates were coming down in Western populations as a whole, the decrease was unacceptably gradual, especially among certain subgroups (e.g., those of lower socioeconomic status). Community and organization-wide programs were subsequently developed, as exemplified by the Minnesota and Pawtucket Heart Health Programs.[7] These community-wide programs recognized that very few adults use formal cessation programs to improve their chances of quitting, but instead generally "quit on their own," if at all. Therefore, incentives to accelerate this process were used in "Quit and Win" and similar lottery-based efforts. At the same time, prevention programs based on earlier refusal skills efforts continued to proliferate and were adopted and implemented by entire school systems. Nevertheless, the domestic and international marketing of tobacco products continued relatively undiminished with laissez-faire governmental policies coinciding with the pro-business governments of the U.S., U.K., Germany, and elsewhere. In other words, the freedom of the tobacco industry to promote its product continued unabated, while public health and tobacco control efforts were spotty, at best.

The 1980s witnessed an awakening of societal forces which sought to reimpose restrictions on the tobacco industry and promote smoke-free societies more aggressively. During this decade, 500 ordinances restricting smoking in restaurants, stores, and workplaces were passed in the U.S.[8] A major notch on the anti-tobacco gun was carved in 1987 with the smoking ban on domestic airline flights. In Scandinavian countries, the concept of the smoke-free class of 2000 was promoted in an attempt to rid these nations of the tobacco epidemic by the turn of the century. Other nations, as well, are interpreting "Health for All by the Year 2000" as equivalent to "Freedom from Tobacco by the Year 2000." In the U.S., groups such as Doctors Ought to Care (DOC), The Advocacy Institute, Americans for Non-Smokers' Rights, and

Stop Teenage Addiction to Tobacco (STAT) coordinated anti-tobacco activities nationwide while supporting or even enjoining lawsuits against tobacco companies by plaintiffs or their representatives who were seriously ill or had died from tobacco use. Although somewhat more difficult to coordinate, these groups also joined in the international outcry against U.S. policies which promoted the sale of tobacco products abroad, especially in underdeveloped countries.

Local community organization activities hold even greater promise for immediate anti-tobacco successes. For years, students at Niles North High School in Skokie, Illinois, have not been allowed to smoke on school grounds. However, the fact that faculty could smoke flew in the face of their own policies and educational efforts to prevent tobacco use among students, and it took a student effort to point out this hypocrisy. Students collected 1,600 signatures on a petition to ban smoking in the faculty lounge (which primarily was a hiding place for teachers who wanted a cigarette). They wrote numerous editorials about this issue and presented their petition to the school board. The board voted 6–0 to impose the ban. A school staff member complained, "I don't think it's a good idea for the kids to think they took something away from us. They're not 21." A student countered, "It's difficult for students to feel like they're part of decision-making, and this is a nice feeling."[9]

In spite of all cessation, prevention, and societal-level initiatives, Western countries, and especially the U.S., still comprise "tobacco cultures." In the U.S., billboards and magazines are dominated by the Marlboro Man, the Camel "Smooth Character" and their friends, while insidious presentations of ads frequently appear in the background of Hollywood movies and other popular media. Adults and youth alike have ready access to cigarettes through sales from vending machines, convenience stores, and nearly every other conceivable retail outlet. (A recent study in eighteen U.S. communities showed that an average of 50 percent of youth under the legal age to purchase cigarettes were nevertheless successful at doing so.) Although cigarettes remain inexpensive, many retailers sell them singly (and illegally) for the convenience of those who do not have enough disposable income to purchase an entire pack, or those trying to quit and want "just one more." In spite of their relative inexpensiveness

and the salutary public health effect of increasing taxes, tobacco taxes are seldom increased in the U.S. or by its constituent states, and cigarettes remain affordable to the bulk of the population.

Proposition 99 and Assembly Bill 75: The California Experience

In California, voters realized that strong, government-sponsored anti-tobacco efforts were unlikely, given that the tobacco industry is a major contributor to nearly every legislator's and government executive's campaign fund. Therefore, following the leadership of major voluntary health organizations, **in 1988 the voters opted to increase the tax on a pack of cigarettes from the low level of 10 cents to 35 cents. Moreover, this voter-initiated proposition ("Prop. 99") mandated that one-fourth of the tax revenues realized in this increase would be spent on anti-tobacco education and tobacco-related disease research.** This $150 million per year for the state of 25 million people was especially important, given the relative decline of federal funding for such types of research and educational efforts. In spite of the fact that the tobacco industry spent well over ten times as much in anti-Proposition 99 media advertising as spent by the coalition promoting the proposition, the proposition was passed by the voters by nearly a 2 to 1 margin.

The effects of the increased tax were immediate. Consumption dropped nearly 10 percent from the previous year in spite of the fact that the actual anti-tobacco campaign had not yet begun. Recently the educational effort has shifted into high gear with extensive mass media, local health department-sponsored, school based-sponsored, and innovative individual and community initiatives. A good example of a locally initiated program funded by Proposition 99 is Project TRUST ("Teens and Retailers United to Stop Tobacco"), which is a county-wide educational effort designed to encourage supermarkets, gasoline stations, convenience stores, liquor stores, and independently owned retailers to: (1) decrease tobacco sales to children under eighteen years of age, (2) decrease access of tobacco products by children under eighteen, and (3) decrease tobacco advertising inside and outside stores. Volunteer adults and teens have teamed up with Project TRUST staff to

EXHIBIT 16–1

WHAT WORKS WELL ON THE WEST COAST DOESN'T ALWAYS TRAVEL WELL EASTWARD

Anti-tobacco activists in Montana attempted to emulate the success of California's Proposition 99 with their own "Initiative 115," which attracted only 41 percent of the votes in the November 1990 election. Montana voters apparently thought that the revenues raised would create additional wasteful bureaucracy, an opinion reinforced by the tobacco industry outspending the tobacco control proponents by $1.4 million to $40,000. Specifically, the designers of Initiative 115 encountered six "pitfalls" which contributed to its lack of success:

1. Voters doubted that the allocation of revenues toward tobacco control in education would actually be spent wisely and appropriately.
2. There was a general perception that wasteful bureaucracy would increase without more efficiency in government, which voters really want.
3. The designers of Initiative 115 failed to get endorsements from important organizations such as the Montana Medical Association and the Montana Education Association.
4. There was a lack of national sponsorship by nationwide health organizations.
5. Tobacco control marketing was underfunded and ineffective.
6. Finally, volunteers were sparse and overworked, and by election time they were unable to put the necessary energies and resources into developing effective coalitions and other efforts necessary for victory.*

*R. W. Moon & M. B. McFarland. (1991). Failed Tobacco test plan offers valuable lessons. *Chronic Disease Notes & Reports, 4*(2/3), 14–16.

develop a strategy whereby these children under eighteen (who are legally barred from purchasing tobacco) go into stores and attempt to purchase cigarettes. In baseline purchasing attempts, 75 percent of these 12–17-year-olds purchased cigarettes with "no questions asked." An intervention is currently in progress whereby stores which refuse to sell tobacco to minors will receive free advertising for their high level of social responsibility, while clerks and owners of all tobacco-selling stores will be given special training to check for identification and how to refuse politely to sell tobacco to teens. Finally, continuing violators will be warned by county officials that they are breaking the law.

Other programs funded by Proposition 99 include highly aggressive anti-tobacco media campaigns; large-scale smoking cessation and preven-

tion contests; policy changes promoting increased restrictions on public consumption of tobacco; and efforts specifically targeting the Latino, African-American, and Asian communities which are heavily targeted by the tobacco industry. Minorities are shown how the tobacco industry attempts to exploit them. For example, an African-American rapper cants:

> . . . We used to pick it
> now you want us to smoke it?
> yeah, right—you must be jokin'!

The refrain points out the parallel between the slavery of the pre-Civil War U.S. and the slavery to tobacco experienced by today's smokers.

The proliferation and increased aggressiveness of the anti-tobacco efforts in California (and to a

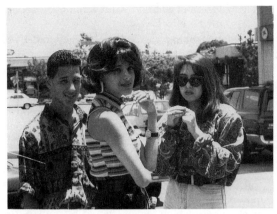
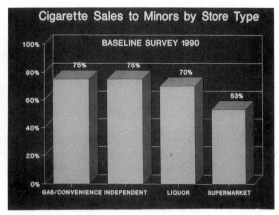

FIGURE 16–4.   These teens working with Project TRUST prepare to go on some "stings" by trying to buy cigarettes in gas stations and convenience stores. Before the TRUST intervention, they were almost always successful. *Photos courtesy of Project T.R.U.S.T.*

lesser extent throughout the U.S.) conflict with the laissez-faire, business-oriented philosophy of the U.S. and California governments. Policies which seek to restrict or prohibit the advertisement of tobacco have been implemented in Canada and are encountering stiff opposition, not only in the U.S. (which is a large producer of tobacco), but also in the European Economic Community. As Michael Leach, mouthpiece for the British tobacco industry, puts it, "an EC advertising ban . . . strikes at our freedom of expression and allows our personal choices to be removed by those who think they know best."[10] Ironically, anti-tobacco policy initiatives also bring us into occasional conflict with civil libertarians who fear violation of an individual's "freedom of choice" when the purchase or use of tobacco is restricted or incentives are offered to avoid or quit the use of tobacco. For many, aggressive tobacco control efforts conjure images of totalitarian governments and heavy-handed (or at least paternalistic) health policies.

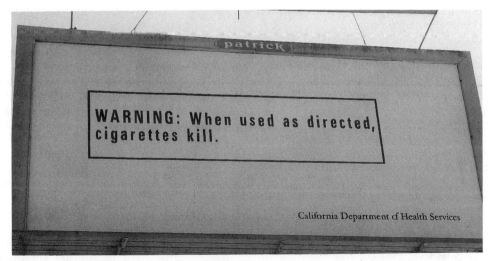

FIGURE 16–5.   California fights back: this billboard sponsored by the "Prop 99" effort is one of many uses of media in this aggressive campaign. *Photo courtesy of Betsy Clapp.*

Those of us involved in community organizing for tobacco control must be prepared for occasional negative reactions to our efforts and select organizational strategies accordingly. These strategies parallel Rothman's locality development (largely consisting of the coordination of tobacco control efforts), social planning (the development and enforcement of policy), and social action (or "activism").

Categories of Organizational Strategies

Coordination. In most communities and regions, some coordination of prevention, cessation, and other programs is already occurring. Generally, representatives from voluntary health organizations (such as the American Lung Association, the American Cancer Society, and the American Heart Association), governmental offices (e.g., county and regional health departments and school officials), professional associations (e.g., medical societies), and others meet formally or informally to discuss existing activities and plan new initiatives. Such groups are immeasurably important for long-term community ownership and success in tobacco control. Nevertheless, they can often benefit from fresh ideas and new directions.

In order to improve the coordination and enhance the effectiveness of existing tobacco control efforts, local smoking control groups should consider the following questions:

1. Is the community truly represented among the group's membership? For example, do blue-collar workers, high-risk teens, women, and minorities have a voice in developing directions and priorities? In other words, does this effort represent effective and appropriate locality development?
2. Is the smoking control council aware of current research developments in tobacco control? Well-meaning groups have been known to adhere to approaches which have been ineffective.
3. Does the group know what the tobacco industry is up to in their community?
4. Are anti-tobacco activists represented in communication with the group? Are sufficiently aggressive policy and activism strategies being considered in addition to prevention, cessation, and media efforts?

Social Planning and Policy. Policy initiatives may have two components: *development* of new tobacco control policies and *enforcement* of existing policies. Much of policy-related tobacco control is designed to "protect the innocent." Young people, whose exposure to tobacco advertisements and access to purchase the product, either through vending machines or over-the-counter, may be well along the way to addiction before they are sufficiently mature to consider the consequences. Other nonsmoking individuals may suffer from passive smoking at the worksite or elsewhere which legally should be smoke-free areas. Indeed, research in the U.S. has shown passive smoking to be the #3 preventable cause of death.[11] Restricting advertisements, eliminating access and sales to youth, and protecting nonsmokers from passive smoke are priorities for policy development and enforcement.

Going beyond the enforcement attempts of California's Project TRUST, the Health Authority for Wales (U.K.) has sought to educate merchants regarding existing proscriptions on selling to under-age youth (defined in Wales as fifteen-years-old or younger). A flyer reminds them of the law and the fine enforced for violation (equivalent to U.S. $700). Rather than asking for identification, merchants in the U.K. may refuse to sell to anyone who looks younger than sixteen. To make this awkward situation easier to deal with, the Health Authority distributes cards (see Fig. 8–9) to merchants which read, "This is to show, I have to say no. The law says it is illegal for me to sell cigarettes to anyone under the age of 16. Since I am not sure what age you are, I will have to say no. This law applies even if you are buying cigarettes for someone else." Thus, both negative reinforcement and response facilitation have improved the probability of compliance with this progressive policy.

Finally, our overall tobacco control efforts cannot be complete without recognizing the need for further restrictions on the international trade of tobacco. Phillip Morris, R. J. Reynolds, British American, and others make huge profits promoting their products abroad, increasingly in underdeveloped countries. As the populations of these regions often have neither the knowledge nor power to restrict tobacco imports and marketing, those of us in tobacco-exporting countries are obligated to lead the way.

Social Action.   A minister of a church in Harlem was disgusted with the excessive amount of alcohol and tobacco billboard advertising near his church and the local public schools. He and his parishioners took to the streets with paint and brushes, and at the end of a long day, many of these ads had disappeared. The "Bugger Up" efforts in Australia promoted a similar concept, resulting in the defacement of tobacco ads throughout the country.

Recently, a group of Latino health promoters and students, armed with cameras and anti-tobacco fliers, appeared at a Chicano festival in a San Diego park, correctly anticipating that representatives of Camel cigarettes would be there in force. First, they followed "roamers" walking around the park giving out free packs of Camels, placing the anti-tobacco fliers in the hands of people who had just received a pack and taking pictures of the process. Feeling harassed, the roamers eventually gave up and returned to a central promotional stand. At this location, people were lined up to spin a wheel which yielded "prizes" of Camels and promotional products. The protesters continued to snap pictures (with flashes) of the process from a distance of only a few feet, inviting complaints and derisive comments from the Camel representatives operating the stand. Frustrated, one of them pushed a camera into a protester's face, an act which was widely seen by observers, including his supervisor. After a brief staff conference, the Camel team decided to pack up their promotion (and their hundreds of cartons of cigarettes) and leave (see Fig. 4–3).

None of the above efforts resulted in a lasting decline of the sleazy marketing being confronted. Instead, social action strategies can: (1) generate free publicity around a particular controversial topic; (2) invite an industry counter-response, which may backfire and elicit even more public sympathy for the anti-tobacco cause; and (3) crystallize public opinion for — or against — the cause. While social action is energizing, it can also be exhausting, and it requires a tremendous amount of dedication and work to be effective. And even with this commitment, care must be taken to prevent specific actions from backfiring and producing greater sympathy for the industry.

In summary, community organizational strategies include coordination of anti-tobacco efforts, development and implementation of policy, and anti-tobacco activism. These efforts hold the greatest potential for meeting the threat to our health posed by tobacco (or more appropriately, the tobacco industry). We can be assured of the validity of this assertion by the vigorous counterattacks conducted by the tobacco industry against policy and activism, while they ignore (or even express support for) cessation and prevention efforts. A note of caution is therefore appropriate: our anti-tobacco activism slingshots will continually be met with the industry's nuclear counter-strikes. Very careful community assessment, research, and the integration of complementary prevention, cessation, and marketing efforts are a must if tobacco is to be eliminated in our culture.

NEEDS/RESOURCES ASSESSMENT IN TOBACCO CONTROL

Before launching a new community tobacco control effort or integrating or modifying existing ones, careful attention needs to be given to a community's existing tobacco control profile and its potential for further change. Key informant interviews, archival research, clinical data, and surveys should help answer some of the following questions which, in turn, establish intervention and research priorities:

1. Who are the "movers and shakers" in local tobacco control efforts? Who represents various health-related organizations at tobacco control meetings and how high up are they in their respective hierarchies? Who is not represented, and why?
2. How familiar is the community and its health and sociopolitical leadership with the tobacco problem and state and national priorities for its resolution?
3. Which past local efforts have succeeded or failed? To what new ideas might the community be receptive?
4. What is the tobacco industry doing in the community? What points of vulnerability does it have?

PRIORITY SETTING

Healthy People 2000 establishes the following objectives related to tobacco control in the U.S.

1. Reduce cigarette smoking to a prevalence of no more than 15 percent among people age 20 and older (from 29.1 percent in 1987).

2. Reduce the initiation of smoking by youth to no more than 15 percent as measured by the prevalence of smoking among people ages 20–24 (from 29.5 percent in 1987).

3. Increase to at least 50 percent the proportion of current smokers age 20 and older who made a serious attempt to quit smoking during the preceding year with one-third or more of these attempts resulting in abstinence for at least three months.

4. Increase smoking cessation during pregnancy so at least 60 percent of women who are cigarette smokers at the time they discover they are pregnant will quit smoking and maintain abstinence for the remainder of their pregnancy.

5. Reduce to no more than 25 percent the proportion of children age 6 and younger who are exposed to cigarette smoke at home.

6. Reduce smokeless tobacco use to a prevalence of no more than 4 percent among men ages 18–24.

7. Increase to at least 85 percent the proportion of adolescents ages 12–17 who perceive social disapproval and great risk or harm to their health from smoking cigarettes.

8. Increase to at least 75 percent the proportion of all primary care providers who routinely advise cessation and provide assistance and follow-up for all their tobacco-using patients.

9. Include tobacco use prevention in the curriculum of all elementary, middle, and secondary schools, preferably as part of comprehensive school health education.

10. Increase to at least 75 percent the proportion of worksites with a formal smoking policy that prohibits or severely restricts smoking in the workplace.

11. Enact in all states comprehensive laws on clean indoor air that prohibit or strictly limit smoking in enclosed public places.

12. Enact and enforce in all states laws prohibiting the sale and distribution of tobacco products to youth younger than age eighteen.

13. Eliminate exposure to tobacco product advertising and promotion among youth younger than age eighteen.

14. Ensure that all tobacco product packages and advertisements provide information on all major health effects of tobacco use, including addiction, and will identify product ingredients and the harmful tobacco smoke constituents.

15. Increase to at least 80 percent the proportion of people with time- and/or cost-limited health insurance coverage for services to overcome nicotine addiction.

Naturally, these objectives are set for the entire nation and will need to be adjusted based on information gathered during the needs and resources assessment (N/RA) phase. In any case, they represent points of departure for establishing local priorities. In setting such priorities, it should be noted that national objective-setting by its nature involves compromise and often results in positions more conservative than necessary, especially for states and communities with strong anti-tobacco track records.[12] Using principles of shaping, communities can gradually build their own version of a tobacco-free society.

What are the critical priorities for developing a tobacco-free society? How far can we go? Do we really expect tobacco use to be wiped out eventually? In the U.S., we are often reminded by smokers (and the tobacco industry) of the failure of Prohibition — the period between World War I and the Franklin Roosevelt administration, when the legal sale of alcohol was banned. This, in turn, contributed to large-scale illegal distribution and sales and, naturally, to an increase in organized crime. Although this argument at best is flawed (and its proponents suspect), we are unlikely to see tobacco disappear in our lifetime. Realistic goals should be selected and priorities set which will minimize both the short- and long-term prevalence of regular tobacco use. Organizations should weigh the pros and cons of different categories of priorities presented in Table 16–1 to decide on their own best course of action.

RESEARCH, MONITORING AND EVALUATION

Research efforts focus on the differential effectiveness of the above strategies and the particular form for a particular intervention process. Research can also be used to (a) set the stage for monitoring and evaluating by identifying those markers of change which are sensitive to intervention efforts and (b) represent valid indications that the tobacco problem is getting under control.

For example, "reducing the number of deaths due to lung cancer" is a socially valid goal and indeed represents a hopeful accomplishment. It is unlikely, however, that even years of effort in a community will yield much change in this index. "Reducing over-the-counter sales to minors" is far more attainable in a short period of time, but will require a type of "sting operation" or other complicated assessment approach to monitor progress. "Reducing access of minors to vending machines" is simultaneously valid (assuming many youth buy their cigarettes in this way), easily measured (only the physical location of machines need be determined), and potentially sensitive to policy or activism efforts.

Priorities and research activities will in turn dictate which counter-measures are to be monitored and which will be selected for additional evaluation at a selected interim or end point of a tobacco control intervention. As in any other health promotion effort, monitoring of progress toward a given tobacco control goal should emphasize a variable easily measured and sensitive to change. For example, it may be easier to send adolescent "spies" into selected stores to buy cigarettes, even though they are under age, in order to determine (on an ongoing basis) what percentage of stores will sell to these adolescents without asking for identification. These data may prove far superior to monitoring the number of citations given by police departments or health officials for illegal sales to minors, since citation data may be difficult to access or may not represent a valid picture of tobacco control in the community. Conversely, sending these adolescent spies into grocery stores may not only be controversial, but fairly time-intensive as well. At any rate, the method selected for monitoring the effectiveness of tobacco control should be compatible with the ideal of frequent yet long-term measurement.

INTERVENTIONS

Cessation Programs

During the 1970s, two distinct approaches to smoking cessation, which addressed the addiction process, emerged in response to a growing consumer demand for giving up "the habit." **Fading** procedures involved gradually reducing the number of cigarettes smoked per day until a quitting day was reached. Fading is assisted through the promotion of a variety of incompatible alternative behaviors, such as exercising, chewing gum or munching low calorie snacks, and various stress reduction activities. Careful self-monitoring is a key component of fading, involving the ABC recording of (a) urges to smoke, (b) the frequency of smoking, and/or (c) the duration of intervals between smoking cigarettes. Permanent product validation of these measures (by counting the number of cigarettes left in a pack or butts in an ashtray) can also be included. Once the fading process begins, the self-monitoring procedure can become part of the intervention (e.g., by having the smoker wrap the data-recording form around the pack of cigarettes) thereby cutting down on "smoking without thinking." Narrative recording data may also be used to help identify and avoid high-risk situations (e.g., bars). Brand changes from regular to menthol or vice versa, and to cigarettes with successively lower levels of nicotine can also be included. A quit day is set for the smoker to cut down to five or so cigarettes per day, whereafter all ashtrays and other smoking paraphernalia are removed from the environment, and an extra emphasis is placed on mobilizing social support from family members and friends. The American Lung Association's Freedom from Smoking program contains many of the above elements.

The other major category of cessation approaches are considered **satiation** procedures,[13] including either aversive smoking or pharmaceutically-assisted cessation. Pharmaceutically-assisted cessation involves the use of gum, a skin patch, or another delivery medium which releases nicotine into the body and presumably reduces withdrawal symptoms. Generally, clinical counseling oriented toward some of the procedures described above are recommended as part of such interventions. Aversive techniques involve having the participant smoke continuously and rapidly in a poorly ventilated space over the course of a half-hour or more, and discarding butts in a highly visible (and presumably disgusting) manner, such as putting them in a jar of water. After several sessions on consecutive days, the smoker is expected to: (1) accumulate a sufficient amount of nicotine in his or her system for forestalling withdrawal symptoms for a period of time, and (2) develop an aversion to cigarettes through unpleasant gustatory, olfactory, and visual sensations.

After the last rapid smoking session, environmental and relapse-prevention interventions like those described above are implemented to help the smoker stay smoke-free.

Cessation programs are probably the least cost-efficient method of doing something about tobacco. Fading procedures require highly trained facilitators, whereas satiation interventions are often either administered or supervised by physicians. Nobody can question that every life of a former smoker saved through a self-help or assisted cessation effort is immeasurably important. Nevertheless, given that: (1) most smokers who quit do so without use of formal cessation programs, (2) most smokers who quit will return to their addiction sooner or later, and (3) many smokers have already damaged their health, we are forced to seek more efficient means of achieving a public health impact.

Although not necessarily in the forefront of public health efforts, reducing the tobacco industry's number of current consumers through getting them to quit smoking rather than watching them die will nevertheless continue to be an important approach to attacking tobacco on the home front. Perhaps the most promising public health approach to cessation is offered through the cessation contest, the most widely used being "Quit and Win."

An effective variation of the cessation contest approach was entitled "Quit Date '88"[14] and was held in Bloomington, Minnesota. Following a recruitment promotion through print and interpersonal channels, smokers were eligible to enter the contest at any point in an eight-month period as long as they pledged a quit date. All participants who had quit in the current or a previous month of the contest were eligible for a $200 prize at the end of each month. At the end, all participants were eligible for a grand prize trip for two to Mexico. Smokers could quit on their own or obtain help through materials or programs offered by the sponsoring Minnesota Heart Health Program.

A total of 918 smokers entered the program (in this city of 85,000), 347 by the first month and 203 in the last month before the grand prize was drawn. An intermediate follow-up showed an abstinence rate of 16.7 percent. Although seemingly low, this rate compares favorably to that found in more intensive programs and was successful given the large numbers of individuals participating in the program.

Preventing Tobacco Use

Beginning with the work of Evans and his colleagues at the University of Houston,[15] researchers began to realize the relative futility of trying to get people to give up a drug (tobacco) to which they were seriously addicted, and thus they shifted their attention to prevent first-time or regular use of cigarettes. Previous *educational* programs had emphasized to children the dangers of smoking (e.g., through slides showing diseased lungs and statistics indicating how much earlier one could expect to die by smoking), but this new generation of programs emphasized the process of beginning to smoke and sought to counter the social influences which lead to smoking. Specifically, these *refusal skills training* programs stem from the belief that most children do not actively seek to try smoking but are pressured to do so by their friends, older siblings, etc. Therefore, programs developed by Evans, McAllister, Perry, and others focused on developing in-school programs to teach children how to refuse an offer of a cigarette. San Diego's Project SHOUT represents a current version of these types of programs.[16]

Project SHOUT. Based on the work of these researchers, Project SHOUT (an acronym for Students Helping Others Understand Tobacco) was launched in junior high schools throughout San Diego County (California) in 1988. This intervention process was designed to work with one multi-school group of students as they progressed from seventh through ninth grade to help them resist offers of cigarettes and smokeless tobacco through this most vulnerable period in their lives. SHOUT uses a combination of educational, skills training, motivational, and community activities to create the optimal environment-behavior relationships for tobacco-free schools.

The intervention was conducted by a large cadre of trained undergraduate students selected to be classroom leaders based on their desire to gain health education experience in return for college course credit. As part of the intervention, the seventh grade participants:

1. Watched a videotape on the health consequences of tobacco use.
2. Discussed social consequences of tobacco use.
3. Became familiar with smokeless tobacco products.

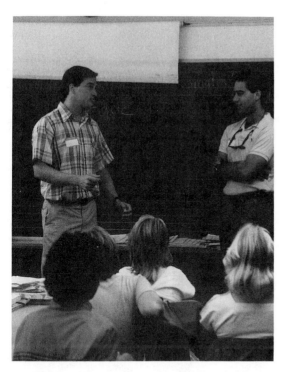

FIGURE 16–6. Two undergraduate students implementing the Project SHOUT intervention role play an offer of a cigarette and a refusal of that offer before middle school students. *Photo courtesy of John Elder.*

4. Discussed antecedents of tobacco use and made public commitments not to smoke.
5. Rehearsed methods of resisting peer pressure.
6. Practiced decision making related to avoidance of tobacco use.
7. Wrote letters to tobacco companies describing their negative opinions of tobacco marketing.
8. Developed and performed a skit for their class-mates in which they were offered and then refused tobacco.

Participation in all of the above activities was reinforced with raffle tickets, exchangeable for a variety of prizes donated by local businesses and organizations (sports equipment, movie passes, t-shirts, record albums, etc.). At the end of the year, a "Fresh Mouth" contest was held as an additional way to win raffle tickets. For this con-test, students wrote their names on a sheet of paper if they had not been smoking or chewing tobacco and wanted to enter the drawing. Stu-dents whose names were drawn received a carbon monoxide test to see whether they indeed had not been smoking. (All students tested showed them-selves to be smoke-free). Fresh Mouth contests were held on a random, unscheduled basis to maximize the effectiveness of this reward contingency.

These same students went through a parallel SHOUT curriculum in their eighth grade, this time with greater emphasis on rehearsing refusal skills over and over again. Community activism took on a more mature flavor, as well, with students join-ing together to encourage merchants located near the schools not to sell cigarettes to minors. Also, students with smoking parents were taught ways to reach out to help them quit.

In its third and final year of tobacco-use pre-vention, many of the target students had trans-ferred to high school. Therefore, SHOUT con-ducted a home-based intervention consisting of bimonthly newsletters mailed to the subjects' homes alternated with phone call conversations (made by a new group of undergraduate leaders) with these students. Newsletters were designed to provide tobacco information as well as opportuni-ties for the students to express their views about tobacco distribution and use. Components of the newsletters included interviews with students (by undergraduate volunteers through the phone con-versations), announcements of birthday and to-bacco-related contest winners, previous contest winners' entries (i.e., cartoons or letters), a column devoted to answering students' questions regard-ing tobacco, articles about opportunities to partic-ipate in anti-tobacco activities, students' opinions on controversial tobacco-related issues (based on the phone conversations), and other miscella-neous tobacco articles. Five newsletters were mailed to the students' homes. In addition, twice during the year parents of each SHOUT student received a newsletter similar in content to the students' newsletters.

Phone call opinion interviews were made be-tween the hours of 3:30–6:30 p.m. and were ap-proximately four minutes in length. Four separate phone call sessions were carried out during the year (two per semester) with each session lasting approximately one month. The undergraduate "volunteer" counselors were given a script to fol-low to ensure that all components were covered, however, paraphrasing was encouraged. It was stressed that the phone calls should be a conver-sation, not just a survey of the students' opinions or a lecture. Components of each phone call included verification of receipt of the most recent newsletter, discussion of specific articles in the newsletters, encouragement to participate in the tobacco activism activity, discussion on a controversial tobacco-related issue to obtain students' opinions, and questions pertaining to educating the students on smoking norms. One feature of this intervention was its low cost, with the only major expenses coming from the printing and mailing of the newsletters (as most phone calls were local).

Prevention programs represent substantial improvement over individually-based cessation programs in terms of potential for public health impact. Not only were these children caught before they became addicted to the use of cigarettes, they were "treated" in group (usually classroom) situations which allowed the target audience to deal with a potential problem in the same context (i.e., in front of other peers) in which it was likely to occur. Moreover, whereas standard cessation programs have implicitly "blamed" individuals for picking up the smoking habit and placed the responsibility on their shoulders for giving it up, this prevention program was based on the assumption that children do not exercise freedom of choice when smoking their first cigarette.

The goal of prevention was to manipulate the peer environment — in other words, to change reinforcement for smoking into reinforcement for not smoking — and develop the students' skills to such an extent that experimenting with cigarettes should become unlikely. However, the end of the 1970s saw these programs still in their experimental phases and not ready for large-scale public health application, at the same time, the tobacco industry cleverly modernized their strategies and began to market products heavily which would appeal to young children, such as smokeless tobacco and tobacco look alike candies and gum.

Social Marketing Strategies

The bulk of early social marketing (and motivational) efforts went into promoting the benefits of smoking cessation and later the importance of not starting. More aggressive messages were withheld from the airwaves through a deal struck with the tobacco industry twenty years ago, whereby they agreed to help write legislation banning cigarette advertising via broadcast media. Gradually, messages became more strident, with posthumous pleas to avoid tobacco from lung cancer victims such as Yul Brynner.

A marketing approach using similar negative reinforcement (or vicarious punishment) strategies was to take advantage of the shared grief society has for tobacco victims. For instance, almost all families have lost one or more members prematurely to smoking, yet only rarely do obituaries (or for that matter, death certificates) mention smoking as the cause. For example, when Amanda Blake (Miss Kitty of the TV series "Gunsmoke") died in 1989, her *Los Angeles Times* obituary read in part, "The 60-year-old actress . . . died at 7:15 p.m. Wednesday of mouth and throat cancer . . . Blake had smoked two packs of cigarettes a day until cancer first struck in 1977 in the form of a tumor under her tongue."[17]

After first developing cancer from her smoking habit, Ms. Blake became an active spokesperson for the American Cancer Society. In her obituary,

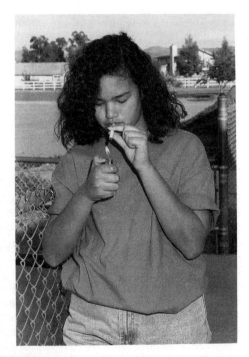

FIGURE 16–7. Although the tobacco industry emphasizes smokers' rights to choose to smoke, most smokers make that "choice" when they are still quite young. *Photo courtesy of Andy Suarez.*

she spoke out against smoking one last time. While personally painful, families should be encouraged to consider including anti-tobacco statements in their loved ones' obituaries. In the late 1960s, *Life* magazine published the pictures of all Americans killed in Vietnam in one specific week, personalizing this tragedy for communities across the country. With the help of sympathetic journalists, community tobacco control specialists should consider publishing the names or pictures of residents who had died from a smoking-related disease in a given week or month. By bringing this slaughter out of the closet, social marketing can make major contributions toward ending it.

Table 16–1 summarizes the advantages and disadvantages of cessation, prevention, and media as tobacco control strategies.

WHERE DO WE GO FROM HERE?

1. Defining "Freedom."   Perhaps we should begin with an agreement on the definition of "freedom," not only for tobacco control, but for all health promotion efforts. However, unlike arguments for protecting a motorcycle rider's "freedom" to decline to wear a helmet—they mainly hurt themselves—recent evidence linking one's tobacco use to another person's illnesses places a refusal to accept proscriptions on tobacco use in the category of refusing to get vaccinated for communicable diseases. Personal health is not the only issue. In any case, while we luxuriate in fascinating discussions about who should decide whether tobacco use is allowable and how far we should go in anti-tobacco efforts, the tobacco industry continues to enjoy the freedom to attract more and more smokers every year to replace the many who are dying from having "chosen" to begin smoking when they were younger.

2. Policy.   Health promoters—especially those involved in trying to counteract the ill effects of well-entrenched and wealthy purveyors of illness—need to look beyond changing individual behavior if we hope to achieve any success at all in reducing death and disease from tobacco, alcohol, and other legally marketed products. First, we need to make sure that laws in effect (e.g., those prohibiting the sale of tobacco to minors) are enforced. Second, even more aggressive efforts to limit tobacco advertising (e.g., allowing only black

and white "tombstone" ads) and legal battles to make the tobacco industry pay for the carnage they inflict on their patrons need to be enjoined. Those of us with expertise in changing health behavior need to target the political behaviors of consumers and target populations who can expand anti-tobacco policy. For the long term, it may prove more effective to get one hundred individuals to turn out for an anti-tobacco rally than to get them to exercise twenty minutes three times per week. Implied by both policy and economic considerations are strategies which would directly attack the tobacco industry and its promoters. Recent research and policy initiatives have advocated consumer boycotts of tobacco-owned subsidiary companies and their products, such as (RJR) Nabisco and, for example, Oreo cookies.[18] In much the same way as the U.S. prosecutes its war on cocaine, trade concessions and restrictions could be applied by non-tobacco growing countries to tobacco-exporting countries (such as the U.S.) for weaning themselves or continuing to profit from selling tobacco.

3. Economics.   How do we pay for these expanded efforts, especially when most Western governments are seeking to spend less on health programs? The recent California experience suggests that not only can smokers be coaxed (and coerced) into paying for efforts to help them give up their habit, but also to help prevent their children from using tobacco. Not only have these revenues been used for some of the most aggressive anti-tobacco programs in the U.S., the increased tax has also reduced tobacco consumption directly by over 5 percent greater than the reduction expected. Clearly, such revenues will eventually be self-limiting: the higher the tax, the fewer cigarettes people will smoke and the lower the overall revenue will be. But with fewer people smoking, there will be less need for health education in this area.

An argument promoted by the tobacco and alcohol industries against such a tax is that it is regressive (or even racist) because it imposes a greater burden on poor people than on the wealthy (who are less likely to be minorities). Yet recent surveys in California showed that poorer minority communities support this tax as much or more than did people with greater economic means. Perhaps they recognized that the illness industry is seeking to exploit them to make up for

TABLE 16-1
Advantages and Disadvantages of Various Tobacco Control Strategies

Priority Area	Example	Advantages	Disadvantages
Cessation	Quit and Win Smoking Cessation Contests	1. Non-controversial	1. Addiction generally firmly in place — high relapse rates. 2. Physical damage to smoker may already have been done. 3. Intensive intervention may be required. 4. Much doubt about public health impact.
Prevention	Project SHOUT	1. Non-controversial 2. Targets children before addiction sets in	1. Some doubt about long-term efficacy.
Media	California ("Prop 99") Tobacco Control Media Campaign	1. Broad reach (in some applications) 2. Can be used to complement any of the other four activities	1. Can be very expensive. 2. Not sufficient by itself.
Policy	Banning smoking at the worksite	1. Potentially highly effective 2. Protects the innocent (i.e., passive smokers)	1. Controversial — likely to provoke response from tobacco industry (e.g., through Smokers' "Rights" Groups), which will need to be countered. 2. Requires support of frequently conservative bureaucracy or elected officials (some of whom may receive financial support from the tobacco industry).
Activism	Doctors Ought to Care	1. Can be highly visible — creates own media through news coverage, etc. 2. Can be effective — establishes cutting edge for others to follow	1. Highly controversial. 2. May include activities of questionable legality. 3. May offend some elements of the public or be seen by them as the "radical fringe."

a loss of profits from white Anglos, or more simply they do not want more health problems in their communities. To borrow a tobacco industry strategy, it is suggested that future special tax designations include provisions to designate certain communities for special health promotion projects funded by the tax, thereby reinforcing them for supporting the political actions necessary to enact the tax, while at the same time providing a direct health benefit.

SUMMARY

The public health profession has been slow to respond to the tobacco epidemic. Initial efforts to control tobacco use emphasized smoking cessation. Eventually, greater emphases were placed on apparently more cost-effective prevention, media, and policy interventions. California's "Prop 99" tobacco control campaign represents a unique blend of educational, motivational, social marketing and policy interventions funded through a twenty-five cents per pack increase in cigarette taxes.

Health promotion efforts for taking on tobacco need to consider the tobacco industry's strategies in order to be truly effective. The "industry" combines efforts at protecting their niche in our sociocultural fabric with aggressive promotions to increase consumer markets for tobacco and subsidiary products. Public health strategies should anticipate these strategies and attack and counter-attack with policy and other more effective interventions accordingly. Without truly aggressive tobacco control approaches, the incredible loss of life worldwide due to tobacco use will continue unabated.

EXERCISE

The Miller Brewing Company recently developed a booklet entitled *Responsible Drinking: It's Up to You* (available from the Miller Brewing Company at 3939 West Highland Boulevard, Milwaukee, WI 53201). Chapters in this booklet include "How to drink most responsibly," "Understanding alcoholism and alcohol abuse," "Separating beer from illicit substances," "Talking with our children about beer," "Possible questions from kids," "Guide to family discussions,"

and "Corporate responsibility at work." In this booklet the authors discuss how to set up a designated driver system, how to stop people from driving drunk, and other clearly straightforward and non-controversial healthful tips. Also included are sections differentiating beer from illicit drugs (the only true valid distinction they make is that beer is legal and illicit drugs, of course, are not, and that you can drink beer in front of children without directly or indirectly encouraging them to do the same). On the controversial side, the booklet states that one aspect of being a "positive role model" for children is feeling "at ease drinking in front of child."

Analyze the above points (or better yet, obtain a copy of the booklet from Miller Brewing Company) and express your opinion on these topics. Should a major brewing company be promoting "responsible drinking"? If so, what form should this promotion take? How is this similar or dissimilar from the promotion of tobacco products and the excuses the tobacco industry uses for advertising in marketing defense and offense operations?

ADDITIONAL REFERENCES

Keep Your Fire Extinguisher Loaded with These Tobacco Control Resources.[19]

(This section, extracted from their "Resource Guide," was developed as part of the California Statewide Tobacco Control Program. It provides a list of organizations offering programs, services, and materials for tobacco control activities. The organizations are listed alphabetically and are numbered. Under each listing are specific programs and their names, publications, and other materials for prevention, cessation, policy, and activism in the U.S.)

  1. **Action on Smoking and Health (ASH)**
     2013 H Street, N.W.
     Washington, DC 20006
POLICY: ASH provides information on legal action (lawsuits) and policy issues; *Smoking and Health Review*—newsletter; and a source list of products and services.
  2. **The Advocacy Institute**
     1730 Rhode Island Avenue, N.W., Suite 600
     Washington, DC 20036-3118
POLICY: This is a resource and support organization which tracks the tobacco industry and provides information and strategic counseling for other groups. A computer network SCARCNet (Smoking Control Advocacy Resource Center Network) keeps subscribers in-

formed of developments in the anti-smoking movement.

3. American Cancer Society

Contact the local chapter in your area.

ACS provides resource information and guidance, referrals, self-help and classroom cessation programs, and pamphlets, such as *PREVENTION: An Early Start to Good Health* — grades K–3.

- The Big Dipper — 19-minute video on smokeless tobacco for ages 11–21.
- Smoke-Free class of 2000 Project — joint effort with AHA and ALA starting in 1988 with first-grade students, to be followed up as the students progress through subsequent grades.

CESSATION:

- Can They Stop Smoking? Can You? — pamphlet on smoking cessation designed for Black women.
- Cuando Fuma Mujer — cessation pamphlet in Spanish for women.
- Fresh Start — four one-hour group sessions in a two-week stop smoking group program.
- Nine Quit Smoking Tips — bookmarker with nine self-help smoking cessation strategies.
- Special Delivery — designed to help low-income pregnant women stop smoking; for use by prenatal clinic staff, social services, and schools.

POLICY: A Decision Maker's Guide to Reducing Smoking at the Worksite.

- The Smoke Around You: The Risks of Involuntary Smoking — pamphlet.

4. American Lung Association

CESSATION: Freedom from Smoking Clinic — 8-session group program using a positive behavior change approach with the assistance of a facilitator; includes the Lifetime of Freedom from Smoking maintenance manual and an audiocassette with relaxation and imagery exercises. Designed for middle-aged, middle-class white collar workers, and may be appropriate for pregnant women.

- Freedom from Smoking for Teens — grades 7–12.
- Freedom from Smoking for You and Your Baby — 10-day self-help program on quitting smoking with manual, exercise chart, progress calendar, pattern-breaker chart, and audiocassette featuring aerobic and relaxation techniques for pregnant women with low literacy skills.
- Freedom from Smoking for You and Your Family — 10-day self-help manual on quitting with nicotine addiction test, fold-out quitting calendar, and an "Ex-Smoker's Eating Guide." Designed for blue collar workers, pink collar workers, and smokers with low literacy levels, and also appropriate for mothers of young children, school-age youth and families, and out-of-school youth.
- Freedom from Smoking in 20 Days — self-help manual to quit smoking.
- A Lifetime of Freedom from Smoking — 28-page self-help maintenance manual, with pocket reminder and progress calendar for developing a nonsmoking habit; also appropriate for pregnant women and mothers of young children.

POLICY: Freedom from Smoking at Work: Taking Executive Action; Creating Your Company Policy — two manuals for management and employees to reduce smoking at the workplace.

5. Americans for Nonsmoker Rights (ANR)/American Nonsmokers' Rights Foundation (ANRF)

ANR is a national lobbying and advocacy group protecting nonsmokers from involuntary smoking. ANRF is the educational arm of ANR.

PREVENTION:

- Death in the West — curriculum guide for grades 5–7 to accompany the film Death in the West (available from ETR/TECC and Pyramid Films).

POLICY:

- ANR Update — newsletter.
- Legislative Approaches to a Smoke-Free Society: Vol. 1 (text); Vol. 2 (appendices).
- National Matrix of Local Smoking Ordinances.
- A Smokefree Workplace: An Employer's Guide to Nonsmoking Policies — brochure for instituting a nonsmoking policy in an organization.

MISCELLANEOUS:

- Smokefree Travel Guide — brochure.
- Tobacco Smoke and the Nonsmoker — brochure.
- Also available are stickers, pins, plaques, a fan, etc.

6. Cancer Information Service
National Cancer Institute

Office of Cancer Communications
Building 31, Room 10A24
9000 Rockville Pike
Rockville, MD 20892
(1-800-4 CANCER)

MATERIALS FOR HEALTH PROFESSIONALS:
CESSATION: How to Help Your Patients Stop Smoking: An NCI Manual for Physicians — pamphlet.

- Pharmacists Helping Smokers Quit Kit—to help pharmacists help patients quit smoking. Includes:
- for the pharmacist: A Program Guide for the Pharmacist, plus a counter card with smoking and drug interactions, certificate of participation, posters, and reorder card.
- Guia Para Dejar de Fumar—A guide to quit smoking; pamphlet in Spanish.

POLICY:

- Guide to Public Health Practice: State Health Agency Tobacco Prevention and Control Plans.
- Major Smoking Ordinances in the United States.
- Media Strategies for Smoking Control: Guidelines.

7. **Doctors Ought to Care (DOC)**
   1423 Harper Street
   Augusta, GA 30912

DOC is a coalition of health professionals and other concerned individuals that uses innovation and entertainment to educate the public, especially young people, about the major preventable causes of poor health and high medical costs . . . with particular emphasis on counteracting the promotion of alcohol and tobacco.

- DOC News and Views—newsletter.
- Also available are a tobacco slide presentation and script, stickers, posters, t-shirts, and other items.

8. **Office on Smoking and Health**
   Centers for Disease Control
   Atlanta, GA 30333

- Bulletin on Smoking and Health—bimonthly abstracts of published literature on smoking, tobacco, and health.

9. **Pyramid Film & Video**
   Box 1048
   Santa Monica, CA 90406-1048
   (800) 421-2304

PREVENTION:

- Death in the West—32-minute film or video of six smoking cowboys dying of smoking-induced illnesses, with curriculum guide (also in French, Portuguese, Spanish, and Swedish).

PREVENTION AND CESSATION:

- The Feminine Mistake—film or video for women.
- Hugh McCabe: The Coach's Final Lesson—17-minute video.

CESSATION:

- The Quitter—7-minute film or video.
- Smoking: How to Stop—23-minute film or video.

POLICY:

- On the Air: Creating a Smokefree Workplace—15-minute video to help management develop and implement a smoke-free policy.
10. **San Diego State University**
    Graduate School of Public Health
    AB 75 Tobacco Control Program Evaluation
    San Diego, CA 92182
    (619) 594-1976

SDSU has the contract with California DHS to evaluate the AB 75 tobacco control programs. (You can order the entire list from which this was abstracted.)

11. **Students Helping Others Understand Tobacco (SHOUT)**
    6363 Alvarado Court, Suite 100
    San Diego, CA 92120
    (619) 594-1976

PREVENTION: Social skills and refusal training curriculum for school-aged youth (grades 7–10); shown to be effective with Hispanic youth, delivered in classroom and by phone.

ENDNOTES

1. Blum, A. (1991). The Marlboro Grand Prix: Circumvention of the television ban on tobacco advertising. *New England Journal of Medicine, 324,* 913–916.
2. Miles, R. (1902). *Coffin nails and corporate strategies.* Englewood Cliffs, NJ: Prentice-Hall.
3. USDHHS. (1967). Surgeon General's Report. (1967). *Health consequences of smoking.* Rockville, MD: U.S. Department of Health & Human Services, Smoking Control.
4. Miles actually uses the word "domain" instead of, but synonymously with, "market."
5. Begay, M. & Glantz, S. (1991). *Political expenditures by the tobacco industry in California state politics from 1976 to 1991.* San Francisco: University of California.
6. Of course, the U.S. government continues to back the industry. When Thailand sought to limit these marketing practices, the State Department threatened trade sanctions.
7. Mittelmark, M., Luepker, R., Jacobs, D., Bracht, N., Carlaw, R., Crow, R., Finnegan, J., Grimm, R., Jeffrey, R., Kline, F., Mullis, R., Murray, D., Pechacek,

T., Perry, C., Pirie, P., & Blackburn, H. (1986). Community-wide prevention of cardiovascular disease: Education strategies of the Minnesota Heart Health Program. *Preventive Medicine, 15,* 1–17; and Elder, J., McGraw, S., Abrams, D., Ferreira, A., Lasater, T., Longpre, N., Peterson, G., Schwetfeger, R., & Carleton, R. (1986). Organizational and community approaches to community-wide prevention of heart disease: The first two years of the Pawtucket Heart Health Program. *Preventive Medicine, 15,* 107–117.

8. Tax-fixed drive against smoking in California seen as model effort. *Los Angeles Times,* January 30, 1992.

9. Student Power. *Sacramento Bee,* May 22, 1991.

10. The freedom to sell our brands. *The Gazette* (London), September 20, 1991.

11. Begay, M. & Glantz, S. *Political expenditures by the tobacco industry in California state politics from 1976 to 1991.*

12. The opposite can be true for communities in tobacco-producing states which may look upon national policy as too strident.

13. Lichtenstein, E. & Metmelstein, R. (1984). Review of approaches to smoking treatment: Behavior modification strategies. In J. Matarazzo, S. Weiss, J. Herd, & N. Miller (Eds.), *Behavioral Health* (pp. 695–712). New York: Wiley.

14. Lando, H., Hellerstedt, W., Pirie, P., Fruetel, J., & Huttner, P. (1991). Results of a long-term community smoking cessation contest. *American Journal of Health Promotion, 5,* 420–425.

15. Evans, R. I. (1976). Smoking in children. Developing a social psychological strategy of deterrence. *Preventive Medicine, 5,* 122–127.

16. Evans, Ibid; and Perry, C. L., Maccoby, N., & McAllister, A. L. (1980). Adolescent smoking prevention: A third year follow-up. *World Smoking & Health, 5,* 41–45.

17. Rites for Amanda Blake of "Gunsmoke" Planned. *Los Angeles Times,* August 18, 1989.

18. Elder, J. P., Amick, T. L., Sleet, D. A., & Senn, K. L. (1987). Potential consumer participation in a boycott of tobacco-company-owned nontobacco products. *American Journal of Preventive Medicine, 3,* 323–326.

19. Elder, J., Allen, J., & Parra-Medina, D. (1991). *A compendium of effective tobacco control programs.* San Diego, CA: San Diego State University.

Chapter 17

Nutritional Health: You Are What You Shop for, Cook, and Eat

OBJECTIVES

By the end of this chapter, the reader should be able to:

1. Apply the ONPRIME model to the area of nutrition promotion.
2. Discuss the strengths and limitations of legislation restricting nutrient information and claims on packaging and television.
3. Describe four general monitoring and measurement strategies for nutrition-related behaviors.
4. Discuss intervention strategies for changing food content, food accessibility, consumer knowledge about nutrient information, and consumer skills.
5. Contrast current approaches to increasing dietary fiber with current approaches to controlling tobacco use.

INTRODUCTION

Achieving the "optimal" nutritional status of a community is a complex task, because (a) there are numerous vitamins, minerals, and macro-nutrients (e.g., protein, fat), each having their own daily requirements; (b) scientists and/or health agencies may disagree in their nutritional recommendations; (c) the nutrition-related problems of the community may vary widely, depending on the age group, gender, income, ethnic background, and other patterns that may influence nutritional status (e.g., alcohol consumption); (d) nutritional status is mediated by a combination of biological (e.g., metabolic), environmental (e.g., food nutrient content), and behavioral (e.g., food selection) factors; and (e) the elimination of both nutritional excesses (e.g., overconsumption of calories and fat) and deficiencies (e.g., underconsumption of iron or even of calories among malnourished people) may be required.

For this chapter, we define "optimal" nutritional status broadly, as the status associated with health and the absence of nutrition-related diseases. Because the areas of nutrition assessment and promotion are broad, this chapter excludes a large number of sub-topics. For example, we do not include information on the prevention and/or treatment of eating disorders or vitamin deficiencies. Nor do we examine malnutrition, diarrhea control, breast feeding, or other issues more relevant to underdeveloped countries, as these are addressed in chapter 20. Rather, this chapter applies selected components of the ONPRIME model of intervention primarily to two nutrition-related endpoints: an increase in dietary fiber and a decrease in dietary fat for the general population.

Why did we choose these endpoints? First, both of these goals have been put forward as high priority objectives by the Department of Health and Human Services. Specifically, in *The (1988) Surgeon General's Report on Nutrition and Health,* the foreword stated that "Of highest priority among these changes is to reduce intake of foods high in fats and to increase intake of foods high in complex carbohydrates and fiber."[1] More recently, in *Healthy People 2000,*[2] specific objectives regarding these goals were stated; they are discussed below. These dietary priorities are based on scientific evidence (a combination of correlational and experimental studies) linking high fat diets (or low fiber diets) to a variety of chronic diseases. For example, high fat diets have been associated with coronary heart disease (CHD), obesity, and certain types of cancer, and

low fiber diets are associated with colon cancer and diverticular disease.[3] Thus, these goals are important from a primary prevention perspective, particularly given the high rates of CHD, obesity, and certain types of cancer in many industrialized countries. A second reason for focusing on these goals, while excluding others, is that they provide clear, fairly simple illustrations of the behavior change principles discussed in the introductory chapters, as well as a straightforward application of the ONPRIME model.

Promoting changes in the overall dietary patterns of a community is no simple task. Food preferences are acquired fairly early in life and food selection remains fairly consistent over time among adults. Food choices reflect individuality and cultural identity. In addition to providing essential nutrients to promote growth and life, eating functions as an important social behavior, serving to punctuate daily routine activities. In this chapter we address the complexity of promoting changes in eating behavior by including intervention and assessment strategies at multiple levels.

Conceptually, promoting dietary change provides an interesting contrast to promoting the elimination of smoking. While health professionals agree that tobacco use in all forms is detrimental to the users and those around them, debate abounds in the dietary arena regarding such topics as the strength of the data on diet–disease relationships and the stringency of the objectives. The goal of a "smoke-free" society is discrete and clear cut, since *any* exposure may be detrimental. On the other hand, dietary objectives must consider that consumers will continue to (a) eat, (b) be exposed to a wide variety of foods, and (c) be exposed to a variety of promotional messages from both the food industry and health agencies. Thus, campaigns to provide nutritional changes may be relatively "tame" compared to some of the tobacco campaigns. Selected organizational and policy-based efforts for achieving nutritional objectives are described in the next section.

ORGANIZING FOR NUTRITION INFORMATION REFORM

Organized social action to reduce undernutrition receives much attention in the lay press (e.g., soup kitchens for the homeless, "Meals on Wheels" for low-income elderly and/or disabled

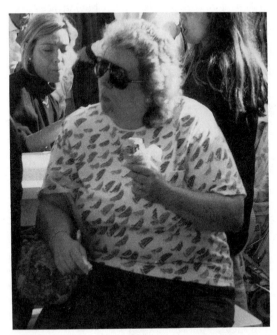

FIGURE 17–1. Excessive consumption of foods high in fat and calories are major risk factors for heart disease, cancer, and other chronic illnesses. *Photo courtesy of Betsy Clapp.*

adults). Nevertheless, in recent years, activism to promote a lower fat diet by Americans has been generated by national organizations such as the Center for Science in the Public Interest (CSPI), as well as the national offices and local affiliates of the American Heart Association and the American Cancer Society. The CSPI was one of the groups instrumental in lobbying Congress to pass the Nutrition Labeling and Education Act of 1990 (H.R. 3562),[4] which will attempt to ensure that consumers are provided with clear, accurate information on a variety of nutrients on product packaging. Consequently, in the fall of 1991, the Food and Drug Administration (FDA) who enforce the act, released the proposed regulations for response by the public. The Act was to be enforced by May, 1993, but on March 19, 1992, it was announced that meat and poultry packaging was granted an extra year to comply. Other postponements may follow. The regulations will attempt, as one component of many, to reduce the extent of misleading package claims related to fat content. For example, food manufacturers are currently allowed to state the relative fat content of products by weight rather than by the percentage of calories it comprises. Although fat can be light in weight, it is dense in calories, with 9 calories per gram of fat (versus 4 calories per gram of protein or carbohydrate). Thus, ice cream that may have 85 percent of its calories from fat may be described as "97% fat free," and this claim is allowed under present regulations. A health-conscious consumer, who has taken seriously the message to reduce dietary fat, may well be misled by this claim.

The FDA has authority over the package content of all non-beef and non-poultry items, the U.S. Department of Agriculture (USDA) has authority over the package content of beef and poultry items, and the Federal Trade Commission (FTC) has authority over the content of all television advertisements. Thus, the contents on the box of a frozen cheese pizza is regulated by the FDA, the contents on the box of a frozen pepperoni pizza is regulated by the USDA, and the contents of the TV ads for both products are regulated by the FTC. To make matters more confusing (and frustrating from the health promotion specialist's perspective), although the FDA's function is primarily protective and regulatory, the USDA's goals include both regulation and promotion of the beef industry.

The Labeling Act described above, which applies to all packages (including those under USDA authority), does not have a direct impact on TV ad content. This is problematic, because of the relatively strong reach and power of televised ads. Additionally, discrepancies between claims on TV versus actual product packaging lead to even greater confusion among consumers. Consequently, groups such as CSPI lobbied Congress to pass a law (H.R. 1662, the Food Advertising Coordination Act of 1991) to synchronize the nutritional information regulations of each agency.

Fat, cholesterol, and sodium content were the targets of a program launched nationally in 1990 by the American Heart Association (AHA) to promote the manufacture and sale of "heart-healthier" products by using special AHA endorsed labels. The program, called "Heart Guide," was to operate by (a) charging food companies to test the contents of their product(s) and (b) allowing the manufacturer to use the AHA endorsement on the package and printing brochures (for in-store dissemination) of "approved" products. A toll-free number for consumers was also proposed. The "Heart Guide" program had the potential to encourage the modification of existing products and the development of new ones, assuming that companies wanted to participate. However, the program's impact could not be evaluated because the program was never fully implemented. Its failure to thrive was due, in part, to the FDA, which had objections to the use of a "seal of approval" by a third party.

Although food boycotts may be an effective way of influencing the behavior of food producers, distributors, and products related to specific brands or food categories (e.g., grapes), a boycott against all products that make misleading claims would not be feasible.[5] Depending on one's definition of misleading, nutrition claims related to fat and cholesterol are over 50 percent within certain food categories, as discussed in Exhibit 17–1.

To what extent will labeling and advertising restrictions have an impact on what consumers purchase and ultimately eat? Certainly, it is intuitively appealing to provide consumers with accurate and comprehensive nutrition information. However, information on the package might not be sufficient to promote dietary change. Other intervention strategies are discussed later in this chapter.

EXHIBIT 17–1

Advertisers Use Fat and Cholesterol Claims to Promote Products

Although surveys have indicated that the American public has become more knowledgeable about serum cholesterol, consumers are confused about the specific roles of dietary fat, dietary cholesterol, and other nutritional factors in the prevention and treatment of high cholesterol. Food manufacturers commonly promote their products using claims related to cardiovascular health. In order to quantify the extent of these claims both in television commercials and on product packaging, one of the authors (JM) and her students conducted two studies.[1]

Initially, consumers' beliefs that specific claims indicated that a food would prevent high cholesterol were evaluated in a survey (e.g., "no cholesterol"; "97% fat free"). Consumers endorsed the majority of these claims. In Study 1, a representative sample of television time slots indicated that of all food commercials, 39 percent made at least one health claim; 58 percent of the commercials that made health claims made a target claim (i.e., one that consumers associate with high cholesterol prevention). Forty-one distinct target claim commercials were observed.

We were particularly interested in determining the prevalence of commercials making claims consumers associate with low cholesterol content about products actually high in fat. Thus, we categorized a claim as potentially misleading when the product derived more than 30 percent of its calories from total fat. The results were disturbing but not surprising: 51 percent of the target commercials made at least one claim that was potentially misleading, using our definition. In Study 2, we applied this definition to snack cracker packaging, and found that 58 percent of the products whose package contained a target claim were potentially misleading. As laws are passed and enforced to regulate nutrition information and claims, data such as these will provide a baseline to which future data can be compared.[2]

---

[1]J. A. Mayer, G. Flynn-Polan, P. Orlaski, & J. Workman. (1992, March). *These shoes contain no cholesterol: The prevalence of deceptive nutrition claims.* Paper presented at the 13th Annual Meeting of the Society of Behavioral Medicine, New York.
[2]U.S.D.H.H.S. (1990). *Healthy People 2000.* D.H.H.S. Publication No. (PHS) 91–50212, Washington, D.C.; and U.S.D.H.H.S. (1988). *The surgeon general's report on nutrition and health,* DHHS (PHS) Publication No. 88–50210, Washington, D.C.

PRIORITY SETTING

Healthy People 2000 includes objectives specific to fat and fiber, as well as more general, yet relevant, objectives. We have categorized the objectives by food content, food access, nutrient information, and consumption; each factor is addressed later in the sections on intervention and evaluation.

Food Content

1. Increase to at least 5,000 brand items the availability of processed food products that are reduced in fat and saturated fat (from 2,500 items in 1986).

Food Access

2. Increase to at least 90 percent the proportion of restaurants and institutional food service operations that offer identifiable, low-fat, low-calorie food choices, consistent with the *Dietary Guidelines for Americans* (about 70 percent of fast food and family restaurant chains with 350 or more units had at least one low-fat, low-calorie item on their menu).

3. Increase to at least 90 percent the proportion of school lunch and breakfast services and child care food services with menus that are consistent with the nutrition principles in the *Dietary Guidelines for Americans*.

Nutrient Information

4. Achieve useful and informative nutrition labeling for virtually all processed foods and at least 40 percent of fresh meats, poultry, fish, fruits, vegetables, baked goods, and ready-to-eat carry-away foods (from 60 percent of sales of processed foods regulated by FDA in 1988; baseline data on fresh and carry-away foods unavailable).
5. Increase to at least 85 percent the proportion of people aged 18 and older who use food labels to make nutritious food selections (from 74 percent in 1988).

Consumption

6. Reduce dietary fat intake to an average of 30 percent of calories or less and average saturated fat intake to less than 10 percent of calories among people aged two and older.
7. Increase complex carbohydrates and fiber-containing foods in the diets of adults to five or more daily servings for vegetables (including legumes) and fruits, and to six or more daily servings for grain products (from two and one-half servings of vegetables and fruits and three servings of grain products for women aged nineteen through fifty in 1985).[6] (The National Cancer Institute recommends 20 to 30 grams of fiber daily, not to exceed 35, from a baseline of approximately 11).[7]

Currently, the *Dietary Guidelines for Americans*[8] which were referred to in two of the above objectives are:

1. Eat a variety of foods.
2. Maintain healthy weight.
3. Choose a diet low in fat, saturated fat, and cholesterol.
4. Choose a diet with plenty of vegetables, fruits, and grain products.
5. Use salt and sodium only in moderation.
6. If you drink alcoholic beverages, do so in moderation.

Guideline 3 recommends 30 percent or less of calories from total fat and less than 10 percent of calories from saturated fat. Guideline 4 recommends at least three daily servings of vegetables, two of fruit, and six of grain products.[9]

The specific numbers and proportions noted in the above objectives will need to be adjusted, depending on the base rates in the target community (or part thereof). For example, a particular ethnic group may differ from the community as a whole on purchase/intake of some foods (and nutrients), but not others, as a function of culture, acculturation, income, and availability and promotion of specific food items.

RESEARCH, MONITORING, AND EVALUATION

The choice of research and evaluation strategies in nutrition promotion is determined by the specific endpoint of interest (e.g., mean percentage of calories from fat vs. mean grams of fat vs. number of people selecting a low-fat product), the focus of the intervention (e.g., monitoring product content vs. label content vs. product availability), the level of the intervention (e.g., changes in individuals vs. groups), and the scope of the intervention (e.g., an eight-week class vs. a three-year, broad-based community program). Four general categories of monitoring strategies (self-report, direct observation, biochemical, and indirect) are discussed below.

Self-report data via interviews and questionnaires are commonly relied upon for information on food/nutrient consumption. Several national surveys are implemented on an ongoing basis, including the National Health and Nutrition Examination Survey (HANES), and the National Health Interview Survey. The National Cholesterol Education Program, sponsored by the National Heart, Lung and Blood Institute (in conjunction with the FDA), have beem conducting cholesterol awareness surveys among the public and physicians since 1983.[10] Surveys such as these can be used with communities or smaller groups. Using them may be advantageous because (a) they provide validated, previously tested items (and procedures), and (b) they give us the opportunity to compare our target group to the national norms when adjusting priorities and evaluating progress.

The assessment of individual food intake to determine overall nutritional status is generally accomplished by twenty-four-hour recalls (usually via interview) or food frequency/history question-

---

EXHIBIT 17–2

Food Purchase Patterns in a Latino Community

In one study, the purchase patterns in grocery stores of predominately Latino versus Anglo customers were compared.[3] Because a computerized inventory system was not available, observers recorded purchases of selected items at various time intervals at two large supermarkets and one smaller grocery store in each community. Within each food category under study, a proportion was computed which was the number of "healthy" choices divided by the number of all choices within that category. In the milk category, all milks with 2 percent fat or less were combined. Of all milk purchases, "less fat" purchases comprised only 27 percent in the predominantly Latino stores and 68 percent in the comparison community. Lard comprised 43 percent and 13 percent of cooking fat purchases, respectively, in the Latino and comparison stores.

These data do not describe food and nutrient intake of the populations under study. However, if we assume that (a) the customers observed are representative of each community in their food purchasing patterns and (b) the relationship between purchases and intake was the same between the communities, the data indicated differences that should be considered when defining priorities for each group.

[3]R. M. Delapa, J. A. Mayer, J. Candelaria, N. Hammond, S. Peplinski, C. deMoor, G. Talavera, & J. Elder. (1990). Food purchase patterns in a Latino community: Project Salsa. *Journal of Nutrition Education, 22,* 133–136.

---

naires or interviews. The choice of a self-reported food intake strategy is determined by (a) availability of trained staff, (b) reading and recall level of your participants, (c) need for data representative of long-term intake (vs. a "snap-shot" approach, and (d) other resources (e.g., time, space, staff to score and analyze data).

Observational procedures, although relatively labor-intensive, can provide valuable information on eating or food purchasing behaviors in the natural environment. For example, in the study described in Exhibit 17–2, a computerized inventory system was not available. Additionally, observation at shelves and freezers was not time-efficient, and a manual inventory of specific items (e.g., number of milk cartons missing prior to restocking) was not feasible. Consequently, unobtrusive observations near the check-out line appeared to be the best method for evaluating the purchases of the several items of interest. Comparable observation procedures have been used to monitor food selection in cafeterias and restaurants.[11]

A third general strategy for monitoring nutrition-related behaviors consists of biochemical measures (forms of "permanent products"). These measures might be used either to replace or to verify and supplement self-report measures. Examples include serum cholesterol and fecal fat (fat intake), and urinary sodium (sodium intake). The use of these and other biochemical measures should be preceded by investigating their relationship with the target behavior or nutrient, their half-life, their sensitivity and specificity, their cost, and their acceptability to program participants.

A final group of measures overlapping with the previous categories are indirect measures. These include archival data (e.g., lists of low-fat products available from food manufacturers), behavioral by-products (e.g., amount of "plate-waste" in a school cafeteria), and physiological-based measures (e.g., scale weight). As with the other measurement categories, the use of these measures should be determined by research objectives.

INTERVENTION STRATEGIES FOR CHANGING FOOD CONTENT

The factors of food content, food accessibility, nutrient information and consumer nutrition skills may be conceptualized as links in the chain that leads to nutrient intake. These links provide logical targets for intervention. Ideally, interventions involving *all* factors are desirable. The community programs for reducing risks of cardiovascular disease provide examples of comprehensive, community-based approaches to "heart-healthier" eating (e.g., lowered fat intake), including building coalitions; making healthier food choices available in schools, restaurants, supermarkets, and work settings; and educating and motivating citizens through mass-media, organization, group, and individual procedures. The sections below describe a Pawtucket Heart Health Program (PHHP) community intervention and Project LEAN, a national campaign.

The Pawtucket Heart Health Program[12]

The Pawtucket Heart Health Program (PHHP) emphasized both food vendor interventions and weight loss programs among its nutritional interventions. The PHHP's aim was to influence Pawtucket residents to consume less sodium, less fat, and less cholesterol. The overall plan of attack involved (1) increasing the availability and marketing of heart-healthy foods in Pawtucket, and conversely, decreasing the availability and marketing of unhealthy foods, and (2) increasing consumer demand for heart-healthy foods. The latter strategy was implemented through group and individual self-help programs in nutrition and weight loss.

Increasing the availability of heart-healthy foods involved changes in the community environment. Such interventions provided an additional set of stimuli to promote, enhance, and maintain changes being implemented on the individual level. Food retailers and wholesalers played a key role in determining a community's food supply and in shaping eating habits. The cooperation of the local food vendors was viewed as crucial to the success of the nutrition component of a community heart-disease-prevention effort.

With such a mission in mind, the Pawtucket Heart Health Program formed a committee of representatives from the PHHP staff, local food vendors, and interested consumers. This committee, known as the BEAP or "Better Eating Around Pawtucket Committee," met biweekly. All community-level interventions related to modifying food-marketing practices of local food vendors were planned and implemented through this committee.

The first task of the BEAP committee was to interview at least eighteen "key informant" food vendors or related-interest individuals. The purpose of this activity was (1) to announce PHHP goals and presence in the community; (2) to solicit opinions regarding approaches PHHP could take to meet goals; (3) to avoid being viewed as a threat to food vendors' businesses; (4) to stimulate interest in participating in BEAP's activities; and (5) to get food vendors' views on local marketing and purchasing trends.

Six important dimensions were identified for consideration in obtaining food-vendor participation in improving the health-promoting quality of foods offered to the public. Four of these dimensions were sufficiently salient to help develop BEAP's approach to involve the food-vendor sector of the community. Specifically the following conclusions were reached:

1. **Consumer health concerns:** PHHP needed to create a market for heart-healthier food items. Consumers, therefore, were encouraged to request heart-healthy food selections regularly and patronize restaurants that offer such heart-healthy foods.

2. **Motivation for profit:** PHHP needed to recognize that the bottomline for all food vendors is profit. Thus, food vendors were apprised of the increasing trend toward heart-healthier food selections, as well as the increased profitability of certain heart-healthier foods versus unhealthy foods (e.g., chicken versus red meat, fatty red meat versus lean red meat, margarine versus butter), and other profit motives.

3. **Early-adopter strategy:** PHHP had to identify one or two early adopters and then highlight their successful programs to other food retailers in the community, and show retailers how to make changes that were inexpensive and easy. All adopters were provided with as much publicity as possible.

4. **Concerns of customers:** PHHP nutrition programs had to attend to customers' finances as well as to their food preferences in attempting to influence food choices. Participants were educated regarding the economic advantages of poultry, fish, and lean meats, and encouraged to read nutrition information listed on food labels in order to weigh nutritional value with price.

In the process of conducting key-informant interviews, an "early adopter" was identified in the form of a prominent local restaurant. This restaurant volunteered to be the site of a pilot project designed to test the acceptability of three types of menu-item descriptions: (1) health description, (2) taste plus a secondary health message, and (3) a nonspecific message. Results showed an increased trend towards the purchase of items described as both tasty and healthy.

Guided by the results of these assessment activities, the BEAP Committee developed a community-level approach to modifying food-marketing practices that centered around a four-heart rating system, parallel to the five-star rating system used in restaurants. The four hearts represented lower sodium, lower fat, lower cholesterol, and "great taste." Participating food vendors permitted the BEAP Committee to review the choices on shelves or menus and label those that met these criteria with a four-heart logo. Brochures, table tents, and posters throughout the restaurant or store explained the labeling program and encouraged folks to choose designated items not only because they were labeled heart healthy, but also because they were inexpensive and good tasting. Such a labeling system was designed to highlight and encourage the purchase of heart-healthy items already available, as opposed to requiring costly changes in menu items, food-preparation techniques, etc. The expense of maintaining such a system was minimized by use of PHHP volunteers.

This intervention program was flexible to be easily tailored to the needs of each restaurant. For example, one restaurant with a carry-home menu opted to create a separate menu insert that included standard menu items meeting the four heart criteria plus additional menu items that required only slight modification. Another restaurant opted to create coupons for 10 percent off four-heart meals. Still another restaurant instituted a contest to increase awareness of four-heart menu items.

The simplicity of the program ensured that BEAP members without specialized nutrition training were able to implement the program in any Pawtucket restaurant. The simplicity of the approach helped ensure the program was easily adopted and used by customers.

In order to give visibility to four-heart restaurants, the BEAP Committee regularly advertised four-heart restaurants and grocery stores in the local newspaper, at various PHHP community and organizational functions through billboard campaigns, and through various other Pawtucket mass- and mini-media channels. "A guide to heart-healthy eating in Pawtucket," listing all four-heart food vendors was developed and distributed throughout Pawtucket. The four-heart program was implemented in many Pawtucket restaurants and supermarkets, and in one wholesale dairy.

Project LEAN

Project LEAN (Low-fat Eating for America Now) is a multi-component national program initiated in 1988 by the Henry J. Kaiser Family Foundation. Its objectives are (a) to reduce dietary fat intake to 30 percent of calories by 1998, (b) to increase the availability of low-fat foods in supermarkets and eating establishments, and (c) to increase collaboration among national and community organizations committed to reducing dietary fat. Program components include (a) a media (electronic and print) campaign to increase the public's awareness of the dangers of dietary fat that links consumers with a toll-free number for obtaining further information, (b) actions directed toward "food influentials" (e.g., food manufacturers, grocery retailers, etc.) to increase the availability of lower fat foods, and (c) community-based programs coordinated through state or local agencies. Approximately ten community programs received funding from 1989 to 1991. Additionally, Project LEAN has developed a collaboration among at least two dozen co-sponsors, called Partners for Better Health (e.g., Centers for Disease Control; National Cancer Institute; American Heart Association; American Public Health Association; American Medical Association; American Association of Retired Persons; Produce Marketing Association).

INTERVENTION STRATEGIES FOR CHANGING FOOD CONTENT

In addressing food *content*, the idea of a food supply that is likely to provide an adequate amount of nutrients without excessive calories, fat, sodium, and sucrose is attractive to many. However, in the U.S. marketplace, this desire results in the addition of "healthy" products to the existing supply of products rather than removal (or "recall") of "unhealthy" products. Thus, a tour through most supermarkets reveals an incredibly large amount of variability in food categories with respect to nutrient content, from cookies with no fat to cookies which derive over 50 percent of their calories from fat. As part of the North Karelia Project, a cardiovascular risk-reduction program in Finland, manufacturers of a traditionally-eaten (and unhealthy) sausage were influenced into replacing the standard product with a lower-fat, lower-sodium version.[13] In the U.S., however, additions to the number of processed food products have been more prevalent than replacements. The new Nutrition Labeling and Education Act of 1990 may indirectly promote the development of new products. For example, if a company's product can no longer meet the FDA's criteria for claiming "low fat" using a standardized serving size, the company may lower the fat content. Product development will also be influenced by consumer demand.

INTERVENTION STRATEGIES FOR CHANGING FOOD ACCESSIBILITY

Access to lower fat and higher fiber foods should be determined for a given target group. For example, a calorie labeling intervention in a St. Louis, Missouri, worksite cafeteria did not result in a significant reduction in the mean caloric lunch intake.[14] An inventory of the options revealed a likely explanation: employees had few low-calorie, appetizing items to choose from. Through a committee of interested volunteers, these employees then approached the cafeteria vendor to request the addition of lower-calorie items. In a large company in San Diego, California, the costs of the employee recreation association, including the health and fitness programs, are subsidized by vending revenues. Until recently, only "mainstream" candy bars and sodas were available; fruit juices and more healthful snacks have now been added.

An environment that supports newly acquired nutrition awareness and skills by making tasty, nutritious food available is crucial to the maintenance of healthy eating. Strategies to increase availability and access include promotion of grass-roots organizing and lobbying at the local, state, and/or national level (e.g., Parent-Teachers Associations organizing to demand lower-fat, higher-complex carbohydrate school lunches), en-

dorsing supermarkets and restaurants that offer low-fat choices through positive publicity, and publicly embarrassing restaurants and supermarkets that offer only higher-fat products. For high-literate groups, lists and pamphlets can be developed to specify local supermarkets that facilitate "lower-fat" shopping (e.g., using color-coded labels), healthy products by brand name, restaurants with healthy options, and healthier options within fast-food chains. Both low- and high-literate participants can benefit from small group supermarket tours.

INTERVENTION STRATEGIES FOR CHANGING CUSTOMER KNOWLEDGE ABOUT NUTRIENT INFORMATION

Interventions should also target consumer awareness and knowledge. Using information campaigns, projects such as the National Cholesterol Education Program, LEAN, and Five-a-Day attempt to educate the public about (a) relationships between certain eating patterns (e.g., high fat, high cholesterol) and diseases (e.g., cardiovascular disease), (b) foods low and high in the targeted nutrients, and (c) ways to modify one's diet slowly (e.g., with shaping and fading procedures). The results of surveys show that consumer awareness has risen in the last decade.[15] However, consumers continue to be confused about the relative importance of dietary fat vs. dietary cholesterol, and about the sources of various types of fats. During the needs assessment phase, the knowledge level of the target population should be evaluated.

In recent years, point-of-choice (or point-of-purchase) instructional strategies have been popular. These have consisted primarily of labeling procedures in supermarkets and cafeterias that provide information in a descriptive way (e.g., providing fat content) or in a prescriptive way (i.e., directing consumers to "preferred" products such as low-fat items).[16] Labeling strategies have been effective in promoting more nutritious food selections in dining establishments (see Exhibit 17–3).

Of the supermarket point-of-choice interventions, results were mixed. The successful programs used brand-specific information, prescriptive strategies, and nutrient-avoidant rationales

EXHIBIT 17-3

Encouraging Cafeteria Customers to Choose Low-Fat Entrees

What would it take to entice a hungry cafeteria customer, whose mouth is watering for the fried chicken, to choose the broiled chicken or baked fish? We might guess money, a discounted dinner, or free movie or baseball tickets. However, in one controlled study,[4] all it took was a "stimulus control" approach with a simple poster and labeling strategy.

Across the phases of the study, the entree items (around 16 daily) were the same. However, during the intervention phases, (a) a large, colorful poster was placed at the entrance to the cafeteria line, and (b) low-fat entree menus were placed in the entree section. The poster contained a rationale for a low-fat diet, recommended broiled and baked foods and chicken and fish, and stated that day's low-fat entrees. Approximately three low-fat entrees were offered each day. The proportion of entrees purchased that were low-fat increased significantly when the intervention was implemented, from baseline levels of 20-27 percent to intervention levels of 34-37 percent (a relative increase of 85 percent).

This simple intervention provided a cost-effective method to influence point-of-choice eating behavior. However, when the researchers implemented the procedures at a second cafeteria, the intervention was ineffective. Observations of the customers revealed that the layout of the second cafeteria caused them to walk next to the food on the way to getting their tray; the customers' eyes were focused on the food rather than the poster. Unfortunately, there was no alternative placement for the poster (without remodeling the establishment). This failure pointed out the importance of the interplay between the physical environment and the point-of-choice strategy for influencing behavior.

[4]J. A. Mayer, J. M. Heins, J. M. Vogel, D. C. Morrison, L. D. Lankester, & A. L. Jacobs. (1986) Promoting low-fat entree choices in a public cafeteria. *Journal of Applied Behavior Analysis, 19,* 397-402.

(e.g., eating less vs. more of something). However, because these characteristics were not examined systemically (using control groups), we cannot know if they were responsible for the interventions' successes.

Supermarkets provide a challenging arena for intervention because of the many competing displays, some of which conflict with a health promotion message. Nevertheless, their potential as an intervention target is great because of the number of consumers who get repeated exposure to the information at the time and place where they make purchase decisions. Simple, prescriptive labels (e.g., blue shelf labels under low-fat items) in conjunction with package nutrient information, help consumers make more informed choices.

INTERVENTION STRATEGIES FOR CHANGING CONSUMER SKILLS

Finally, interventions can increase consumer skills related to choosing, preparing, and cooking healthier foods. The strategies for promoting these behaviors are usually targeted at the individual and group levels (chapters 12 and 13), and primarily include instructions, modeling and shaping, feedback, and positive reinforcement. However, as discussed in an earlier section, needs assessment and monitoring of the target behavior(s) should be conducted prior to implementing skills training in order to assess the participant's perceptions and values and baseline characteris-

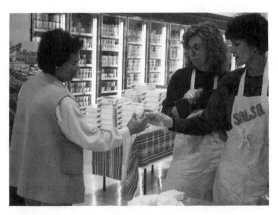

FIGURE 17–2. Point-of-choice interventions can be used to promote healthy grocery purchases. Here, a shopper is given a sample of "licuado," a refreshment made with low-fat milk. *Photo courtesy of Proyecto salsa.*

tics of the behavior. Subsequently, the baseline data should be used to set reasonable goals. For example, if we wish to include a label-reading component in a grocery store tour, it is important to know how naive or sophisticated about label-reading the target population is. Specifically, what is their reading level? Will they know the difference between saturated and unsaturated fat? How much practice will they need to accurately compute the percentage calories from fat once they are instructed to multiply the number of fat grams by 9 and then divide this product by the number of calories, and multiply by 100? Prior to a shaping procedure to promote consumption of non-fat milk, we should assess what kinds of milk the participants are currently drinking, what kinds of milk they have been exposed to previously, and their barriers to drinking non-fat milk (e.g., perceiving that it tastes like water). Often, self-monitoring procedures themselves require skills training in order to obtain accurate data. For example, participants completing food records should be trained a priori in how to report detailed information validly and reliably about the foods, serving sizes, etc. Furthermore, self-monitoring procedures, and their associated skills (e.g., determining the average grams of daily fiber) can serve to promote the target behavior. This type of measurement reactivity could occur, for example, when a participant becomes aware (e.g., receives

feedback from consulting a nutrient-value brochure) that removing the skins of certain fruits and vegetables results in a 20 percent reduction in daily fiber intake. Nevertheless, although self-monitoring and increased awareness may be adequate to motivate some changes for some people, more labor-intensive strategies are typically required.

In our experience, training at the group level and training via videotape provide potentially cost-effective formats for promoting changes in food selection (e.g., shopping), preparation, and cooking. As alluded to earlier grocery-store purchases determine in large part what is eaten at home. Thus, an intervention addressing the interaction between environmental (i.e., point-of-choice, food/labels) and person-related variables (i.e., skills, motivation) aimed at grocery shopping can have a substantial impact on a family's food consumption. The environmental half of the interaction was addressed previously. In addressing the skills half of the equation, the following questions, and others like these, should be asked when developing interventions. How might consumers take advantage of clearer, more informative food labels and/or color-coded shelf markers, that highlight "healthier" selections? Furthermore, how might consumers learn to identify labels that are (still) misleading (e.g., state the percentage of fat by weight) and to select the most nutritious products (e.g., fresh vs. frozen vs. canned vegetables)?

Grocery store tours, which have become more popular in recent years, provide an excellent format for training shopping skills. Typically conducted in groups, tours offer opportunities for both general and specific instruction, modeling (by the leader, other participants, and passersby), and feedback with positive reinforcement (usually in the form of verbal praise). Groups should be large enough to be cost-effective but small enough for participants to ask questions and receive some individualized feedback. For example, in a tour in which one of the authors (JM) participated, participants (approximately 7) were each asked to choose a package of cheese, to compute the percentage of calories from fat (the instructions of which had just been delivered by the leader), to form a line according to the fat content, and to describe the type of cheese and its fat content.

This exercise required practice of a skill previously taught (and corrective feedback if the calculation was inaccurate) and information from co-participants about the fat content of a variety of cheeses. Selecting the items from the shelves (vs. observing them in a classroom) more closely resembled an actual shopping session, and thus, the skills were more likely to generalize to participants' next shopping trip. To familiarize tour participants with new products that have qualities the tour leader promotes (e.g., low fat, cholesterol, and/or sodium), taste-testing is recommended to supplement label reading. In general, a relatively active approach (vs. passivity on the part of participants) results in higher interest level and greater learning of the information and skills. However, pamphlets and brochures that reiterate and/or add to the content covered in the tour can be used as hand-outs.

To train skills related to food preparation and cooking once the food is purchased, demonstration by a skilled cook with practice by and feedback to the learner is ideal, and can be cost-effective if implemented with groups. Moreover, participants have the opportunity to sample the finished products, which may serve as positive reinforcer and result in future preparation of those items. For reaching larger numbers of people on a wider scale, video taped cooking demonstrations are recommended. Although they cannot provide the direct feedback of in vivo training, they can provide influential modeling of the target skills and allow viewers to practice the procedures in an ongoing way throughout the session. For example, Project Salsa produced a Spanish-language videotape featuring a woman who had recently acquired skills for cooking heart-healthier foods demonstrating these skills in her kitchen to an initially skeptical friend. Finally, print materials such as cookbooks can be valuable in imparting food preparation and cooking skills if the language, reading level, and recipes are appropriate for the target population.

In determining which format or channel to use for training specific skills, we should keep in mind the skill level we wish the participants to attain and the training potential of each format. For example, a videotaped demonstration of shopping skills might not be as effective as an actual tour because (a) the store featured in the videotape may differ substantially from the viewer's own store in terms of merchandise, lay-out, etc., making generalizability less likely, and (b) the viewers do not have the opportunity for corrective feedback.

Two principles of behavior change particularly relevant to promoting healthier eating-related skills are shaping and stimulus control. These principles are common to strategies promoting shopping, preparation, cooking, and eating. Shaping is important because drastic changes in eating habits may produce immediate aversive consequences and thus have a low probability of being maintained. For example, increasing fiber intake by consuming large quantities of bran may result in flatulence, frequent bowel movements, and/or aversion to a "saw-dust" like taste or texture. Or, decreasing fat by switching from whole milk to nonfat milk may result in aversion to the "watery" taste or texture of the nonfat milk. Consequently, it is critically important to maintain the "enjoyability ratings" of eating and eating's social and cultural functions, while minimizing potential negative physical and economic consequences of the new eating patterns.

Following through with the examples presented above, bran would be added to the diet in small quantities. It might be added to one's favorite cereal, initially in the amount of one teaspoon with systematic increases over time. In home-baked goods, bran and/or whole wheat flour might be substituted for a small quantity of white flour, with gradual increases in the amount used. For a person who is familiar only with whole milk, low-fat (i.e., 2 percent) milk may be aversive even though the goal may be to "drink only nonfat milk." Consequently, the person might be instructed initially to mix whole with 2 percent in an acceptable proportion until the beverage is entirely 2 percent, then to mix 2 percent with either 1 percent or nonfat, and so on.

Stimulus control strategies typically involve changing the antecedents of the behavior and/or the environment in which the behavior occurs. In contrast to tobacco control objectives, living in a "fat-free" or "fiber-rich" environment may not be feasible. However, control over what foods are available at home is possible (i.e., "out of sight-out of mind"). Furthermore, restaurants offering healthier choices can be frequented. At home, preparation methods that increase the likelihood of eating healthier items are valuable (e.g., pre-mixing bran with cereal in bulk quantities; pre-chopping vegetables and having frozen vegetables on hand when fresh vegetables are not available).

SUMMARY

Interventions for changing nutritional behavior related to reducing dietary fat and increasing dietary fiber might address: the actual content of prepared foods, accessibility to/availability of certain foods, consumer knowledge of nutrient information of certain foods (e.g., point-of-choice displays), and development of consumer skills for reaching the dietary targets; an intervention that addresses all of these factors is ideal. The specific intervention strategies described in this chapter would be most effective in an environment that supports the changes. Clearer, more comprehensive and accurate messages on commercials and packages will be a step in the right direction to creating that environment, but should not be viewed as a panacea. The variables influencing eating behavior are many and complex, but if approached systematically using the principles and strategies described in this text, the objectives of the year 2000 specific to fat and fiber are achievable.

ADDITIONAL READINGS

Between the spices and sauces, keep these references handy:

1. D. Nieman, D. Butterworth, & C. Nieman. (1990). *Nutrition.* Dubuque, IA: William C. Brown.
2. California Department of Health Services. (1990, April). *The California daily food guide: Dietary guidance for Californians.* Sacramento: California DHS.
3. S. Gershoff. (1991). *The Tufts University guide and total nutrition.* New York: Harper Collins.

ENDNOTES

1. U.S.D.H.H.S. (1988). *The surgeon general's report on nutrition and health,* DHHS (PHS) Publication No. 88-50210, Washington, D.C., p. v.
2. U.S.D.H.H.S. (1990). *Healthy people 2000,* DHHS Publication No. (PHS) 91-50212, Washington, D.C.
3. U.S.D.H.H.S. *The surgeon general's report on nutrition and health.*
4. U.S.D.H.H.S. (1990). Food and Drug Administration Food Labeling: Health messages and label statements; reproposed rules. *Federal Register, 55,* 5176–5192.
5. However, see chapter 21 for a discussion of the highly successful Nestle-Boycott.
6. U.S.D.H.H.S. *Healthy people 2000.*
7. U.S.D.H.H.S. (1987). PHS, NCI. *Diet, nutrition and cancer prevention: The good news.* NIH Publication No. 87-2878, Bethesda, MD.
8. U.S.D.A. & U.S.D.H.H.S. (1990). *Nutrition and your health: Dietary guidelines for Americans.* Home & Garden Bulletin No. 232.
9. Ibid.
10. Schucker, B., Witter, J. T., Santanello, N. C., et al. (1991). Change in cholesterol awareness and action: Results from national physician and public surveys. *Archives of Internal Medicine, 151,* 666–673. For a comprehensive listing of nutrition monitoring activities in the U.S., please refer to *Nutrition monitoring in the United States: The directory of federal nutrition monitoring activities.*
11. Mayer, J. A., Dubbert, P. M., & Elder, J. P. (1989). Promoting nutrition at the point of choice: A review. *Health Education Quarterly, 16,* 31–43.
12. Elder, J. P., Abrams, D. B., Beaudin, P. A., Carleton, R. A., Lasater, T. M., Lazieh, M., Peterson, G. S., & Schwertfeger, R. Behavioral community psychology and the prevention of heart disease: Community-level application of the Pawtucket Heart Health Program. *Perspectives on Behavioral Medicine, 3,* 1988.
13. Nissinen, A., Tuomilehto, J., Elo, J., et al. (1981). Implementation of a hypertension control program in the county of North Karelia, Finland. *Public Health Reports, 96,* 503–513.
14. Mayer, J. A., Brown, T. P., Heins, J. M., & Bishop, D. B. (1987). A multi-component intervention for modifying food selections in a worksite cafeteria. *Journal of Nutrition Education, 19,* 277–280.
15. Schucker, Witter, & Santanello, Change in cholesterol awareness and action, results from national physician and public surveys.
16. Generally, supermarket point-of-choice strategies do not refer to the actual package labeling referred to earlier, but to additional posters and shelf labels near the products.

Chapter 18

Preventing Injuries and Deaths from Vehicle Crashes

OBJECTIVES

By the end of this chapter, the reader should be able to:

1. State reasons for considering vehicle safety belt use a priority health behavior.
2. Design a community-based and corporate-based intervention program for increasing safety belt use on a large scale.
3. Specify real-world environmental factors that increase or decrease the risk of drunken driving.
4. Design a server-intervention program for decreasing the risk of drunken driving.
5. Evaluate the effectiveness of a community-based or corporate-based program to increase the use of vehicle safety belts or child safety belts.
6. Recommend ways to increase the beneficial impact of ongoing community programs designed to increase vehicle safety or decrease the frequency of drug-impaired driving.

INTRODUCTION

Injury is the primary cause of lost person-years of productive life in the U.S.[1] The number of years lost annually to injuries of Americans exceed those lost from cancer by 2.4 million years and heart disease by 2.0 million years of life.[2] And, of the total number of injuries in the U.S., injury from motor vehicle crashes accounts for approximately 45 percent.[3] Although the highway fatality rate in 1990 reached a historic low of 2.1 deaths per 100 million miles of travel, that year there still were more than 44,000 fatalities and 400,000 serious injuries from vehicle crashes. In 1985 alone, approximately 43,800 people in the U.S. died in traffic accidents, and 3.5 million were injured.[4] Vehicle crashes are the single leading cause of death and injury to Americans between the ages of four and thirty-five,[5] and cost our country more than $100 million annually,[6] ranking second only to cancer.[7]

The 1979 report from the Surgeon General identified people and their behavior as the major contributor to poor health, injuries, and death.[8] The basic idea is that unhealthy or injury-prone lifestyles result from excess unhealthy (or unsafe) behaviors and deficient healthy (or safe) behaviors.[9] One particular behavioral excess and one particular behavioral deficit have been identified as contributing most to injuries and fatalities from vehicle crashes: too much alcohol consumption and too little safety belt use. In the U.S., alcohol is estimated to have contributed to 50–55 percent of fatal vehicle accidents and 18–25 percent of injury-producing crashes.[10] The use of shoulder and lap belts is the single most protective measure that can be conveniently taken to reduce the risk of death or injury in a vehicle crash. In fact, it has been estimated that 55 percent of all fatalities and 65 percent of all injuries from vehicle crashes would have been prevented if safety belts had been used,[11] yet observational surveys have indicated that about 75 percent of adults and 50 percent of children (0 to 4 years) fail to use a vehicle safety belt or child safety seat.[12] An increase of only 10 percent safety belt use nationwide would prevent as many as 30,000 injuries, save 1,500 lives and $800 million in direct costs.[13] Studies of the hospital costs resulting from vehicle crashes have shown such costs to be twice as high for unbelted as for belted vehicle occupants.[14]

LOCALITY DEVELOPMENT AND SOCIAL PLANNING

From a policy or legal perspective, significant steps have been made in recent years to reduce alcohol-impaired driving and increase use of safety belts and child safety seats. Stricter penalties for driving under the influence of alcohol (DUI), liability legislation for the servers of alcoholic beverages, and increased enforcement of anti-drunken driving legislation (including police roadblocks for DUI checks) are commonplace throughout the U.S. Moreover, 41 states have increased the minimum legal drinking age to 21.[15] In the domain of occupant protection, all 50 states and the District of Columbia have now passed legislation requiring young children (from 0 to 4 years in most states) to be protected in child safety seats[16]; and at the time of this writing, 34 states had enacted mandatory safety belt use laws (BUL) for adults.[17]

The legislative attempts to reduce drunken driving and increase the use of vehicle safety belts and child safety seats have made beneficial differences in injuries and fatalities from vehicle crashes, but much more behavior change is necessary. Actually, the deterrence effects of stricter DUI laws and increased enforcement have been generally mild and transitory, largely because of the low risk of punishment—about one DUI arrest per 5,000 miles of drunken driving.[18] Raising the legal drinking age has significantly reduced injuries and deaths in the age group affected,[19] but this impact is actually minuscule considering the overall drunken-driving problem.[20]

Safety belt use has increased dramatically in virtually every state that passed a belt use law (BUL). For example, during the last six months of 1985, observations of safety belt use by front-seat occupants in 17 states without a BUL revealed 21.6 percent buckled up,[21] whereas the mean post-BUL belt use across 27 states was 48 percent.[22] However, safety belt use following a BUL has declined rather markedly after the media attention and has rarely stabilized above 50 percent in the U.S. Therefore, legislation has not been sufficient to change the U.S. deficit of vehicle safety belt use. In fact, it is generally believed that the safest drivers are the first to comply with a BUL, and therefore the most prominent decreases in injuries from vehicle crashes will not occur until the second 50 percent buckle up—those currently disregarding belt use laws.[23] Although the rate of buckling infants and toddlers in child safety seats has increased dramatically in the U.S. as a result of child restraint laws,[24] a study of the pre- vs. post-law fatality rates among young children in 11 states showed minimal differences.[25] This outcome was partially due to ineffective use of available safety seats by as many as 70 percent of the users.[26] It is also likely that parents at the highest risk for a vehicle crash are least likely to protect their children in an appropriate safety seat.

School and college settings often represent the last important opportunity for increasing group awareness of drinking and driving issues and teaching a socially responsible approach to alcohol consumption. In fact, alcohol awareness groups based at high schools, e.g., Students Against Drunk Drivers (SADD) and colleges have been among the most innovative and active in encouraging socially responsible drinking. Obviously, no single approach is sufficient to prevent injuries and fatalities from drunk driving and nonuse of safety belts. There is, in fact, an urgent need for a comprehensive nationwide attack on these behavioral problems by politicians, corporate leaders, employee groups, health and medical professionals, educators, media writers and producers, grass-roots agencies, civic and service clubs, and family members. The good news is that many grass-roots groups, government agencies, enforcement officials, and treatment professionals are available to help implement effective behavior change interventions to reduce DUI risk and increase safety belt use. Unfortunately, the combined social action and social planning focus of these groups has been on the development and enforcement of ineffective contingencies for punishing the alcohol-impaired driver and the non-user of vehicle safety belts. Striking a better balance between "carrot and stick" (i.e., reward vs. penalty approaches) in the interventions of these groups is yet another pressing challenge for the behavior change professional who wants to make a difference in road safety.

ASSESSING NEEDS AND RESOURCES

The Needs/Resources Assessment (N/RA) phase starts with a look at some of the organizations working in this area and the activities they are undertaking. Do Mothers Against Drunk Drivers (MADD), Students Against Drunk Drivers (SADD), and similar organizations exist in the target community? If so, for how long have they been active, and what have they accomplished? Where are they headed?

Other youth-oriented resources can be assessed in local high schools. What are the quality and extent of their driver education courses? What other programs exist in the school? Is there a college nearby? Are there any "responsible drinking" initiatives in the local schools or colleges? Conversely, what promotions are sponsored by the alcohol industry, either on a college campus or in the community in general?

Police, hospital, and death records should provide adequate sources of local accident rates as well as causal or contributing factors. Police can also provide DUI arrest records and tickets given for not using safety belts and child safety seats.

Although safety belt promotions by the auto industry are generally conducted on a large scale, local dealerships should be contacted to see what they or others (e.g., the American Automobile Association) are doing to promote motor vehicle safety. If bartender organizations exist, their leadership may be able to provide an opinion as to the potential for server intervention training in the area, as well as providing access to bartenders and

wait personnel to receive the training. Medical associations or their pediatric subgroups should be able to give an estimate of the amount of promotion taking place among these potential intervention agents.

Finally, the health professional can simply use his or her own eyes to see the prevalence of safety belt use by looking for that familiar diagonal silhouette to the outside of any driver or passenger seated by a door. On a more systematic basis, this observational procedure can be used to monitor and evaluate the impact of a given program to increase safety belt use.

PRIORITIES

The challenge for everyone who could receive an unintentional injury at home, at the workplace, or on the road is to focus on prevention. However, motivating individuals to act for prevention is most difficult because rewards to support such behavior are usually not available. Instead, the unsafe or unhealthy alternatives are often followed by immediate pleasures. Therefore, not only do prevention behaviors usually lack immediate reinforcing consequences, they often compete with alternative unsafe or unhealthy behaviors which are reinforced. This chapter reviews interventions to change two of the most critical behaviors responsible for unintentional injury — nonuse of vehicle safety belts and driving a vehicle while under the influence of alcohol (DUI).

Compared to most prevention strategies that require repeated responding in order to be preventive (e.g., exercising regularly, wearing protective work clothing, brushing teeth, eating nutritious food), using a vehicle safety belt is not only most convenient, it is also most likely to pay off in substantial dividends. Since safety belt use requires minimal response cost and is intuitively protective (once certain myths about belts and crashes are dispelled), basic principles of large-scale behavior change are directly applicable; and because safety belt use or non-use can be readily observed in field settings, it is possible to evaluate the ongoing efficacy of different applications of behavior change principles. Indeed, a number of strategies have been developed for increasing safety belt use in a variety of community settings, including schools, universities, industries, banks, churches, and naval bases. It is encouraging that most of these interventions can be successfully delivered by indigenous personnel or volunteer groups, and they have been willingly sponsored by both the private and public sectors.

Attacking drunken driving with behavior change interventions has not been nearly as straightforward as intervening to increase safety belt use. To decrease inappropriate behavior, behavior change specialists typically focus on increasing the occurrence of behaviors incompatible with the undesired behavior. This is a more appropriate approach to DUI prevention than the current punishment strategies receiving increased attention in the U.S. Because it has been impossible to administer the kind of punishment contingency for DUI that works — one with a consequence that is frequent, consistent, immediate, and adequately severe — catching an alcohol-impaired driver is usually not corrective nor rehabilitative, and the threat of such punishment for DUI is not a long-term deterrent.

The initial challenge for a positive reinforcement approach to DUI prevention is to define situations and behaviors that decrease the risk of DUI. In particular, certain environmental conditions have been studied as potential facilitators or inhibitors of excessive drinking (e.g., the size of drinking groups and drink containers, the availability of breathalizers for blood alcohol concentration feedback, "happy hour" incentives, labels on beer kegs). In addition, one mechanism has been studied for applying the results of this research to prevent DUI (i.e., through server intervention). It is clear, however, that DUI prevention research is only in its infancy.

The following are among the *Healthy People 2000* objectives for unintentional injury control in the U.S. relevant to the present chapter.

1. Reduce deaths caused by unintentional injuries to no more than 29.3 per 100,000 people.
2. Reduce deaths caused by motor vehicle crashes to no more than 16.8 per 100,000 people (30 percent of which would come from reductions in motorcycle, bicycle and pedestrian deaths).
3. Reduce deaths caused by alcohol-related motor vehicle crashes to no more than 8.5 per 100,000 people.
4. Increase the use of occupant protection systems to 85 percent of motor vehicle occupants.

5. Extend to 50 states legal blood alcohol concentration tolerance levels of .04 percent for motor vehicle drivers aged 21 and older and .00 percent for those younger than 21.

As can be seen, these objectives range from the very specific to the general, and apply behavior change, policy and engineering strategies. The present chapter shows how these divergent areas can be integrated into single health promotion efforts.

RESEARCH ISSUES

Motivating Safety Belt Use

Because many cost-effective techniques for increasing safety belt use have been identified, it cannot be assumed that continued research on safety belt promotion is any less important than work on DUI prevention. In fact, the opposite is true. Much of the safety belt research reviewed in this chapter raises important empirical questions. For example, in order to increase the greatest number of safety belt users over the longest period of time, it is necessary to study: (a) various schedules for delivering and fading buckle-up reinforcers; (b) different combinations of incentives and commitment procedures[27]; (c) differential effects of various intervention strategies on adults vs. children, blue-collar vs. white-collar workers, and employees vs. retired persons; (d) comparative cost-effectiveness of implementing safety belt programs at corporations, schools, recreational facilities, churches, and local businesses; (e) long-term effects of combining behavior change strategies such as incentive/reinforcements programs for safety belt use and disincentive/punishment strategies for non-use of safety belts; and (f) tactics for mobilizing groups of people and resources for implementing community-wide programs for safety belt promotion.

Engineering Innovations

Although the installation of airbags in new car models is increasing and automatic safety belts are nearly universal, reliance on the behavior of the occupants to protect themselves and their children passengers will continue into the foreseeable future. For example, the lap belt is more protective against fatalities[28] than shoulder belts and airbags, yet many automatic systems only include shoulder belts. Most lap belts still require manual buckling.

Buzzer-light reminders in contemporary vehicles, a common method of prompting safety belt use, generally consist of only a panel light and a pleasant chime that initiates when the ignition key is turned on if the driver is not buckled up and terminates in four to eight seconds. When people start their vehicle before buckling up it is not possible to avoid the reminder tone, which was the case for about 50 percent of 1,492 field observations. This prompted General Motors Research Laboratories to loan one of the authors (E.S.G.) a research vehicle (i.e., a 1984 Cadillac) that provided any one of the following reminder systems: (a) the standard 4–8 second buzzer or chime that initiates upon engine ignition; (b) a 4–8 second buzzer or chime that initiates 5 seconds after engine ignition; (c) a voice reminder ("Please fasten your safety belt") that initiates 5 seconds after engine ignition and offers a "Thank you" after the driver's belt is buckled; and (d) a second reminder option whereby the 4–8 second buzzer, chime, or verbal prompt initiates if the driver is not buckled when the vehicle makes its first stop after exceeding 10 miles per hour.[29]

Two consistent findings from research comparing these types of prompts were that the vocal reminder in lieu of the buzzer or chime increased belt use prominently in three out of five cases,[30] and the second reminder was effective at increasing belt use in two out of seven subjects.[31] Delaying the buzzer reminder 5 seconds after engine ignition had no impact. However, much more research with this and alternative reminder systems is needed before reliable conclusions can be made.

Server Intervention

Although current research in the area of teaching bar personnel to prevent intoxication among customers indicates promise, much more research and development of this concept is needed. For example, the impact of any training program will be transitory if the behaviors taught during the training are not supported by the environmental context in which they are to occur. Thus, trained competencies to monitor alcohol consumption for potential DUI-risk will not be used consistently unless reinforced by natural or contrived contingencies. The policy in some bars, for example, is to provide wait personnel a guaranteed 15 percent gratuity if a drinker must be "cut-off" from excessive consumption or forcibly prevented from driving a vehicle. Geller et al. reported a natural contingency that might be particularly effective in maintaining the behaviors taught during server intervention training; namely, customers' gratuities tended to be higher after the wait personnel received server intervention training.[32] Further field research along these lines is critically needed, as well as comparative studies of different techniques to teach and maintain server intervention behaviors to decrease DUI risk.

The rationale for this server intervention is based on the behavior analysis principle that the optimal time to intervene for behavior change is at the place where the target behavior has an opportunity to occur. Server intervention is a DUI prevention strategy that meets this behavior change criterion, in contrast with the standard DUI education and awareness messages which are typically delivered to persons when they are sober and remote from the milieu that sets the occasion for DUI risk.

INTERVENTIONS FOR PROMOTING VEHICULAR SAFETY

Prompts

Vehicle Reminder Systems. Over the years, a variety of buzzer-light reminder systems have been included in motor vehicles. Most intrusive was the buzzer that continued to sound until the front-seat safety belts were buckled. Such "unlimited" buzzer reminders, as well as the ignition interlock system that required front-seat safety belts to be buckled for the vehicle to start, were undermined by a majority of vehicle owners either by disconnecting the buzzer or by sitting on a buckled belt.[33] Thus, these intrusive systems were short-lived.

Buckle-Up Reminder Stickers. Simple buckle-up stickers are available in various formats for exhibition on vehicle dashboards. Thyer and Geller studied the behavioral impact of a 1.5" x

2.5" sticker with the message "Safety Belt Use Required in This Vehicle" by asking 24 graduate students to keep systematic records of the safety belt use of passengers traveling in the front seat of their vehicles before, during, and after sticking the reminder to the passenger-side dashboard of their vehicle.[34] This intervention doubled safety belt use (from 34 percent to over 70 percent). Rogers found similar dashboard reminders to increase safety belt use by approximately 400 percent (i.e., from 10 percent to 38 percent) among drivers of state-owned vehicles.[35]

The "Flash for Life" Reminder.   About a decade ago, Geller developed a "Flash for Life" approach to safety belt promotion, whereby a person displayed to vehicle occupants the front side of an 11" x 14" flash card that read, "Please Buckle Up—I Care."[36] If the vehicle occupant buckled up after viewing this message, the "flasher" flipped the card over to display the bold words, "Thank You for Buckling Up." For the first evaluation of this behavior change tactic, the "flashee" was in the front seat of a stopped vehicle and the "flasher" was the driver of an adjacent, stopped vehicle. The flash card was shown to 1,087 unbuckled drivers, and of the 82 percent who looked at the flash card, 22 percent complied with the buckle-up request on the spot.

Education.   Over the years, educational strategies for prompting safety belt use have been numerous, varying from simple television prompts to comprehensive public education campaigns involving countrywide dissemination of signs, billboards, radio and TV advertisements, school programs, films, slide shows, and pamphlets. Typically, the impact of these educational efforts on safety belt use has been negligible, whether applied in employee safety programs,[37] through home television,[38] or throughout an entire community in varied formats.[39]

Modeling

People set both appropriate and inappropriate examples, and in the process influence the behavior of observers. Sometimes the number of observers can be numerous, and therefore the behavioral influence can be large scale. For example, when TV stars buckle-up, some viewers learn how to put on a safety belt, others are reminded that they should buckle-up on every vehicle trip, and still others realize that safety belt use is normative behavior. On the other hand, the frequent non-use of safety belts on TV can create or support the attitude that certain types of individuals (e.g., macho males or sexy females) do not use safety belts.

Contracting

Commitment and goal-setting tactics request verbal or written statements from individuals or

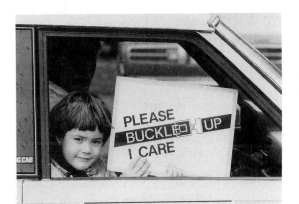
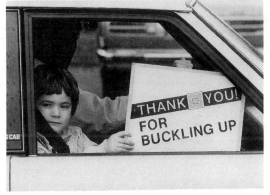

FIGURE 18–1.   In the "Flash for Life" intervention, Karly (age three and one-half) combines stimulus control and positive reinforcement for promoting seatbelt use among passengers in other cars stopped next to her father. *Photo courtesy of Scott Geller.*

groups promising they will perform a certain behavior (see chapter 12). Substantial increases in safety belt use were observed after buckle-up pledge cards were distributed and signed at an industrial site,[40] a community hospital,[41] during a church service,[42] and throughout a university campus.[43]

The Geller et al. study[43] was a long-term and large-scale investigation conducted on the Virginia Tech campus with 22,000 students. During the spring and fall academic quarters, 1986 buckle-up pledge cards were available throughout the campus (10,000 in the spring and 18,000 in the fall). Signing this pledge card implied a commitment to use vehicle safety belts for an entire academic quarter. Depositing a detachable portion of the pledge card in one of several raffle boxes located throughout the campus enabled entry into weekly random drawings of prizes donated by local merchants. The remainder of the pledge card was designed for hanging from a vehicle's inside

rear-view mirror or radio knob as a reminder of one's commitment to buckle-up.[44] By requesting pledge card signers to write the vehicle's license plate number on the pledge card and by recording vehicle license plate numbers during systematic observation of campus safety belt use, Geller was able to dichotomize the belt observations according to whether the driver had signed a pledge card. Since parking decals were also recorded during belt audits, it was possible to categorize the belt use data according to whether the vehicle driver was faculty/staff or a student.

During each phase of the study, faculty/staff drivers used safety belts significantly more often than students. Those who signed a buckle-up pledge were buckled up more often than those who did not. During both the spring and fall pledge-card lotteries, faculty/staff pledgers ($n =$ 208) went from a high pre-pledge belt use level of 56.4 percent to a post-pledge level of 75.9 percent, and students who signed pledge cards ($n =$

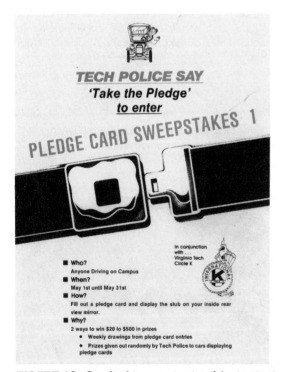

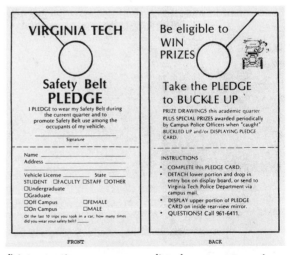

FIGURE 18–2. In this organizational (or institutional) intervention, a campus police department used a series of motivational procedures whereby students, faculty, and staff pledged to use their safety belts and were thereby eligible for cash prizes in weekly raffles of signed pledge cards. *Photos courtesy of Scott Geller.*

252) increased their belt use from a pre-pledge use of 49.3 percent a post-pledge level of 69.8 percent.

Positive Reinforcement to Increase Safety Belt Use

Promoting safety belt use by reinforcing individuals for signing a buckle-up pledge card has been termed an *indirect* reinforcement strategy, in contrast to the *direct* approach of reinforcing an individual directly for using a safety belt.[45] Reinforcers are *direct* and *immediate* response consequences when vehicles are stopped and occupants are reinforced on-the-spot for being buckled up. On the other hand, vehicles with occupants using safety belts can be identified (e.g., by recording license plate numbers) and the occupants can be contacted later to receive reinforcing consequences for being buckled up. This is a *direct* and *delayed* reinforcement strategy. According to principles of reinforcement, the direct and immediate approach should be most effective at increasing safety belt use, and the indirect reinforcers should be least effective. However, reviews of the literature have generally shown these reinforcement strategies to be equivalently effective at motivating the use of safety belts.[46] This may be the case partly because buckling a vehicle safety belt is a relatively convenient response chain and readily becomes a habit.

Direct and Immediate Reinforcers. On-the-spot consequences for direct and immediate reinforcement programs have usually been inexpensive and have varied widely in type (e.g., flowers, candy, balloons, baseball caps, trinkets, lottery tickets, silver dollars, or coupons exchangeable for money or food). It has been particularly worthwhile to solicit donations for prizes from community businesses. This reduces the program expense while involving the local community in a worthwhile safety effort. Most community merchants appreciate the special goodwill advertising available for their support of a local safety belt program.[47] Whether implemented at industrial sites,[48] shopping malls,[49] bank exchange windows,[50] high schools,[51] or universities,[52] direct reinforcers for safety belt use have at least doubled the baseline percentage of those buckled up in target vehicles. Although belt use has dropped substantially after the removal of an incentive/re-

inforcement program, in most cases the post-treatment follow-up levels of belt use have remained significantly higher than the pre-treatment baseline levels.

None of the direct and immediate reinforcement programs referred to so far targeted young children, perhaps the most critical age group for developing a buckle-up habit. Michael Roberts and his colleagues have successfully applied direct and immediate reinforcers to protect children in vehicles by reinforcing parents with lottery tickets redeemable for prizes if their children (ages 0.5 to 6 years) were appropriately buckled up when arriving at day-care centers,[53] by reinforcing preschool-age children directly with colorful stickers when they arrived at day-care centers,[54] and by teaching PTA volunteers to reinforce elementary school children with lapel stickers, lottery tickets for pizzas, bumper stickers, and colorful books if all vehicle occupants were buckled up when arriving at school.[55] In all of these child-directed studies, the use of safety belts or child safety seats increased dramatically, from baseline buckle-up averages as low as 5 percent[56] and 11 percent[57] to usage levels of 70 percent and 64 percent, respectively, during the intervention program. When these reinforcement programs were withdrawn, safety belt use declined but remained prominently higher than the initial baseline levels, as with the reinforcement programs that targeted adults.[58] Actually, the residual effects of the child-directed programs have been notably higher than typically found with safety belt programs that targeted adults (i.e., high school students, college students, and company employees).

Direct and Delayed Reinforcers. Sometimes reinforcers for safety belt use must be delayed because vehicles cannot be stopped conveniently and safely for behavioral observation and reinforcement delivery. For this type of program, shoulder belt use is observed as vehicles enter or exit the plant, and without stopping the vehicles, the license plate number of vehicles with buckled occupants are recorded for a subsequent prize drawing. The winning license plate numbers are publicly posted, and the owners of the identified vehicles claim their prizes at an announced location. Kalsher et al. adapted this delayed reinforcement strategy for the largest naval base in the world (with approximately 75,000 vehicles entering the base daily) by using the navy base police to collect license plate numbers for weekly prize lotteries.[59] The use of indigenous personnel (i.e., police officers) to administer the large-scale navy base programs was particularly advantageous. Even though the police officers collected a substantial number of license plate numbers (i.e., 20 officers recorded a total of 16,000 raffle entries during the four-week navy base program), none of the officers reported disruption in their daily duties. This suggests that a police-administered, delayed reinforcement program for safety belt promotion is feasible for communitywide or even statewide application. It is likely that such a program would make the enforcement of a state mandatory belt use law more palatable to both the police and the public, and would increase the number of safety belt users.

Geller et al. compared the impact of six corporate-based, direct and immediate reinforcement programs for safety belt promotion with the results of five direct and delayed programs and found no significant differences.[60] The six immediate reinforcement programs increased safety belt use among employees an average of 137 percent above baseline, and the five delayed programs increased employee belt use an average of 101 percent above the baseline levels. Those programs that included long-term follow-up assessment (i.e., four immediate and four delayed reinforcement programs) found steady declines in belt use but with some residual effects. The follow-up records of the immediate reinforcement programs (taken 1 month to 2 years after the program; *Mean* = 7.0 months) showed an average belt use 62 percent above the pre-intervention baseline levels. The residual effects for the delayed reinforcement programs averaged only 15 percent above the initial baseline levels, however.

Indirect Reinforcement. The pledge card strategy discussed earlier as a personal commitment intervention is considered an indirect reinforcement technique when reinforcers are given for signing the buckle-up pledge.[61] For these programs, reinforcers were not given directly for individual safety belt use; rather, individuals signed buckle-up pledge cards in order to enter raffle drawings. Thus, the behavior of making a personal commitment to buckle-up was reinforced. For example, it was impossible to develop an equitable system for choosing winners among the 6,000 potential safety belt users entering or exiting the six gates across two work shifts at the General Motors (GM) Technical Center and, therefore, an indirect reinforcement strategy was developed and implemented. Every employee was given a chance to enter the GM "Seatbelt Sweepstakes" if they signed a buckle-up pledge card committing the signer to use vehicle safety belts for one year. This program increased safety belt use at the GM Tech Center from 36 percent to an average belt use percentage of 60 percent two years after the program was terminated.[62]

Group-Level Reinforcement. Besides the individual pledge-card contingency, the GM "Seatbelt Sweepstakes" included a group contingency to motivate safety belt use. Specifically, the group (i.e., the entire work force of 6,000 employees) had to reach a certain percentage of safety belt use (i.e., the group goal) before each of three successive prize drawings were held in which a new automobile was the first prize. Employees reported incidents of peer pressure to buckle up in order to achieve each goal, and the successively increasing goals per raffle of 55 percent, 65 percent, and 70 percent belt use were, in fact, reached.

Another group-based reinforcement contingency was implemented by Geller and Hahn to increase the impact of their corporate-based safety belt program.[63] For this direct and delayed reinforcement program, a single cash prize was raffled off each week from the pool of license plate numbers collected from daily observations of safety belt use. The amount of the cash award for each weekly raffle was determined by the average percentage of safety belt use by the work group during the preceding week (i.e., the cash prize amounted to one dollar per percentage point). A feedback chart displayed the mean safety belt use each day and reminded the workers of their group-based reinforcement contingency. This public posting of daily group progress probably had motivating properties of its own, as found in a variety of community-based programs for motivating behavior change.[64]

INTERVENTIONS FOR DRUNKEN DRIVING PREVENTION

Excessive alcohol consumption and drunken driving are target behaviors influenced by certain environmental events or conditions which precede and follow these responses. For example, incentives might be available to encourage excessive drinking (e.g., 2-for-1 prices during "happy hour") or the assignment of sober individuals to do the driving (e.g., free food and soft drinks for a "designated driver"). Alternatively, a disincentive could discourage alcohol consumption (e.g., the checking of ID cards by police officers) or Driving Under the Influence (DUI) (e.g., the announcement of a police roadblock). Likewise, certain consequences can encourage continued alcohol consumption (e.g., peer support and social attention for participating in drinking games) or discourage future alcohol-impaired driving (e.g., being stopped at a DUI checkpoint). In addition, the efficacy of particular intervention strategies to prevent DUI (e.g., feedback of Breath Alcohol Content (BAC), DUI-prevention training for the servers of alcohol, the availability of safe driving alternatives) depend upon the antecedent conditions and the reinforcing or punishing consequences. The remainder of this chapter highlights intervention research that targeted the critical societal problem of alcohol-impaired driving.

The DUI problem is substantially more complex and difficult to influence than the problem of low safety belt use, and thus requires more than an antecedent-behavior-consequence analysis. For example, the impact of a behavior change intervention for DUI prevention is influenced by a number of individual factors (e.g., age, gender, genetics, attitudes, and drinking history) that predispose a person to drink excessively or DUI. In other words, one cannot assume that a given set of marketing, educational, and behavior change interventions will have the same effect across individuals.

Feedback Interventions

Some have argued that drinkers are not always aware of their alcohol impairment, and that receiving personal feedback about one's BAC may reduce the possibility of DUI.[65] Feedback regarding a drinker's level of intoxication impairment can be readily available at bar and party settings in the form of: (a) a BAC chart called a "nomogram," (b) a breath alcohol test that can be self-administered, or (c) through one's performance on certain field sobriety tests.

BAC Nomograms.   Nomograms are graphs with a set of three parallel lines, one for each of three variables. When a straightedge connects two of them, information from the third unknown variable can be obtained. Body weight and the number of drinks consumed within two hours can be readily used to estimate BAC. For example, a 120-pound individual who consumes four 12-oz. beers in two hours could have a maximum BAC of .10 percent.[66] Nomograms have been printed on key chains and bar napkins and have been widely distributed as part of some anti-drunk driving campaigns, but they are not fool proof. Although these scales were derived from carefully controlled studies, nomograms may lead individuals to over or underestimate their BAC substantially.[67] In the case of underestimation, nomograms can be a menace to DUI prevention. Therefore, it has been suggested that nomograms be removed from circulation and a better index of alcohol impairment developed.[68]

Self-Testing BAC Meters.   Minimal effort is required to obtain accurate BAC measurements from the relatively inexpensive, portable BAC meters.[69] Such devices can be placed in drinking establishments to provide immediate, individualized BAC feedback for guiding individuals in their drinking/driving decisions. However, research assessing the utility of BAC meters has not been completely favorable. For example, in a field study with drinking and driving information provided to bar patrons, Oates reported that subjects who received BAC feedback were no more likely to use the public transportation services (i.e., taxi or bus) than were non-participants.[70]

Calvert-Boyanowsky and Boyanowsky placed BAC meters in several bars in British Columbia to study whether BAC feedback influenced DUI of bar patrons.[71] They administered questionnaires to assess the driving plans of those patrons who volunteered to take the breath test. The authors concluded that although breath testing was popular, knowledge of BAC did not deter the majority of alcohol-impaired subjects from driving.

A particular concern of this approach to DUI prevention is that BAC feedback might actually exacerbate alcohol consumption, because drinkers may view the feedback as a game score rather than information to prevent DUI. Support for this notion was observed in a study conducted at a university fraternity party.[72] During the party, a few students actually urged others to obtain higher BAC levels, cheering enthusiastically as "players" successively increased their BAC levels. The BAC measures taken of all students when they left the party actually showed significantly higher mean BAC among those who used the BAC meter at least once during the party. It is likely, however, that this finding resulted from a self-selection sampling bias, with those who consumed more alcohol being more apt to assess their BAC during the party.

Field Sobriety Tests. Given that alcohol affects performance adversely along several dimensions, including reaction time and standing steadiness,[73] behavioral tests of impairment might be useful in a social context for determining a person's level of intoxication. The validity of this thesis was studied by asking students at college beer parties to participate in simple behavioral tasks that might indicate alcohol impairment.[74] Subjects were asked, for example, to catch a ruler as it dropped between their thumb and forefinger. The number of inches it fell was used as an indication of reaction time. The subjects were also asked to participate in a five-step, progressive body balance task. Participants were given points for maintaining their balance at each increasingly difficult level of the task.

Performance on both the ruler drop and body balance tasks contributed significantly to the prediction of actual BAC. Many subjects reported that poor performance on these tasks would dissuade them from driving. However, such favorable reaction to the field sobriety tests decreased significantly as the participant's BAC increased. More research is needed to investigate how simple performance tests can be used to convince alcohol-impaired individuals not to drive. Indeed, field sobriety tests may be more valid than BAC as an index of performance deficits related to driving.[75] Furthermore, simple sobriety tests could be administered by party hosts, drink servers, or friends to increase a respondent's awareness of the debilitating effects of excessive alcohol consumption.

The Drinking Milieu

The party or social gathering of friends and acquaintances is an ideal setting in many respects for introducing techniques that reflect socially responsible drinking. For example, such events could provide opportunities to serve low-alcohol or non-alcoholic beverages, or to administer field sobriety tests, or to make BAC feedback meters available. Interactive discussions can evolve naturally among friends to provide the rationale and support for appropriate server intervention strategies. Indeed, such discussions may result in practical refinements of procedures to control drinking and driving.

The Bar Environment. Sommer identified several factors likely to attract a patron to a bar and influence subsequent drinking behavior, including bar location, room decor, and drink prices.[76] The availability of recreational and entertainment activities, such as watching sports on a large television screen, dancing, and live band music, may also influence the risk of DUI in particular ways. Whereas bar entertainment prolongs the time spent in a bar and thus increases the amount of alcohol consumed,[77] certain activities (e.g., dancing) may detract from excessive drinking and increase "sobering up" time.

From an investigation of 185 bars in Vancouver, Graham concluded that intoxication and aggression were directly related to larger seating capacity, rows of tables, no decor theme, and lower standards of furnishings and upkeep.[78] Graham also suggested that the decor and upkeep in a bar may convey a message to patrons about the kinds of behavior expected. Other activities and general atmosphere characteristics he identified as significant determinants of intoxication included the type of entertainment, availability of food, ventilation, noise, and crowding. Additional naturalistic studies of relationships between alcohol consumption and setting variables are urgently needed.

The "Happy Hour." The "happy hour" typically refers to a period of time after the workday has ended and before the evening meal. In order to attract a greater volume of business during this "off-peak" period, some entrepreneurs offer alcohol at bargain prices. As many as sixteen states actually prohibit happy hours or other forms of sales promotion, and twenty-two additional states have proposed such legislation.[79]

The effects of reduced drink prices on individual drinking patterns were explored by monitoring the same persons as they drank in experimental

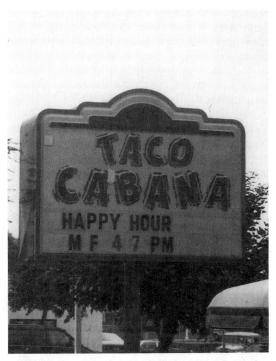

FIGURE 18-3. Low alcoholic beverage prices offered over long periods of time reduce barriers to excessive drinking and drunken driving. *Photo courtesy of Betsy Clapp.*

and natural settings.[80] In both settings, reduced prices (during happy hour) significantly increased the frequency of drinking episodes and the amount of alcohol consumed among both casual and heavy drinkers. In a controlled setting, Babor, Mendelson, Greenberg, and Kuchnle observed that during periods of reduced drink prices, male volunteers increased their alcohol consumption eightfold compared to a control group without a happy hour, and the increased alcohol drinking during the happy hours was not a substitute for consumption at other times of the day.[81] Furthermore, Babor et al. found that the patterns of drinking influenced by the happy hour (i.e., gulping drinks, massing successive drinks, and consuming straight drinks) were likely to be learned and repeated at other times. The same function of lower beverage cost and increased consumption was found in the general population.[82]

Size of Drinking Group. Sommer observed isolated male drinkers sitting alone in thirty-two Edmonton beer parlors and contrasted their drinking behavior with that of drinkers in groups.[83] He found that isolated drinkers ordered an average of 1.69 drinks, whereas individual drinkers in groups ordered 3.51 drinks. The data suggested that the reason persons in groups drank more than isolated drinkers was not because they drank faster, but because they remained in the barroom longer.

Rosenbluth, Nathan, and Lawson also observed that male and female college students drank more beer in groups than in dyads.[84] An intriguing finding from these field observations requiring follow-up research, was that same-gender dyads showed less rapid beer consumption than mixed-gender dyads.

Glasses Versus Pitchers. There is convincing evidence that the sale of beer in pitchers may contribute to excessive alcohol consumption and subsequent risk for DUI. In one study, the most beer was consumed per person when it was ordered by the pitcher (i.e., mean per capita beer consumption was 35.2 oz. from pitchers, 15.1 oz. from bottles, and 10.0 oz. from cups).[85] But *rate* of drinking did not vary significantly as a function of drink container, because those who ordered their beer by the pitcher stayed in the bar significantly longer (mean of 66 minutes) than those ordering beer by the bottle (mean of 34 minutes) or by the cup (mean of 23 minutes).

The Barroom Server. The server of alcoholic beverages (i.e., bartender, waitress, or waiter) is an especially critical aspect of the drinker's social environment. In response to "Dram Shop" Laws which permit holding tavern owners liable if they serve alcohol to an intoxicated patron who later causes an accident while DUI, servers of alcoholic beverages receive special training aimed at preventing their customers from DUI.[86] Most intervention training programs teach servers to identify the specific warning signs that indicate when a customer may overindulge. Then servers learn to use a variety of tactics, including delaying alcoholic drink service, offering food, serving non-alcoholic beverages, and suggesting that the patron not drive. Some programs include the use of video vignettes and role-playing to help servers evaluate customers' behavior and to practice intervention skills.

Drinking at Parties. In one study the impact of beer brand labels on alcohol consumption was demonstrated.[87] At an initial fraternity party, the three beer kegs were not labeled according to the three different beers available — Budweiser, Bud Light, and LA. Then, at a second party one month later, the three kegs were labeled according to brand name. At the first party the drinking preferences during the party matched the results of the taste preference tests obtained at the start of both parties (i.e., Budweiser was most preferred and selected most often, LA was least preferred and selected least often). When the beer kegs were labeled according to brand name, the subjects (151 males and 220 females) showed significant preference for Bud Light over Budweiser.

The LA beer was only consumed to any extent at the party with unlabeled kegs, suggesting a social stigma attached to ordering a low alcohol drink. The preference for Bud Light over Budweiser implies a powerful influence of marketing strategies. Indeed, it is possible that most individuals perceive light beers as having only less calories and not less alcohol. Would Bud Light have been more popular than Budweiser if the kegs had been labeled according to their alcohol content as well as brand name (i.e., 3.8 percent alcohol for Budweiser and 2.8 percent alcohol for Bud Light)?

Although low alcohol beer is not typically the "beer of choice," it may reduce the risk of alcohol impairment and DUI if served at a party (perhaps near the end of the evening) without the guests being informed. Geller and Kalsher researched this empirical question with the general party observation procedures described above.[88] At two fraternity parties, both mixed drinks and beer were available at no cost to the subjects. At the start of the party, each participant was required to select one drink alternative (beer or mixed drinks) and to continue with that choice throughout the evening. For one party (64 males and 43 females), the only beer was Budweiser, whereas at the other party (70 males and 48 females), the beer was LA. Subjects were unaware of the brand of beer being served. The BAC levels at the end of the parties were significantly lower among those students who drank LA beer than for those who drank Budweiser ($p < .01$), and no one complained about either beer. Also, those who drank beer (approximately half of the persons at each party) did *not* drink at significantly higher rates or get more impaired than those who chose mixed drinks. This finding contradicts the conclusion from interview research that beer drinkers get more impaired than those who consume mixed drinks.[89]

SUMMARY

The challenge for everyone who could receive an unintentional injury at home, at the workplace, or on the road, is to focus on prevention. Motivating individuals to act for prevention, however, is most difficult because reinforcers to support such behavior are usually not available. Not only do prevention behaviors usually lack immediate reinforcing consequences, they often compete with alternative unsafe or unhealthy behaviors which are reinforced. This chapter reviewed research that focused on the development and evaluation of interventions to change two of the most critical behaviors responsible for unintentional injury — nonuse of vehicle safety belts and driving a vehicle while under the influence of alcohol (DUI).

Compared to most prevention strategies that require repeated responding in order to be effective (e.g., regular exercise, daily use of protective work clothing, brushing teeth, proper nutrition), using a vehicle safety belt is not only most convenient, it is also most likely to pay off in substantial dividends. Since safety belt use requires minimal response cost and is intuitively protective (once certain myths about belts and crashes are dispelled), basic principles of large-scale behavior modification are directly applicable; and because safety belt use or nonuse can be readily observed in field settings, it has been possible to evaluate the relative efficacy of different applications of behavior modification principles. As a result, a number of antecedent and consequence strategies have been developed for increasing safety belt use in a variety of community settings, including schools, universities, industries, banks, churches, and naval bases. It is encouraging that most of these interventions can be successfully delivered by existing staff or volunteer groups, and they have been willingly sponsored by both the private and public sectors.

In order to increase the greatest number of safety belt users over the longest period of time, it is necessary to study: (a) various schedules for delivering and fading buckle-up rewards; (b) different combinations of extrinsic incentives and

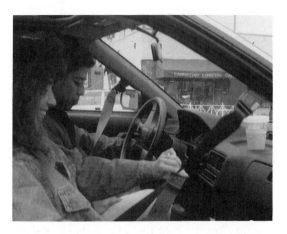

FIGURE 18–4. Occupant safety devices in newer automobiles involve both automatic and manual protection systems. *Photo courtesy of Betsy Clapp.*

intrinsic commitment procedures; (c) the differential effects of various intervention strategies on adults vs. children, blue-collar vs. white-collar workers, and employees vs. retired persons; (d) the comparative cost-effectiveness of implementing safety belt programs at corporations, schools, recreational facilities, churches, and local businesses; (e) the long-term impact of combining behavior change strategies such as incentives/reinforcers for safety belt use and disincentives/punishers for safety belt nonuse; and (f) techniques for mobilizing groups of people and resources to implement community-wide programs for safety belt promotion.

Attacking drunken driving with behavior modification has not been nearly as straightforward as intervening to increase safety belt use. To decrease inappropriate behavior, behavior change specialists typically focus on increasing the occurrence of behaviors incompatible with the undesired behavior. This is a more appropriate approach to DUI prevention than the current punishment strategies receiving increased attention in the U.S. Because it has been impossible to administer the kind of punishment contingency for DUI that works—one with a consequence that is frequent, consistent, immediate, and adequately severe. Catching an alcohol-impaired driver is usually not corrective or rehabilitative, and the threat of such punishment for DUI is not a long-term deterrent.

The initial challenge for a positive reinforcement approach to DUI prevention is defining situations and behaviors that decrease the risk of DUI. The possibilities for study seem endless, however, there has been only a minimal amount of research related to this essential aspect of DUI prevention. There have been some promising beginnings, and these were highlighted in this chapter. In particular, certain environmental conditions have been studied as potential facilitators or inhibitors of excessive drinking (e.g., size of drinking groups and drink containers, the availability of BAC feedback meters, "happy hour" incentives, labels on beer kegs), and one mechanism for applying the results of this research to prevent DUI (i.e., through server intervention) has been addressed. Many grass roots groups, government agencies, enforcement officials, and treatment professionals are available to help with a positive, behavior modification approach to reducing DUI risk. Unfortunately, the focus of these groups has been on the development and enforcement of ineffective contingencies for punishing the alcohol-impaired driver. Changing the intervention approach of these groups is yet another pressing challenge for the public health professional who wants to make a difference.

ENDNOTES

1. Waller, J. A. (1986). State liquor laws as enablers for impaired driving and other impaired behaviors. *American Journal of Public Health, 76,* 787–792.

2. National Academy Press. (1985). *Injury in America: A continuing public health problem.* Washington, D.C.: National Academy Press.

3. Sleet, D. A. (1987). Motor vehicle trauma and safety belt use in the context of public health priorities. *Journal of Trauma, 27,* 695–702.

4. Curry, J. R. (1991, Summer). Safety achievement —Prelude to progress. *Auto & Traffic Safety, 1,* p. 1.

5. McGinnis, J. M. (1984). Occupant protection as a priority in national efforts to promote health. *Health Education Quarterly, 11,* 127–131.

6. Graham, J. D. (1988). Injury control, traffic safety, and evaluation research. In J. D. Graham (Ed.), *Preventing automobile injury* (pp. 1–23). Dover, MA: Auburn House.

7. Hartunian, N. S., Smart, C. N., & Thompson, M. S. (1981). *The incidence and economic costs of*

major health impairments: *A comparative analysis of cancer, motor vehicle injuries, coronary heart disease and stroke.* Lexington, MA: Lexington Books.

8. Califano, Jr., J. A. (1979). *Healthy people: The surgeon general's report on health promotion and disease prevention.* Washington, D.C.: U.S. Government Printing Office.

9. Gelfand, D. M. & Hartmann, D. P. (1984). *Child behavior analysis and therapy* (2nd ed.). New York: Pergamon.

10. Fell, J. C. (1982). Alcohol involvement in traffic crashes. *American Association for Automobile Medicine Quarterly Journal, 4,* 23–42.

11. *Federal Register.* (1984, July). Federal motor vehicle safety standards: Occupant crash protection, Final Rule, 48 (No. 138). Washington, D.C.: U.S. Department of Transportation.

12. Ziegler, P. (1986, January). Observed safety belt and child safety seat usage at road intersections: 19-city survey results. *Research Notes.* Washington, D.C.: Office of Driver and Pedestrian Research, National Highway Traffic Safety Administration, U.S. Department of Transportation.

13. Sleet, D. A. Motor vehicle trauma and safety belt use in the context of public health priorities.

14. Ibid.

15. Steed, D. K. (1988, February). *Administrator.* Washington, D.C.: National Highway Traffic Safety Administration, U.S. Department of Transportation.

16. Steed, D. K. (1987, November–December). National Highway Traffic Safety Administration. *Proceedings of the 1987 Conference on Injury in America,* U.S. Department of Health and Human Services, Public Health Service, *102,* 667–668.

17. Steed. *Administrator,* February, 1988.

18. Ross, H. L. (1987). Reflections on doing policy-relevant sociology: How to cope with MADD mothers. *American Sociologist, 18,* 173–178.

19. Wagenaar, A. C. (1983). *Alcohol, young drivers, and traffic accidents.* Lexington, MA: D. C. Heath.

20. Ross, H. L. (1985, December). *Deterring the drinking driver: Legal policy and social control.* Lexington, MA: D. C. Heath, 1982; and Russ, N. W. & Geller, E. S. Changing the behavior of the drunk driver: Current status and future directions. *Psychological Documents, 15,* 1–30.

21. Ziegler, P. Observed safety belt and child safety seat usage at road intersections: 19-city survey results.

22. Campbell, B. J., Stewart, J. R., & Campbell, F. A. (1987). *1985–1986 experience with belt laws in the United States.* Chapel Hill, NC: UNC Highway Safety Research Center.

23. Ibid.

24. Steed. National Highway Traffic Safety Administration. *Proceedings of the 1987 Conference on Injury in America.*

25. Wagenaar, A. C., Webster, D. W., & Maybee, R. C. (1987). Effects of child restraint laws on traffic fatalities in eleven states. *Journal of Trauma, 27,* 726–731.

26. Cynecki, J. & Goryl, M. E. (1984). *The incidence and factors associated with child safety seat misuse.* (Final Report DOT-HS-806-676). Washington, D.C.: National Highway Traffic Safety Administration, U.S. Department of Transportation; and Shelness, A. & Jewett, J. (1983). Observed misuse of child restraints. *Proceedings of the 27th Stapp Car Crash Conference: Child Injury and Restraint* (pp. 207–216). Warrendale, PA: Society of Automotive Engineers.

27. Geller, E. S. & Lehman, G. R. (1991). The buckle-up promise card: A versatile intervention for large-scale behavior change. *Journal of Applied Behavior Analysis, 24,* 91–94.

28. Evans, L. (1991). *Traffic safety and the driver.* New York: Van Nostrand Reinhold; and von Busek, C. R. & Geller, E. S. (1984). *The vehicle safety belt reminder: Can refinements increase safety belt use?* Technical Report for General Motors Research Laboratories, Warren, MI.

29. Berry, T. D. & Geller, E. S. (1991). A single-subject approach to evaluating vehicle safety belt reminders: Back to basics. *Journal of Applied Behavior Analysis, 24,* 13–22.

30. Geller, E. S. (1988). A behavioral science approach to transportation safety. *Bulletin of the New York Academy of Medicine, 64,* 632–661.

31. Berry, T. D. & Geller, E. S. A single-subject approach to evaluating vehicle safety belt reminders: Back to basics; and Geller, E. S. (1988). A behavioral science approach to transportation safety. *Bulletin of the New York Academy of Medicine, 64,* 632–661.

32. Geller, E. S., Russ, N. W., & Delphos, W. A. (1987). Does server intervention training make a difference? An empirical field evaluation. *Alcohol, Health & Research World, 11,* 64–69.

33. Geller, E. S., Casali, J. G., & Johnson, R. P. (1980). Seat-belt usage: A potential target for applied behavior analysis. *Journal of Applied Behavior Analysis, 13,* 669–675; and Robertson, L. S. (1975). Safety belt use in automobiles with starter-interlock and buzzer-light reminder systems. *American Journal of Public Health, 65,* 1319–1325.

34. Thyer, B. A. & Geller, E. S. (1987). The "buckle-up" dashboard sticker: An effective environmental intervention for safety belt promotion. *Environment & Behavior, 19,* 484–494.

35. Rogers, R. W. (1984). *Promoting safety belt use among state employees: The effects of prompting, stimulus control and a response-cost intervention.* Unpublished doctoral dissertation, Florida State University, Tallahassee.

36. Geller, E. S., Bruff, C. D., & Nimmer, J. G. (1985). "Flash for Life": Community-based prompting for safety belt promotion. *Journal of Applied Behavior Analysis, 18,* 145–159.

37. Geller, E. S. (1982, January). *Development of industry-based strategies for motivating seat-belt usage: Phase II.* (Quarterly Report for DOT Contract DTRS5681-C-0032). Blacksburg: Virginia Polytechnic Institute and State University; and Phillips, B. M. (1980, June). *Safety belt education program for employees: An evaluation study.* Opinion Research Corp. (Final Report for Contract DOT-HS-01707). Washington, D.C.: U.S. Department of Transportation.

38. Robertson, L. S., Kelley, A. B., O'Neill, B., Wixom, C. W., Eiswirth, R. S., & Haddon, W. (1974). A controlled study of the effect of television messages on safety belt use. *American Journal of Public Health, 64,* 1071–1080.

39. Cunliffe, A. P., DeAngelis, F., Foley, C., Lonero, L. P., Pierce, J. A., Siegel, C., Smutylo, T., & Stephen, K. M. (1975, September). *The design and implementation of a seat-belt educational program in Ontario.* Paper presented at the Annual Conference of the Roads and Transportation of Canada, Calgary.

40. Geller, E. S. & Bigelow, B. E. (1984). Development of corporate incentive programs for motivating safety belt use: A review. *Traffic Safety Evaluation Research Review, 3,* 21–38; and Horne, T. D. & Terry, T. (1983). *Seatbelt Sweepstakes—An incentive program.* SAE Technical Paper Series (No. 830474). Warrendale, PA: Society of Automotive Engineers.

41. Nimmer, J. G. & Geller, E. S. (1988). Motivating safety belt use at a community hospital: An effective integration of incentive and commitment strategies. *American Journal of Community Psychology, 16,* 381–394.

42. Ibid.

43. Geller, E. S., Kalsher, M. J., Rudd, J. R., & Lehman, G. R. (1989). Promoting safety belt use on a university campus: An integration of commitment and incentive strategies. *Journal of Applied Social Psychology, 19,* 3–19.

44. Ibid.

45. Geller, E. S. (1984). Motivating safety belt use with incentives: A critical review of the past and a look at the future. *SAE Technical Paper Series* (No. 840326). Warrendale, PA: Society of Automotive Engineers; and Geller, E. S. (1985). *Corporate safety belt programs.* Blacksburg: Virginia Polytechnic Institute and State University.

46. Geller, E. S. Motivating safety belt use with incentives: A critical review of the past and a look at the future; and Geller, E. S. & Bigelow, B. E. Development of corporate incentive programs for motivating safety belt use: A review.

47. Geller, E. S. *Corporate safety belt programs,* 1985; and Streff, F. M. & Geller, E. S. (1986). Strategies for motivating safety belt use: The application of applied behavior analysis. *Health Education Research: Theory and Practice, 1,* 47–59.

48. Geller, E. S. (1983). Rewarding safety belt usage at an industrial setting: Tests of treatment generality and response maintenance. *Journal of Applied Behavior Analysis, 16,* 189–202; Geller, E. S., Davis, L., & Spicer, K. (1983). Industry-based rewards to promote seat belt usage: Differential impact on white collar versus blue collar employees. *Journal of Organizational Behavior Management, 5,* 17–29; Spoonhour, K. A. (1981, September–October). Company snap-it-up campaign achieves 90 percent belt use. *Traffic Safety,* 18–19, 31–32; and Stutts, J. C., Hunter, W. W., & Campbell, B. J. (1984). Three studies evaluating the effectiveness of incentives for increasing safety belt use. *Traffic Safety Evaluation Research Review, 3,* 9–20.

49. Elman, D. & Killebrew, T. J. (1978). Incentives and seat belts: Changing a resistant behavior through extrinsic motivation. *Journal of Applied Social Psychology, 8,* 72–83.

50. Geller, E. S., Johnson, R. P. & Pelton, S. L. (1984). Community-based interventions for encouraging safety belt use. *American Journal of Community Psychology, 10,* 183–195, 1982; and Johnson, R. P. & Geller, E. S. Contingent versus noncontingent rewards for promoting seat belt usage. *Journal of Community Psychology, 12,* 113–122.

51. Campbell, B. J., Hunter, W. W., & Stutts, J. C. (1984). The use of economic incentives and education to modify safety belt use behavior of high school students. *Health Education, 15,* 30–33.

52. Geller, E. S., Paterson, L., & Talbott, E. (1982). A behavioral analysis of incentive prompts for motivating seat belt usage. *Journal of Applied Behavior Analysis, 15,* 403–415.

53. Roberts, M. C. & Turner, D. S. (1986). Rewarding parents for their children's use of safety seats. *Journal of Pediatric Psychology, 11,* 25–36.

54. Roberts, M. C. & Layfield, D. A. (1987). Promoting child passenger safety: A comparison of two positive methods. *Journal of Pediatric Psychology, 12,* 257–271.

55. Roberts, M. C. & Fanurik, D. (1986). Rewarding elementary school children for their use of safety belts. *Health Psychology, 5,* 185–196; and Rob-

erts, M. C., Fanurik, D., & Wilson, D. (1988). A community program to reward children's use of seat belts. *American Journal of Community Psychology, 16,* 395–407.

56. Roberts, M. C. & Fanurik, D. Rewarding elementary school children for their use of safety belts.

57. Roberts, M.C. & Turner, D. S. Rewarding parents for their children's use of safety seats.

58. Geller, E. S. Motivating safety belt use with incentives: A critical review of the past and a look at the future, 1984; and Geller, E. S. (1982). *Corporate incentives for promoting safety belt use: Rationale, guidelines, and examples.* Washington, D.C.: U.S. Department of Transportation.

59. Kalsher, M. J., Geller, E. S., Clarke, S. W., & Lehman, R. R. (1987) Safety belt promotion on a naval base: A comparison of incentives vs. disincentives. *Journal of Safety Research, 20,* 103–113.

60. Geller, E. S., Rudd, J. R., Kalsher, M. J., Streff, F. M., & Lehman, G. R. (1987). Employer-based programs to motivate safety belt use: A review of short- and long-term effects. *Journal of Safety Research, 18,* 1–17.

61. Geller, E. S., Kalsher, M. J., Rudd, J. R., & Lehman, G. (1989). Promoting safety belt use on a university campus: An integration of commitment and incentive strategies. *Journal of Applied Social Psychology, 19,* 3–19.

62. Horne, T. D. Workshop presentation at the Michigan Life Savers Conference. Boyne Mountain, MI, November, 1984.

63. Geller, E. S. & Hahn, H. A. (1984). Promoting seat belt use at industrial sites: An effective program for blue collar employees. *Professional Psychology: Research & Practice, 15,* 553–564.

64. Geller, E. S., Winett, R. A., & Everett, P. B. (1982). *Preserving the environment: New strategies for behavior change.* Elmsford, NY: Pergamon Press.

65. Geller, E. S., Altomari, M. G., Russ, N. W., & Harwood, M. K. (1985, June). Exploring the drinking/driving behaviors and attitudes of college students. *Resources in Education,* Ms. No. ED252756; and Geller, E. S. & Russ, R. W. (1986). Drunk driving prevention: Knowing when to say when. In *Alcohol, accidents, and injuries* (No. P–173), Warrendale, PA: Society of Automotive Engineers.

66. U.S. Department of Transportation. (1975). *A message to my patients* (DOT-HS-804-089). Washington, D.C.: National Highway Traffic Safety Administration.

67. Waller, J. A. State liquor laws as enablers for impaired driving and other impaired behaviors. *American Journal of Public Health, 76,* 787–792.

68. Dubowski, K. (1984, June). *Absorption, distribution, and elimination of alcohol: Highway safety aspects.* Paper presented at the meeting of the North American Conference on Alcohol and Highway Safety, Baltimore, MD.

69. Picton, W. R. (1979). An evaluation of a coin-operated self-tester. In I. R. Johnston (Ed.), *Proceedings of the Seventh International Conference on Alcohol, Drugs, and Traffic Safety* (pp. 327–331).

70. Oates, J. F. (1976). *Study of self-test drivers.* (Final Report, DOT-HS-5-01241). Washington, D.C.: National Highway Traffic Safety Administration.

71. Calvert-Boyanowsky, J. & Boyanowsky, E. O. (1980). *Tavern breath testing as an alcohol countermeasure.* Ottawa, Ontario: Technical Report: Ministry of Transport.

72. Harwood, M. K. (1984). *New directions toward increasing awareness of alcohol impairment.* Unpublished senior research paper, Blacksburg: Virginia Polytechnic Institute and State University.

73. Carpenter, J. A. (1962). Effects of alcohol on some psychological processes: A critical review with special reference to automobile driving skill. *Quarterly Journal of Studies on Alcohol, 23,* 274–314.

74. Geller, E. S. & Russ, N. W. Drunk driving prevention: Knowing when to say when; and Russ, N. W. & Geller, E. S. (1982). Using sobriety tests to increase awareness of alcohol impairment. *Health Education Research: Theory & Practice, 1,* 255–261.

75. Johnson, D. (1983). *Drunkenness may not be accurately measured by 12 blood-alcohol levels: UCB researchers report* (Public Information Office News). Boulder, CO: University of Colorado.

76. Sommer, R. (1969). *Personal space: The behavioral basis of design.* Englewood Cliffs, NJ: Prentice-Hall.

77. Clark, W. B. (1981). The contemporary tavern. In Y. Israel, F. B. Glaser, R.E. Klant, W. Popham, W. Schmidt, & R. G. Smart (Eds.), *Research advances in alcohol and drug problems* (Vol. 6). Toronto: Addiction Research Foundation; and Schaefer, J. M. (1983, May). *The physical setting: Behavior and policy.* Paper presented at Lifesavers 3 Conference, Orlando, FL.

78. Graham, K. (April, 1984). *Determinants of heavy drinking and drinking problems: The contribution of the bar environment.* Paper presented at the Symposium on Public Drinking and Public Safety, Banff, Alberta.

79. Waller, J. A. State liquor laws as enablers for impaired driving and other impaired behaviors.

80. Babor, T. F., Mendelson, J. H., Uhly, B., & Souza,

E. (1980). Drinking patterns in experimental and barroom settings. *Journal of Studies on Alcohol, 41,* 634–651.

81. Babor, T. F., Mendelson, J. H., Greensberg, I., & Kuchnle, J. (1978). Experimental analysis of the "happy hour": Effects of purchase price on alcohol consumption. *Psychopharmacology, 58,* 35–41.

82. Schmidt, W. & Popham, R. E. (1978). The single distribution theory of alcohol consumption: A rejoinder to the critique of Parker and Harman. *Journal of Studies on Alcohol, 39,* 400–419.

83. Sommer, R. (1969). *Personal space: The behavioral basis of design.* Englewood Cliffs, NJ: Prentice-Hall.

84. Rosenbluth, J., Nathan, P. E., & Lawson, D. W. (1978). Environmental influences on drinking by college students in a college pub: Behavioral observation in the natural environment. *Addictive Behaviors, 3,* 117–121.

85. Geller, E. S., Altomari, M. G., Russ, N. W., & Harwood, M. K. (1985, June). Exploring the drinking/ driving behaviors and attitudes of college students. *Resources in Education,* Ms. No. ED252756.

86. Mosher, J. F. (1979). Dram shop liability and prevention of alcohol-related problems. *Journal of Studies on Alcohol, 40,* 773–798; and Peters, J. E. (1986). Beyond server training: An examination of future issues. *Alcohol, Health & Research World, 10,* 24–27.

87. Kalsher, M. J. & Geller, E. S. (1992). *Beer consumption at university parties: Stimulus control of brand labels.* Unpublished manuscript. Blacksburg: Virginia Polytechnic Institute and State University.

88. Geller, E. S., Kalsher, M. J., & Clarke, S. W. (1992). *Beer versus mixed-drink consumption at fraternity parties: A time and place for low-alcohol beer. Journal of Studies on Alcohol, 52,* 197–204.

89. Berger, D. E. & Snortum, J. R. (1985). Alcoholic beverage preferences of drinking-driving violators. *Journal of Studies on Alcohol, 46,* 232–239.

Chapter 19

Adolescent Sexual Behavior: Control of Pregnancy, Sexually Transmitted Diseases, and AIDS

OBJECTIVES

By the end of this chapter, the reader should be able to:

1. Describe the means of transmission of the AIDS virus.
2. Describe the behaviors that must be avoided and the role of condoms in the prevention of AIDS and STDs.
3. Explain the determinants of AIDS risk/protective behavior.
4. Describe the importance of metacontingencies in the control of AIDS risk behavior.

INTRODUCTION

The U.S., other developed countries, and underdeveloped countries are sharing very serious epidemics. In the U.S., the rate of teenage pregnancy exceeds that of all other Western countries.[1] The rate of sexually transmitted diseases **(STDs),** such as syphilis, has remained high, and the relatively newly discovered acquired immune deficiency syndrome (AIDS) is no longer limited to the African continent or the gay male population but has been established in the heterosexual community, as well. This has resulted in serious compromises to individuals' health and the health of the population within which a prematurely pregnant or infected individual lives. These problems are caused by certain types of sexual behavior in addition to other means of transmission of pathogenic organisms. The prevention and control of these epidemics require a behavioral analysis of sexual practices, as well as co-risk factors for pregnancy or transmission of pathogenic organisms. This chapter reviews the basic epidemiology of these "conditions" and the role of behavior in their etiology, prevention, and control. Emphasis will be placed on the environmental and social factors that determine sexual behavior, co-risk behaviors, and the use of learning theory and the ONPRIME process to design possible AIDS prevention and control procedures for adolescents in developed countries.

Public Health Significance

Unplanned Teenage Pregnancy and Population Control.   In Western nations, the rate of teenage pregnancies has been uncontrolled for decades. In the U.S., one million teenagers become pregnant each year. The pregnancy rate in the U.S. is twice that of Canada and as much as seven times that of the Netherlands.[2] Young women who become pregnant face traumatic decisions regarding abortion, adoption, or the arduous task of raising a child in the absence of life experience, food, shelter, and general education for the child or the mother. Pregnant adolescent women (for those who deliver), their babies, and the nation suffer by paying for the compromised welfare of both the mother and baby for life. The U.S. now expends almost $17 billion each year for public health, medical, and social services to pregnant adolescents, their babies, and families.[3] In the context of reliable and affordable technologies for controlling births, this epidemic is inexcusable. However, our basic understanding of the development of sexual relationships is so shallow that all efforts to prevent or control teenage pregnancies are compromised by a lack of basic theory and research.

World Population Control.   Teenage pregnancy is a serious epidemic in the U.S. and other Western nations. High birth rates among adults tend not to be a problem in Western countries. Indeed, a few nations have reached a stable or slightly negative growth rate. The reasons that birth rates have declined in developed nations relative to underdeveloped nations is not fully understood. Speculation places the "cause" of declining birth rates on such factors as universal education, relatively high income for all members of the population, and increasing equality for women.

Though some nations have achieved stable or declining birth rates, the birth rates for underdeveloped nations and the world overall is increasing at an alarming rate. Given the demography of developing countries, much of the increased birth rate is due to relatively young people having babies; however, it is not limited to teenagers. In many countries a single family may have many more than two children. In cities like Mexico City or Rio de Janeiro, children and *their* children live on the fringe of human society. The resources of these nations are so limited that few individuals or families can afford the basic resources to sustain normal or healthy lives. They lack shelter, live in cardboard shacks, or have no home at all; food is limited and rarely includes meat or high protein staples; sanitation is compromised and infections are common. In the most severe cases, frequent famines kill thousands each year from starvation. The population size in these nations may be so much greater than available food and other resources that diseases and death are commonplace.

The public health significance of overpopulation and uncontrolled growth rates is obvious for persons living in crowded underdeveloped countries. These consequences and the birth rates, specifically, are a function of sexual behavior. Yet few studies have been conducted to better understand the specific sexual practices in these countries.

The Public Health Significance of World Population for Developed Nations.   The severe conditions of life in a developing country, especially if overpopulated, are obvious to anyone who has the opportunity to observe them. The impact of overpopulation in developing countries on developed nations and the world overall is much less obvious. Spaceship Earth is a finite globe with limited resources, and some of the more critical resources are delicately balanced. The destruction of the world's rain forests is largely a function of developing nations' desperate need for income and developed nations' voracious appetite for wood products. The destruction of rain forests extinguishes many animal and plant species, thereby increasing the fragility of life in general. It also depletes the world's primary source of oxygen in the atmosphere. Ultimately, changes in ecology, in large part due to the overpopulation of the world as well as the maldistribution of populations and wealth, threaten the very survival of humankind and possibly life in general (See in chapter 22).

To enhance the humanity of the developing nations as well as protect the well-being of developed nations—and ultimately life in general—worldwide population must be controlled. To do so requires an in-depth understanding of sexual practices and the use of birth control, including abortion.

Sexually Transmitted Diseases (STDs) and AIDS

STDs. Sexually transmitted diseases have been around since the beginning of time. **The most common are gonorrhea, syphilis, chlamydia, herpes, and genital warts. These are caused by viruses or bacteria, and the primary means of transmission is through sexual contact.** These diseases differ in prevalence and incidence in the population. For example, 50,223 cases of syphilis were reported in 1980, an increase of 9 percent in one year.[4]

By 1985 the incidence had increased to the highest level since 1949. Clearly, available treatment has not prevented the epidemic. An earlier report concluded that present efforts to control STDs and meet the objectives for the nation were inadequate for almost all STDs.[5] Rates of STDs are high and increasing for urban and minority populations. Of course, these rates are probably underestimated because these diseases are not reported reliably to physicians, or from physicians to the public health service. However, a serious problem exists. These diseases can cause both debilitation and death. Syphilis, for example, can cause a form of senility as the infection spreads to the brain and destroys the central nervous system (CNS). In women, these diseases can increase the risk of cancer and cause sterility. Perhaps the most serious medical consequence of STDs is that they increase the likelihood of exposure to and infection with the viruses that cause AIDS.

Acquired Immune Deficiency Syndrome (AIDS). Exposure to the human immunodeficiency viruses (HIV) can lead to infection and subsequently to the acquired immune deficiency syndrome (AIDS). AIDS was first recognized and reported in 1981 and is caused by the human immunodeficiency virus. AIDS is insidious because it attacks the immune system of the body — the very system designed to protect the body from infections. Various cells of the immune system are designed to attack invading organisms, including viruses. For instance, when a virus enters the body, a macrophage detects the virus and triggers the production of T-cells. Different kinds of T-cells are then produced. One kind of T-cell produces a B-cell, which multiplies and produces antibodies to attack the invading virus. With HIV infection, the virus invades the T-cells, blocking their ability to stimulate B-cells, thereby preventing the normal immune response to attack the invading virus (HIV) or other microorganisms. HIV goes on to change the T-cell into a home where additional human immunodeficiency viruses can be reproduced. This destroys the immune system and makes the individual likely to acquire "opportunistic diseases," which normally would have been killed by the immune system. These opportunistic diseases ultimately result in death.

HIV is transmitted only by exchange of bodily fluids, predominantly blood and/or semen. This is not easy to accomplish, and the viruses are most likely transmitted through injections or sexual intercourse — especially anal intercourse. Though increasing numbers of people have been exposed and infected without developing AIDS, even after ten years the disease syndrome is considered fatal in all instances of infection.

Approximately 8 million to 10 million people are infected worldwide; about 1.3 million people have AIDS, and by the year 2000 it has been estimated that over 30 million people will be HIV infected. In the U.S., over 200,000 individuals have AIDS and are dying.[6] Presently, AIDS has become the leading cause of death for people with hemophilia, for whom blood transfusions are required, and for persons using illegal drugs by injection (IV drug addicts). AIDS is the second leading cause of death among men twenty-five to forty years of age — second only to injury.[7]

AIDS is insidious in many ways, and one way concerns its incubation period. A person can be exposed to one of the viruses and acquire the infection, but not develop AIDS for up to ten years. It is possible for a person with the virus which has not yet developed into AIDS to transmit the virus to other healthy people. In other words, you can contract the virus from people who are apparently healthy, but infected.

AIDS and the Gay Community. AIDS was initially linked to the gay male population in the U.S, and homosexual males accounted for about 60 percent of all cases in 1991. This was due to the common sexual practices, and possibly the higher rates of "co-risk factors," among homosexual and bisexual males. These risk behaviors were anal intercourse, in absence of condoms, and with multiple partners. In the early phase of the epidemic, anal intercourse (possibly with multiple partners) was the norm among the majority of gay males. Anal intercourse is likely to tear tissue and inadvertently "inject" semen or other body fluid into the receptive partner's bloodstream; hence, the risk to gay males.

The use of certain drugs is known to increase the risk of infection and/or susceptibility to infection if exposed, making it a co-risk factor for AIDS. Alcohol use, for instance, may reduce inhibitions and lead individuals to practice unsafe sexual behavior, such as anal intercourse. Similarly, alcohol use can compromise the immune system, potentially increasing the chance of infection once exposed.[8] Alcohol is a commonly used drug among gay males and may have contributed to the epidemic in this subpopulation.[9] Other drugs may have similar immune compromising characteristics, and persons who routinely employ drugs, even if not taken by injection, are at risk of infection.

AIDS and Injection Drug Use.   The use of injected drugs can be especially dangerous in terms of exposure to HIV. Intravenous (IV) drug users accounted for about 20 percent of AIDS cases in 1991. Users often acquire their drugs from illegal sources under conditions of poor sanitation, and their practice of sharing needles leads to the transmission of HIV from infected users to not-yet-infected users. This may be the most serious risk factor for the contraction of HIV, given the addiction to narcotics and the extremes to which addicted individuals will go to sustain their habit. They also represent a reservoir of infected individuals from whom the HIV viruses may be spread to the larger population.

Illegal drug use is not the only means of HIV transmission. Latino and other cultural groups use injected vitamins and folk medicines. If they share needles, the possibility of transmitting the HIV viruses from an infected person to a not-yet-infected person is relatively high.

The re-use of needles by health care specialists in developing countries is another means by which HIV can be transmitted, especially if the health system does not have the resources to sterilize needles prior to re-use. This practice is considered an important contributing factor to the nearly equal rates of HIV infection among men and women in African nations.

Finally, medical care specialists and laboratory technicians who come in contact with blood products are at some risk of accidental injection. Though this is possible, only a few cases of physicians, nurses, or other health care professionals have been infected by accidental occupational exposure.

AIDS and the Heterosexual Community.   The heterosexual community is at risk of acquiring HIV through contact through injected drug use and shared needles, intercourse with an injection drug user, intercourse with a partner of an injection drug user, or intercourse with a bisexual partner or a sexual partner who had contact with a bisexual partner. Among these risks, the most probable is exposure via sexual contact. About two percent of U.S. males with AIDS are thought to have acquired the disease from heterosexual contact. The proportion for women has been increasing. In 1987–88, about 10 percent of AIDS cases were attributed to heterosexual contact; this was 12.5 percent by 1990–91. The exact rates of heterosexually transmitted cases is difficult to estimate since people do not report risk behavior reliably, and individuals may engage in multiple risk behaviors. Thus, estimates should be considered as useful for comparison purposes but not for determining exact numbers or proportions.

Complicating the risk of AIDS in the heterosexual community is the degree to which individuals have multiple partners. The single individual who may have two or more lovers has an increased chance of acquiring HIV from one partner and then transmitting it to his/her additional partners. Among married individuals, the number who have extra-marital sexual contacts is substantial and probably underestimated. These individuals run the risk of acquiring HIV and spreading it to their spouses. The long incubation or latency period for developing AIDS further complicates the risks of infection for heterosexual and all other "risk groups." The person who has had several lovers over a few years and subsequently becomes monogamous with a new partner may have acquired the infection from an earlier partner, perhaps as many as ten years before the initiation of the monogamous relationship. For instance, a young man who marries at age twenty-eight may have acquired the infection at age eighteen and unknowingly transmitted it to his wife-to-be, learning about his HIV positive status only from the blood test required to obtain a marriage license. Thus, a person with multiple partners, either concurrently or sequentially, is both at increased risk of the disease and serving as a conduit for transmission to his/her closest friends and loved ones.

The risk of AIDS among the heterosexual community appears not to be equal for men and women. The mechanics of transmission are such that during sexual intercourse tearing the tissue of a man is much less likely than tearing the tissue of a woman. Thus, vaginal intercourse is more likely to result in the transmission of HIV to a woman than to a man. The probability of tearing tissue on the penis and injecting blood or vaginal fluid into the man's bloodstream is very low, whereas the probability of incidentally tearing the woman's vaginal wall and injecting semen into the bloodstream is relatively high. Moreover, in heterosexual relationships, women can be the receptive partner for anal intercourse, where the probability of incidentally tearing tissue and injecting semen into the bloodstream is even greater. Thus, the mechanical procedures of transmission through sexual contact appear to place women at greater risk of acquisition from an already infected man than vice versa. Epidemiological studies have found relative risks for women versus men as high as 17.5 to 1, which confirm these differential risks of infection during heterosexual contact.[10]

This differential risk of AIDS among women versus men is essentially parallel to the differential risks that have been present for pregnancy all along. Therefore, to ensure the lowest risk of infection possible, women will have to take primary responsibility for safe sexual practices, including abstinence.

Testing for AIDS. It can take up to six months from acquiring HIV until the HIV antibodies show up on an HIV test. Therefore, a person who is tested two or three months after a sexual contact/infected needle use may get an incorrect "negative" test result. *That person needs to be tested again, six months after the INITIAL sexual contact or infected needle use, to obtain an accurate AIDS test.* After six months the test may accurately show a "positive" result, meaning the person does have the HIV inside of them.

Acquisition of Sexual Behavior and Intimacy

The acquisition of love and affection from another person and the ultimate development of sexual behavior are part of physical and psychological developmental processes. Children learn to be social, to follow gender specific social roles, and ultimately to establish mature adult relationships. This developmental learning process is a function of biological development (growth and puberty), with attendant hormonal changes in the body. These biological changes make sexual behavior more likely and reproduction possible. However, biology alone does not enable children and younger adolescents to establish intimate friendships, teach them how to initiate sexual relationships, nor how to perform sexual intercourse. These skills are learned through social processes. The cultural, family, and peer influences come to bear gradually on initial attempts at social relations and sexual behavior to yield the skills that make sexual relationships and intimacy possible.

Among the various social influences that lead children toward competence, both socially and sexually, is practice and feedback. Although verbal instruction, media models, and friends and family teach a great deal, the ultimate refinement in skills requires initial practice, feedback, and additional practice of improved variations in a given behavior. Sexual skills are no different than any other in this regard (see chapter 9). Typically, children discover their own sex organs and function, and ultimately experiment with sexual relations with other children. This experimentation occurs almost as incidental events. Their incidental basis, however, in no way reduces their importance to the ultimate development of mature adult relationship skills and sexual abilities.

Unlike learning to ride a bicycle or sing in a choir, the acquisition of sexual/social skills is shrouded in secrecy, practiced covertly, subject to exaggerated tales of sexual prowess among boys, subject to complete denial of experience or interest among young girls, formally proscribed by almost all important religious groups in the world, and rarely discussed by parents with their children. These conditions are designed to suppress the acquisition of sexual and intimacy skills, or at least to delay the behavior until marriage. This situation leads children to experiment in a world of incomplete and incorrect information about sex, and about intimate relationships. Chance experience determines the kind of sexual behavior learned and the age at which it may be acquired and practiced routinely. In spite of the enormous effort by religion and other cultural institutions, sexual behavior has not been reliably suppressed in youth. The teen pregnancy epidemic in the U.S. illustrates this point. The failure to suppress sexual behavior suggests the natural force involved in the acquisition of sexual behavior and intimacy is very powerful. Perhaps it will be healthier for the population and individuals to better understand sexual development and to promote the healthy acquisition of skills, rather than depend on happenstance in the context of coercive efforts at suppression.

ORGANIZATIONAL ISSUES

To paraphrase former Surgeon General C. Everett Koop, most Americans with AIDS contracted it by doing things of which most other people disapprove. This is summarized by the incredible dilemma faced by health promoters who work in the areas of sexuality and STDs. Women's and gay rights organizations, ACTUP, family planning agencies, and other organizers who work at least in part for health promotion are vocally and often violently opposed within their communities, while quietly shunned by federal funding agencies. Operation RESCUE, although apparently representing a minority of Americans' opinions, never seems to fail to recruit ample numbers of protesters for its social action approach to shut down legal family planning clinics. Revelations that celebrities, such as the late Rock Hudson, had AIDS are met as much with derision as sympathy. Magic Johnson was asked to not participate in the 1992 Olympics by Australia's team physician, and young Ryan White was forced out of elementary school in Indiana as penance for his having received HIV-contaminated blood in the course of medical care. (On the positive side, Elton John, Michael Jackson, and others graciously recognized Ryan's plight and added enjoyment and comfort to his final months of life.)

Whether working with existing organizations or starting from scratch, in no other area is the choice of social planning, local government and agency development, or social action more critical. Depending on needs and resource assessment and research data, the health promoter may be forced into a choice not necessarily of his or her own choosing.

NEEDS/RESOURCES ASSESSMENT

Given the highly controversial nature of programs promoting safer sex, a thorough (and relatively low profile) needs and resources assessment is a must. Key informant interviews and archival research can identify those elements and organizations in the community that promote sexual health as well as the types and sources of opposition they face. Rates of AIDS patients-under-treatment, public school educational services, and epidemiological data concerning risk factors help specify the extent of the problems associated with teen pregnancies, STDs, and AIDS. Surveys can be used to ascertain further the extent of support for and opposition to health promotion programs and policies in this area. These surveys can identify the degree to which myths about STDS and AIDS are ascribed to among special interest subgroups within the population, thereby providing guidance regarding the political competition between professional public health interventions and propaganda aimed at influencing public health service and research.

Knowledge, Attitudes, and Behavior (KAB), and Biology

The conduct of AIDS prevention research is troubled by difficulties in measurement. Relatively large sums of money have been directed to recording precise measures in AIDS research projects. It is not unusual for full physical examinations, including neurological analyses, to be conducted for people with AIDS or for gay males followed for possible conversion to HIV positive status. Although applied programs may not have the same resources for needs assessment or evaluation of outcomes, measurement of process and outcome are at least as important. All health promotion programs should have at least 25 percent of their budgets applied to evaluation purposes. Doing less risks continuation of ineffective and possibly damaging interventions. In short, it is unethical to conduct health promotion programs without ongoing evaluation of effects. In the AIDS prevention domain, this can be a very challenging objective.

Risk Behavior. Traditionally, health education or promotion programs rely on knowledge, attitudes, and behavior (KAB) surveys. Individuals are sent questionnaires or interviewed regarding their risk practices and possible variables that might predict (or influence) risk behavior. The HIV antibody testing counselor asks about the use or non-use of condoms, frequency of anal intercourse, etc. Unfortunately, these measures run the serious risk of being inaccurate and, to some extent, are directed toward concepts that may not contribute much to change in risk/protective behavior. Self-report measures of behavior are notoriously inaccurate due to difficulties with memory, with attention to key behavior at the time it was performed, and remembering what conditions prevailed when the behavior was performed. Surveys of KAB related to AIDS suffer from these sources of error and more.

All sanctioned behavior is at risk of being falsely reported. Asking individuals to reveal illegal or socially punishable behavior is likely to yield underestimates of such behavior. Asking about stealing property or other criminal actions, illegal and socially unacceptable drug use and abuse, and socially sensitive issues such as sexual intercourse, especially if practiced with a partner other than one's husband/wife, is not likely to yield accurate information.

This risk of false reporting has been addressed in this field by using anonymous interview procedures, where possible. Under conditions where the interviewer does not know the identity of the respondent, it is presumed the respondent will reveal sensitive information accurately. This almost certainly helps. Indeed, there is evidence that rates of risk behavior are higher when obtained from anonymous interviews than when confidential interviews are employed.[11] However, as self-reports, these measures continue to be invalidated by error due to memory and inattention.

Confidential interviews are the more common measurement procedures for programs with individuals or small groups in order to tailor a risk reduction procedure. These rely on the rapport developed between a counselor or educator and the respondent(s) and the promise not to reveal private information. Unfortunately, these sources of information may be compromised by a respondent's desire to please the counselor. How can you report that you remain sexually active without the use of a condom when your counselor has worked so hard to encourage you to use a condom each time you have intercourse?

Skills. The interview or survey measurement technology is not the only measurement system important in AIDS prevention. Assessing skills related to risk reduction is very important and lends itself to objective measurement. This has been accomplished by use of observers recording social/assertive skills during role-play "tests," or by observing videotapes of the same. These have the great advantage of objective measures obtained from unbiased recorders. The respondent's perception no longer slants the information obtained. Where possible, these measures represent a critical addition to the more typical KAB survey, and resources should be set aside for such measures in all programs targeting social skills training. However, even these measures are subject to important limitations that the program director must consider.

Skill measures are usually taken during role plays that can create "stage fright" or related anxiety. This makes performance of one's best skills difficult and can lead to underestimation of the individual's actual skill level. The more serious risk to measurement accuracy, however, is the degree to which role-play measures predict what the respondent will actually do in the real situation. Will the adolescent who assertively role-plays asking her partner to use a condom be able to use the same assertive skills with her steady boyfriend? Most likely, her assertiveness will depend on the degree of counter assertiveness exercised by her boyfriend and her "motivation" to avoid risk of AIDS. Actually, her social skill level will be less important than her history of reinforcement. Nevertheless, training and accurately measuring social skills is critical—individuals who lack minimum skills will not be able to request the use of condoms, even if motivated.

Attitudes. It is important to identify consumer satisfaction with the program. Asking participants whether they like certain aspects of a counseling program or if they are comfortable with measurement procedures can be critical for response maintenance. Such measures also direct program changes that may increase the effectiveness or, at least, the attractiveness of intervention strategies. These types of attitude measures may be very useful.

More common and more important are attitudes such as those related to birth control, homophobia, and "macho" and related gender-specific attitudes about sexual behavior. These types of attitudes are measured in most KAB surveys concerning the reduction of AIDS risk. These attitudes almost always correlate positively or negatively with actual risk, and they are frequently the target of education program efforts to "improve" attitudes. Although these attitudes can predict certain actions, such as voting against sex education in schools, it is much less clear whether changing attitudes will reliably result in significant change in actual sexual practices. Indeed, evidence to date suggests that changing attitudes does not reliably change risk behavior and that these same attitudes may be consequences of risk behavior (e.g., rationalizations) rather than causes. Thus, although it may be useful to record some forms of attitudes in the assessment of an AIDS risk reduction program, much less emphasis should be placed on attitude measurement and more circumspect interpretation of such measures should be exercised when they are recorded than has been typical of applied programs to date.

Later in this chapter we discuss other probable influences of risk behavior, and these should be considered as additional important measures to be obtained in the assessment of AIDS prevention programs. For instance, among adolescents, the type and density of peer pressure may be more influential than attitudes per se.

Biology. Medicine and public health suffer from an overwhelming bias towards biological measures. It is not unusual to hear that a study evaluated with only behavioral measures is not science. Whereas biological measures have their place, the ultimate outcome of all medicine and public health programs is to ensure the most competent behavior possible. All AIDS prevention programs should measure behavior as a primary outcome for evaluation. However, this does not preclude the assessment of biological outcomes.

The most obvious measure, and perhaps most controversial, is HIV status. Arguments prevail that HIV antibody testing and feedback can yield important decreases in risk behavior: when respondents learn they are HIV positive, they will almost automatically begin to practice safer sexual behavior. However, this may represent errors in causal logic. At least one report suggested that decreases in risk behavior preceded the decision to be tested for HIV status.[12] It is possible that testing is a consequence of other variables also responsible for changes in risk behavior, and in and of itself does not influence risk behavior dramatically. Alternatively, HIV status feedback may have no important influence on risk behavior, as reported in a recent investigation from a southern community with relatively small numbers of deaths due to AIDS within the gay male community.[13] Indeed, HIV positive individuals do not reliably inform their partners of their status or encourage them to be tested, further raising doubt as to the effects of HIV antibody testing for purposes of behavior change.

Some have even speculated that individuals who have been tested and proved to be HIV positive will react with rage and revenge, trying to infect others. Speculation abounds as to the reactions of tested individuals when they learn that they tested negative, apparently having not developed antibodies for the virus. If these individuals have practiced high rate risk behavior, this may reinforce the continued practice of such behavior. Even if not reinforcing risk behavior, negative results that are not followed up at least once or twice at various intervals with additional HIV status testing does not rule out the possibility that the tested individual had been exposed and/or infected, but had not yet produced sufficient antibodies to be detected as positive. This can convey a false sense of relief.

Others argue that testing is irrelevant, that safe life style behavior is all that is important, and that education and other interventions must be provided, regardless of testing outcomes. Indeed, all individuals should practice safer sex and not abuse drugs nor share needles. Testing outcomes do not change the importance of establishing and maintaining safe sex and other life style behaviors that reduce risk of HIV.

There is some fear that testing can only lead to government prejudicial sanctions, such as quarantine or jail for HIV positive individuals. So, should programs include HIV testing as part of their evaluation? The answer is, "it depends."

If the program is limited to preventing risk behavior among a small sample of people and with limited follow-up, there may be no value in HIV testing. If the program is to be evaluated with long-term follow-up for prevention of AIDS, then HIV testing can be one of many follow-up measures useful for determining whether the program resulted in a lower incidence of infection. Similarly, rates of disease and rates of immune system compromise may be crucial elements of a complete evaluation.

The Importance of Program Evaluation

The business of promoting AIDS prevention education and counseling has been underway for about eight years. With this experience, most casual interventions, in absence of evaluation measures, have been replaced by programs evaluated at least by KAB surveys. However, the next logical step is to begin formal analyses of effectiveness and to discontinue ineffective programs. It will be increasingly incumbent on health promotion directors to demonstrate the effectiveness of their programs in order to sustain funding. More importantly, unless more sophisticated evaluation becomes an inherent part of AIDS prevention intervention, these programs will run the risk of not evolving to more effective means of establishing protective life styles and not reducing deaths due to AIDS. Without vigorous assessment of programs, we cannot know what works and what does not, and AIDS deaths will continue at the same or higher rate.

Myths about the Transmission of HIV

The greatest myth about the risk of acquiring HIV is that it is easy to get the infection. Short of using syringes to inject the viruses, no risk factor will make the acquisition of AIDS very likely. In fact, acquisition of HIV is the least likely among the sexually transmitted diseases to be acquired. It is almost impossible to get the disease from doorknobs, toilet seats, shaking hands, or even kissing. Casual contact with persons who are HIV infected or have AIDS will not result in transmission of the disease to those who live with, care for, or befriend the infected individual. Sensible life styles will guarantee the prevention of AIDS. Table 19–1 shows the known means of transmission of HIV. Assessment of knowledge is a critical component of needs resources assessment (N/RA) in this area.

TABLE 19–1
HIV Transmission Routes

1. Blood transfusion with infected blood
2. Injection with contaminated syringe
3. Semen donation/artificial insemination
4. Organ tissue donation
5. Anal intercourse
6. Vaginal intercourse

PRIORITIES/OBJECTIVES FOR THE U.S.

The following are selected examples of objectives related to domestic family planning, STDs, and HIV infection as set forth in *Healthy People 2000*.[14] It is important to note that reaching these objectives is unlikely and even if reached will not result in complete control of teenage pregnancies or HIV infection in adolescents. Reaching these objectives represents an improvement over baseline, but not complete control of these epidemics.

Family Planning

1. Reduce pregnancies among girls aged 17 and younger to no more than 50/1000 from a baseline of 71.1 in 1985.
2. Reduce to no more than 30 percent the proportion of all unintended pregnancies (from 56 percent in 1988).
3. Increase to at least 90 percent the proportion of sexually active, unmarried people aged nineteen and younger who use contraception, especially combined method contraception, that both effectively prevents pregnancy and provides barrier protection against disease.

HIV Prevention and Control Objectives

1. Reduce the proportion of adolescents who have engaged in sexual intercourse to no more

than 15 percent by age fifteen and no more than 40 percent by age seventeen.

2. Increase to at least 50 percent the proportion of sexually active unmarried people who used a condom at last sexual intercourse.

RESEARCH AND INTERVENTION DIRECTIONS

Technology for Prevention and Control

Pregnancy. The medical interventions and technological procedures now available for the prevention or interruption of pregnancy are numerous. Here, only the most common and/or salient procedures are described. The prevention of pregnancy simply involves the prevention of contact between an ovum and sperm. The most reliable means of effecting no contact is abstinence from vaginal intercourse between men and women. Given the difficulty for most people to sustain abstinence as a means of birth control, alternatives have been developed, most notably, "barrier" methods.

Use of a diaphragm inserted into the vagina by the woman prior to sexual intercourse and removed shortly after intercourse will prevent semen from reaching an ovum in the overwhelming majority of cases. Similarly, the male may use a condom over the penis, within which ejaculation occurs during intercourse. In this instance, the semen is retained inside the condom and thereby prevents contact with an ovum. Both the diaphragm and condom methods can be enhanced by the concurrent use of a spermicide, ointments, or lubrications to kill the sperm. Use of spermicide alone is possible, but this is not considered a reliable means of birth control.

Historically, IUDs (intrauterine devices) have been used for birth control. These were inserted by a physician or nurse into the uterus. This device prevents the fertilized ovum from adhering to the uterine wall and elicits a "spontaneous" abortion in those instances where fertilization has occurred.

The pill, of course, is the best known means of birth control in modern societies. The pill is an oral contraception procedure which involves taking estrogen (a female hormone) to prevent ovulation. Sexual intercourse does not result in fertiliza-

tion of an ovum since no ovum is present. The pill is to be taken daily for the entire period within which the woman does not want to become pregnant.

Day-after pills, and most recently RU 486 (in Europe), are available for women as alternatives to daily estrogen. Day-after pills chemically induce spontaneous abortions if taken within the first few days of conception. To date there is no pill available for men as a reliable means of contraception.

Both men and women can be treated surgically to prevent conception. In women this involves tying the fallopian tubes, which prevents the passage of the ovum into the uterus. In men a vasectomy involves the excision of the vas deferens, thereby preventing the delivery of sperm through the penis. Each procedure is considered essentially permanent and is recommended only for women and men who do not plan to have (additional) children. These procedures are relatively safe and inexpensive to perform, but they are still too expensive to be practical for large portions of the population, especially in developing countries.

Finally, physicians and nurses can perform surgical abortions in order to remove a fertilized egg or a fetus prior to full development and delivery. If surgical procedures are conducted by trained and legally operating medical specialists during the first two trimesters, the risk to the woman is minimal. However, if they are performed later in the development period or under duress (i.e., illegal procedures performed by untrained or unscrupulous practitioners), risks to the woman are very high, and permanent sterilization or death is all too common. Even under normal circumstances, most therapeutic abortions involve anxiety and discomfort for the woman.

With all of the procedures now available for prevention of pregnancy or medication-induced abortion, effective contraception is dependent upon the behavior of women in most cases and men in some. The most likely reason for any of these methods to fail is that the individuals involved did not employ the procedure at all or applied them incorrectly. Thus, all of these birth control measures are dependent upon an individual's behavior. In addition, the ready availability of birth control devices or medications, such as the pill, has freed women and men from resorting to abstinence as the only reliable means of preventing births. This has likely increased the rate of sexual intercourse, while decreasing both births and the need for abortion.

Sexually Transmitted Diseases (STDs). The primary treatment for gonorrhea and syphilis are antibiotic medicines, usually penicillin. Treatment is almost always effective, resulting in a complete cure. However, treatment does not prevent reinfection if re-exposure occurs. Antibiotic-resistant strains of gonorrhea and other STD organisms have been identified. The occurrence of these strains raises the concern that uncontrolled epidemics could recur, especially if exposure to the bacteria is not prevented. Most exposure is via sexual contact, once again pointing to the need to understand and affect control of sexual behavior for effective prevention of STDs. Virus-caused STDs (e.g., genital warts) are treated with antiviral agents and, like the bacterial STDs, are not medically preventable. The only means of prevention is elimination of exposure.

Acquired Immune Deficiency Syndrome (AIDS). There is no vaccine or immunization for HIV infection; and as is the case with other STDs, there is no medical prevention of AIDS. Use of AZT and other medications seems to decrease the progress of the disease. However, even AZT does not cure the HIV-infected individual. So far, all infected individuals eventually die from opportunistic diseases due to AIDS-compromised immune systems. Numerous infectious agents cause opportunistic disease in AIDS cases and ultimately cause death.[15] Table 19–2 shows some of these infections. Again, prevention requires avoidance of exposure to the virus. To avoid the virus, major changes are required in the behaviors of injection drug users and the sexual practices of the whole population.

Scientists are working in numerous laboratories to develop an "AIDS vaccine." This has never been achieved for a retro-virus such as HIV and, if possible at all, will take a long time to accomplish. The first human trials of an HIV vaccine are not scheduled before 1994. If successful, a readily available vaccine will not be possible before the year 2000. Once developed, its expense may preclude sufficient dissemination to control the AIDS epidemic in developing nations and poor or minority populations. In short, control of the AIDS epidemic relies heavily on the effectiveness of behavioral science to change risk behavior patterns.

TABLE 19–2
Opportunistic Infections in HIV-Infected Individuals

Aspergillus (fungi)
Atypical mycobacteria
Candida (fungi)
Cryptococcus (fungi)
Cryptosporidium (a protozoan)
Cytomegalovirus
Herpes Simplex
Histoplasma (fungi)
Isospora (a protozoan)
Mycobacterium Tuberculosis
Pneumocystis Carinii
Toxoplasma Gondii (a protozoan)

Development of Sexual/Social Behavior

Evolutionary Foundations. People are highly social animals. We tend to congregate in groups, and we tend to form relatively long-lasting partnerships with the opposite sex. Love relationships and sexual relationships are tied together intimately. Clearly, procreation is necessary to sustain the population. However, procreation does not require love and affection. Yet, most people engage in sexual behavior in the context of loving and affectionate relationships.

Early communities with norms of long-term relationships based on love and affection were presumably more stable than were communities based on casual contact and numerous partners. Indeed, the social support literature suggests that the degree of affective support received may be protective from disease and dysfunction. Loving relationships, including sexual relations, are important for health and well-being. If so, efforts to suppress sexual behavior may be unlikely to succeed and could conceivably increase the risk of morbidity or at least reduce the quality of life.

Understanding Intimacy and Sexual Behavior. The scientific study of intimacy has yet to be developed in a meaningful manner. Sexual behavior has come under scientific study within this century, and most of the attention has been devoted to biology. Investigations of sexual responses from Masters and Johnson's laboratory provided detailed information about arousal and sexual climax in women. These studies represented breakthroughs in the knowledge of sexual responses, even though they did not focus on relationships per se (and most women were recruited from among prostitutes). Most of these studies have not been replicated in representative populations, testimony to the cultural barriers to the study of "normal" people. With the AIDS epidemic, the head-in-the-sand approach to sexual behavior and intimacy is no longer affordable. The barriers to understanding and ultimately influencing sexual behavior and the establishment of healthy intimate relationships must be overcome in order to control the AIDS epidemic, and possibly many other social epidemics which reduce quality of life (e.g., divorce, homicide, suicide, child abuse, spouse abuse, rape, etc.). Unfortunately, many deaths may be required before the political and religious barriers to the study of sexual behavior and intimate relationships are removed.

Teens' Sexual Behavior and Condom Use

Sexual Intercourse. Since 1971 there has been an increase in the proportion of adolescent girls who report having engaged in at least one instance of sexual intercourse. Across all races, rates have increased from about 28 percent to over 40 percent. In 1982, the reported rate of coitus was 64 percent for males and 44 percent for females by age eighteen.[16] Rates of coitus among teen women appear to have risen from just over 40 percent to as much as 52 percent by 1988.[17] These trends suggest that the frequency of sexual intercourse among adolescents is high and increasing. This is especially likely in the context of reporting error, where the reported frequency among women is likely to be an underestimate of the true rate. Males might overestimate their rates somewhat. Interpolation of these data and those recently reported from the Centers for Disease Control suggest that more than 50 percent of all teens have initiated sexual intercourse by age eighteen.[18] Naturally, these rates increase

with age. The mean age of first intercourse is sixteen years, and at least 20 percent of these have had four or more partners.[19]

The ramifications of these data are wide-ranging. First, they imply a natural process that is not successfully suppressed by cultural and religious doctrine or the relative secrecy within the community regarding sexual behavior and intimacy. Second, these data indicate that most teenagers engage in sexual behavior which places them at risk of pregnancy, STDs, AIDS, and emotional upsets in the course of learning mature, person-to-person relationships, including sexual relations. This, of course, assumes that most people eventually acquire a mature and healthy interpersonal relationship and sexual skills.

Condom Use. The only means of preventing AIDS transmission as a result of sexual contact and a common means of preventing pregnancy is continuous use of condoms for all instances of sexual intercourse. Although condoms are not sufficient for preventing all forms of STDs, their use contributes substantially to the prevention of STDs. Thus, the use of condoms while engaging in intercourse is a critical means of prevention. Unfortunately, condom use is not reliable among teens or any other sexually active group. However, since the discovery and publications of the AIDS virus, rates of condom use appear to be increasing.

In 1982, 22.6 percent of sexually active adolescent women reported use of a condom by their male partner during their first intercourse. By 1988, this rate had increased to 47.4 percent. When considered by racial/ethnic groups, white women's partners increased condom use from about 25 percent to 51 percent; African-American women from 18 percent to 35 percent; and Hispanic women from 13 percent to 42 percent.[20] The most recently reported data from CDC confirm these rates, with about 45 percent of high school students reporting use of a condom during their most recent instance of intercourse.[21] These rates are very encouraging, especially for the Hispanic community for whom initial rates were the lowest.

It is critical to point out, however, that these rates of condom use are self-reported retrospectively and are subject to demand bias inflating reports above actual rates. In addition, they are much higher than the rates for continuous condom use for all instances of intercourse. For sexually active teens who reported ever using condoms, only 50 percent reported using them consistently, and of these, 58 percent reported intercourse with multiple partners.[22] These data demonstrate that effective AIDS prevention is not being achieved by reliable use of condoms for the overwhelming majority of sexually active teens, and that many teens are engaging in intercourse with numerous partners, and thereby increase their chance of exposure to HIV.

Patterns of Sexual Behavior and Condom Use.   The patterns of sexual behavior and condom use noted above illustrate that adolescents gradually become sexually active and that some begin to use condoms during intercourse. The patterns also illustrate a wide range of variability among youth. Some initiate intercourse at a relatively young age (e.g., less than sixteen years). A few employ condoms for their first instance of intercourse, but the majority do not. The variability among youth makes it clear that late initiation of sexual behavior can occur and reliable use of condoms can be established. In short, we know it is possible to delay sexual activity and thereby reduce the risk of disease or pregnancy; and for those who are sexually active, it is possible to use condoms reliably. What we do not know is what accounts for the initiation of sexual activity at a given age; what accounts for the frequency or number of partners with whom a given adolescent engages in intercourse, or the determinants of reliable condom use. Theory and theory-based epidemiology can provide some of these answers and point the direction for additional investigations from which these answers are most likely to come.

Theoretical Models of Sexual Behavior and Condom Use

For applied sciences, such as public health, it is important that theories not only point to testable questions, but also that they emphasize potentially modifiable variables. These variables, if confirmed as related to some outcome of importance such as sexual behavior, can be causally related to the outcome and altered to effect change in the outcome (i.e., decrease in the number of sexual partners). For instance, if knowledge of HIV trans-

mission routes is related to HIV risk behavior (e.g., anal intercourse), then training people to understand the means by which certain behaviors lead to increased risk of infection could decrease the practice of the same risk behaviors. Unfortunately, few formal theories of sexual behavior or the reliable use of condoms have been developed. Of those available, most are broad biological or psychosocial models, which tend not to isolate many potentially modifiable variables.[23] These tend to be limited in their potential for directing interventions that might be an effective means of preventing AIDS. Still others point to broad social factors (e.g., income/poverty) which can be changed, but without having the knowledge or ability to change such variables, the practical control of the AIDS epidemic will remain limited.

Rational Cognitive Models.   Most theoretical models designed to explain human behavior rely on some degree of cognition or thinking and a rational weighing of costs and benefits for some action which lead to decision and subsequent action. Two well-known models have been applied to health-related behavior and to contraceptive use in particular. These are the Health Belief Model and the Ajzen-Fishbein Theory of Reasoned Action (see chapter 3).[24] Each of these depends on concepts of thinking/cognition and decision-making which, in turn, lead to overt behavior. The first problem with these models is that the cognitive processes are not objectively measurable. As such, they do not meet one of the requirements for a "good" theory; namely, they provoke questions which are not explicitly testable.

These models assume that an individual weighs the costs and benefits for a given behavior and then proceeds to perform the response that maximizes benefits and minimizes costs. Seemingly foolish behavior, such as riding a motorcycle without a helmet, is presumably a function of inadequate information as to the risks of injury or an inappropriate weighing of risk to benefit. Failure to use a condom during sexual intercourse is presumably a function of not knowing the risks of pregnancy or disease, especially AIDS; or it is due to valuing (an attitude) the sexual pleasure in the absence of condoms more greatly than one fears the risk of disease.

The normal follow-through, given these models, is to provide individuals with appropriate sexual education or counseling to change their knowl-

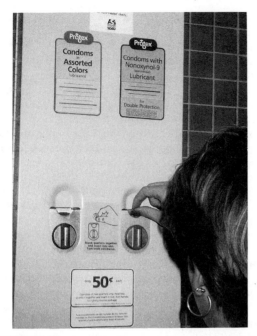

FIGURE 19–1. Condom machines in women's as well as men's restrooms reduce embarrassment and other barriers associated with their purchase. *Photo courtesy of Betsy Clapp.*

edge of risks or to change their attitudes regarding the probability or severity of risks in relation to benefits. Presumably, such education or counseling will lead to more appropriate decisions and lowered risk-taking behavior.

These models have been correlated with intentions to use birth control,[25] when measures of attitudes have been related to intentions to use the pill or condoms. However, when self-reported contraceptive behavior rather than intentions have been used in such studies, the predictive relationship is much weaker.[26] Most studies of these models have been retrospective questionnaires where respondents are asked about their attitudes and "reasons" for using or not using a condom. It has been shown that adolescents will endorse almost any reason for their behavior if given a choice and prompted to do so.[27] These data suggest that correlational support for these types of decision-making models of behavior, especially sexually sensitive behavior, may represent rationalizations after-the-fact; reasons given for not using a condom are those that please an interviewer or avoid criticism. These may have

very little to do with the actual controlling variables, such as reinforcement history or peer pressure. Similarly, when intervention studies based on these models have been tested, results are weaker than the theory predicts.

Results from sex education programs and formal community education services provide persuasive evidence of the limitations of interventions designed to change knowledge and attitudes. Most education programs have resulted in increased knowledge and some change in attitudes.[28] For example, Hillman and colleagues showed that a dramatic live play regarding AIDS risks improved knowledge and liberalized attitudes regarding homosexuality, but did not increase intentions to use condoms.[29] In another study of self-selected and "worried" volunteers reporting for HIV testing, professional and individualized counseling regarding risk behavior increased condom use relative to controls who did not receive the same counseling, but the cumulative rate of condom use did not reach 50 percent for the experimental group. Over half of the counseled group continued to have intercourse in the absence of condom use.[30] Most studies have evaluated only short-term results, and when long-term results were considered, the degree to which people maintained behavior change was marginal. For the studies noted here, it is reasonable to presume that the long-term rates of condom use would be much lower than 50 percent in the long run. These interventions and others strongly suggest that something more than education or counseling is necessary for reliable changes in AIDS risk behavior among most people.[31]

Social Cognitive and Operant Learning Theories. Since Skinner's early work concerning an objective analysis of human behavior and the description of basic principles of behavior, numerous studies have been conducted to verify the validity of the operant model of human behavior.

Overlapping the many operant investigations, Bandura performed related investigations with children, thereby illustrating the relatively great influence of modeling and imitation in child development. Taking his lead from various learning theorists, Bandura promoted "Social Learning Theory," which relied on the same basic principles but placed special emphasis on the role of models and imitation.[32] Social learning theory also reestablished a conceptual role for cognition, or thinking, and, in doing so, drifted toward the rational-decision-making models, such as those noted above (see chapter 3).

In spite of the differences between these two models, their area of overlap is great, especially with regard to implied interventions. As described in earlier chapters of this text, both models assume that principles of reinforcement, including schedules and shaping processes, are responsible for human behavior.

Learning Theory Applications

The use of both operant and social learning theory (chapter 3) to explain some of the critical determinants of sexual behavior and the control of the AIDS epidemic have been described by others.[33] Figure 19–3 shows a highly simplified theoretical schematic for the possible influences that may occur for condom use. When a man and a woman are nearing the point of sexual intercourse, the woman can ask her partner to use a condom. As Figure 19–2 depicts, the immediate consequences of condom use may be quite aversive under the circumstances of love-making. It is possible, especially for the inexperienced teen, to have difficulty putting on the condom, to experience some physical discomfort (e.g., pinching), and to lose his erection. This may result in embarrassment, anger, or social criticism from his female partner, and ultimately a failure to achieve

sexual intercourse or sexual climax. This scenario would be punishing for most people, thereby reducing the probability of condom use in the future, which could even lead to a dissolution of the relationship altogether.

Conversely, Figure 19–3 shows a hypothetical sequence of events that might increase the likelihood of condom use. This scenario assumes past experience with condoms and how to put one on appropriately. The female partner again requests that the male use a condom and he does. The consequences in this case are quite different. There is no pain, no fumbling, and the erection is sustained. Moreover, the erection is sustained longer with the condom than would have been likely in its absence (due to the reduced sensations), thereby enabling the male to hold off climax until his female partner climaxes. This result is likely to be very reinforcing for most people and should lead to condom use in the future.[34] Combined, these scenarios illustrate one of the most important features of these theories, namely, that the probability of future behavior depends on response consequences (i.e., reinforcement or punishment) in one's past experiences. At one point in time and under certain circumstances, the consequences for a given behavior could be very reinforcing; at another time or under other circumstances, the same behavior could be punished.

These examples also point out how difficult it can be to control condom use. The most important reinforcers are likely to be those related to sexual pleasures and partner reactions during and

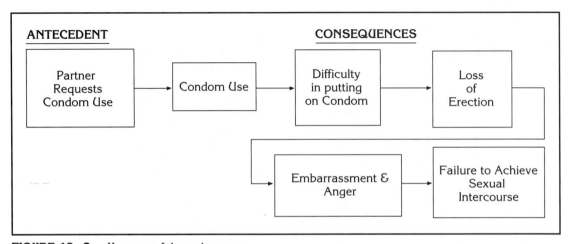

FIGURE 19–2. Unsuccessful condom use

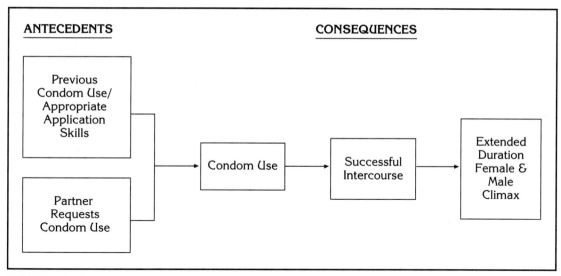

FIGURE 19–3.   Successful condom use

immediately after a sexual experience. The opportunity for parents, religious leaders, or public health professionals to compete with these influences is compromised severely. Nevertheless, indirect interventions may be designed to make condom use more likely.

Comprehensive Interventions to Promote Condom Use

Expanding on the logic initially presented in Figures 19–2 and 19–3, Figure 19–4 shows an expanded model of condom use. This figure depicts a series of distal and proximal antecedents and consequences by major sociological categories. The arrows depict the hypothesized direction of causal influence. Some boxes are shown "causing" some of the other boxes, and these combine to influence the occurrence of condom use. The variables on the left side of the center box (i.e., "condom use") refer to antecedents, while those on the right refer to possible consequences. Although both antecedents and consequences influence the occurrence of condom use, consequences are far more influential.

Gender and Genetics.   The far left side of the figure shows a box depicting gender and genetics. In all likelihood both the specific gender and hor-

monal balance defined by gender, plus unknown genetic variables, set the stage for certain sexual preferences (e.g., homosexual vs. heterosexual) and abilities. For example, the ease or intensity of sexual climax at the conclusion of sexual intercourse can be determined partly by the individual's physical anatomy and general strength. Some people may more easily reach sexual climax and hence are more able to achieve sexual reinforcement. Little research has explored the differences among people in physical or genetic differences that might be related to differential sexual performance. This is an area in need of future investigation.

Culture and Sex Roles.   The general culture within which an individual is born and raised determines the overall rules to be learned and the specific sex roles to be followed.[35] For instance, levels of modesty vary by country and culture. In some Middle East countries it is improper for women to show their faces in public; but as close as a few hundred miles away on the beaches of southern France, it is common to see women topless. Italian, Greek, Russian, and other cultural groups teach men to hug and kiss each other as part of a casual social greeting without implying homosexuality; the same behavior would be considered shocking in Nebraska. Thus, culture defines the general type of behavior learned and

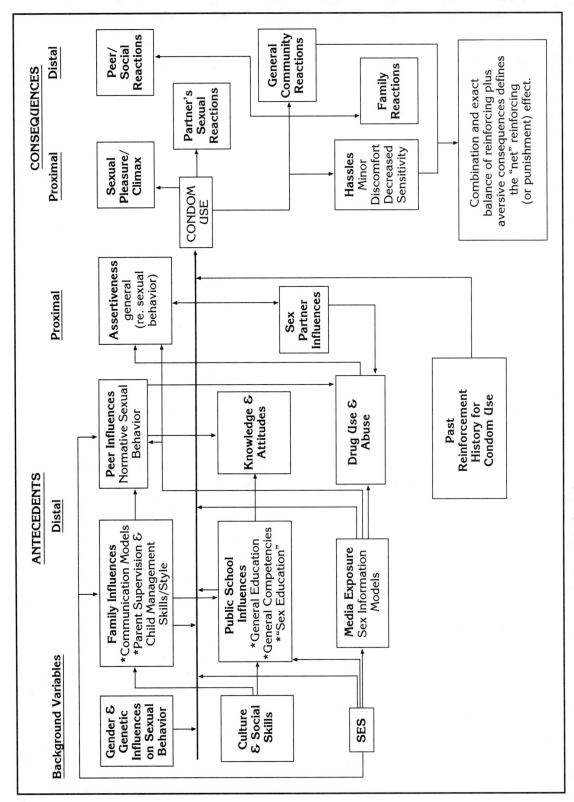

FIGURE 19–4. An operant conceptual model of condom use

expected. Most of the people in a given culture follow the same "rules" and serve as incidental models to be imitated. They also provide incidental feedback, both reinforcing and punishing— depending on the nature of the imitations. These same cultural standards also influence family, schools, and media. Thus, other formal and informal teaching systems provide culturally consistent information and, in turn, differentially promote, reinforce, and punish behaviors consistent with the cultural norms.

How liberal a culture is with regard to sexual behavior influences the frequency of that behavior. However, because sex occurs in private, community sanctions (or reinforcers) are usually indirect, delayed, and often relatively weak in relation to the immediate reinforcers obtained from sexual intercourse. Thus, sexually conservative cultures may have the undesired effect of simply leading people not to admit to their sexual activities. Until the late sixties and early seventies in the U.S., it was not common for homosexuals to be public with their sexual preferences. Such covert behavioral practices complicate the professional community's ability to provide services to control disease. For example, the more conservative community might not permit condoms to be sold without a prescription or in highly public places. Even in relatively "liberal" communities, key officials often maintain conservative policies with regard to AIDS control. Recently, the president of San Diego State University (SDSU) formally opposed the student council when they proposed putting condom machines on campus; in contrast, condom vending machines have been on the Virginia Tech campus since 1989. Undoubtedly the president of SDSU represented many parents' views about sex among college students and, in so doing, inhibited action that might reduce the chance of AIDS transmission among young adult students. The policy at SDSU has changed, however, and condoms can now be bought from machines in men's rooms.

Socioeconomic Status. The subgroups within a given culture vary by education, income, and various subcultures implied by religion, home nationality, etc. Generally, people who represent the very well educated and wealthy have fewer risk factors for morbidity and mortality, have greater access to medical and other community resources, and have the resources to make it possible for their children to achieve similar status in the community. The reverse tends to be true for people at the lower end of the socioeconomic status (SES) continuum.[36] The SES factors defining a given family, influence the neighborhood in which they can afford to live, the neighborhood in which they would prefer to live, and the schools which their children will attend. Thus, the well educated and affluent family can elect to live in a country estate and send their children to select private schools. The poor minority family lives in the inner city, and the children probably attend overcrowded public schools filled with other poor children. Many of the youth in school as well as the general neighborhood are at risk for being recruited into gangs and subsequently engaging in illegal and dangerous behavior. In this manner, the SES of the family determines quality of formal education and other community services, as well as the nature of the peer group with whom a given adolescent will associate. The wealth of the community in general has been associated with condom use among teenagers—the poorer the community, the less the condom use.[37] Therefore, SES determines the background physical and social environment and provides an ecological influence on behavior, including sexual activity.

Family Influences. Families determine the detailed socialization process for children through late adolescence. Parents provide incidental models of general social behavior and, indirectly, sexual behavior. Parents also provide rules and child management contingencies, which make dramatic differences in the child's probable range of behavior. The degree to which parents communicate about sexually sensitive issues or express love and affection in the home can in turn influence the child's ultimate ability to express love and affection. There is little doubt that families influence the sexual behavior of their children. Research concerning family influences has shown that few parents discuss sexually explicit issues with their adolescent children.[38] However, sexually active adolescents are more likely to use contraceptives when their parents discussed sexually sensitive issues with them.[39] More research is needed to determine the degree to which parent-child management influences dating behavior, number of partners, likelihood of sexual intercourse, and use of condoms. The influence of older or younger siblings and their dating patterns has yet to be fully explored, but almost certainly serves as a model to be imitated for some brothers and sisters. In addition, the dating behavior of parents can influence the child's social/sexual behavior patterns. In the latter instance, a parent's behavior might not be consistent with their rules for the adolescent. For instance, a mixed message is evident when a child's mother is having a sexually active relationship with her boyfriend while maintaining rules prohibiting her adolescent daughter from engaging in intercourse prior to marriage. Learning theory predicts modeled behavior to be more influential than instructions.

Family rules and styles of living are influenced to some degree by the neighborhood and the peer group available for an adolescent to join, and vice versa. Parents may allow or disallow certain types of peers into the home, and attempt to control the individuals that their adolescent child is to date or with whom he or she can associate. The balance of these family influences along with peer pressure makes a big difference in an adolescent's sexual behavior and risks for AIDS.

Public Schools.   Perhaps the largest influence schools have on development of sexual behavior is access to a large and varied population of peers —access to youth with whom an individual might have sexual intercourse. Schools also are the place where most youth spend eight or more hours per day with their peers. This enables the development of initial social ties from which dating behavior and eventually sexual behavior evolve. Such extensive exposure to a large peer population also sets the stage for population-specific norms to develop. Styles of dress and interpersonal behavior can become stylized and unique to the school environment or the adolescent community, separate from the broader adult community. Dressing, language and communication fads, as well as standards about sexual behavior, can exert extensive influence over an adolescent's behavior, including dating and sex. It seems that schools are a critical component in the development of peer pressure influence.

Schools also provide general education. Academic skills are likely to make individuals more competent in many areas of life, including social/sexual relations. Grades and academic standing have been related to sexual behavior. However, one of the most powerful influences on sexual behavior is likely to be formal "sex education."

Sex education varies in content, duration, and quality. Early education programs even segregated males and females. Other programs have emphasized the biology of reproduction, with little attention devoted to social or sexual behavior. Some programs have explained the dangers of sexually transmitted diseases, but often without explaining how they are acquired or prevented, short of abstinence. With the development of the AIDS epidemic, improved formal sex education has begun, with increased discussion of sexual issues.[40] However, improvements in contraceptive use in general or condoms in particular has not yet been demonstrated.[41] Implicitly, sex education is predicated on the rational-decision-making models of health behavior, as noted earlier. The new information is supposed to make it possible for adolescents to make intelligent decisions regarding sexual behavior, including condom use. From a learning theory perspective, sex education can provide important information about risks or places to buy condoms, but it is not likely to be sufficient to make big differences in adolescents' sexual behavior. Most programs do not take into account the skills needed for certain outcomes, such as condom use, and none provide reinforcement for specific forms or frequencies of sexual behavior. Although school education programs almost certainly can be improved, they are not likely to make a big difference in sexual behavior as long as they focus on promoting abstinence or are conceptualized as an information dissemination service.

Media.   Television, movies, radio, and print media provide dramatic and vivid models of the overall culture. Moreover, often these models are presented in the context of conditions that make them most likely to evoke imitations; they display individuals similar to their target audience; they display prestigious individuals, and they show heros and heroines as receiving frequent positive reinforcement. There is little doubt that the media influence sexual development and specific forms of sexual behavior.

A number of studies have demonstrated that television contains a considerable amount of information and models concerning sexual issues, and more recently AIDS.[42] These studies have demonstrated that the majority of sexually-related material on TV is erotic and suggestive of sexual pleasure. A small proportion of the content is related to pregnancy or STD prevention, and essentially none of the content demonstrated an individual acquiring a sexually-transmitted disease. Since these studies, there have been dramatic documentaries concerning AIDS and the trials of living and dying with AIDS. However, the popular media continues to present a fantasy version of human sexual behavior, one that promotes sex as a wildly pleasurable activity, free of aversive consequences, and to be performed as often as possible by males, to be resisted, but not too seriously by enticing females, and to be performed on the spur of the moment without planning and without contraception. These models and their pervasiveness in the community probably contribute to the occurrence of sexual activity and the relatively limited use of condoms.

Peers and Sexual Partners.   The generally accepted role of peer pressure as a major influence of adolescent behavior applies to the development and maintenance of social and sexual behavior as certainly as it does to any other. However, because sexual behavior occurs in relative privacy, even within the adolescent subcommunity, the social influence is indirect and imprecise. Youth perform some types of sexual activity at some frequency; but what they are socially applauded for is what they report, and this may be somewhat more or less sexual activity or activity of a different type from that actually performed. Again, the feedback system for sexual behavior remains somewhat imprecise. Nevertheless, female rates of sexual intercourse do correlate significantly with rates reported by their friends.[43] Contraception also is positively related to the rates reported by friends.[44]

From a learning theory perspective, it is presumed that peers provide models of behavior to be imitated. Even if the observed model does not go so far as sexual intercourse, it may serve as a validation of reports of sexual exploits that were not available to public review. In this system, the reports of sexual behavior may serve as a verbal model to be imitated. Unfortunately, imitating reported behavior may lead to an exaggerated view of actual behavior, in that reported sexual activities are likely to be more "positive" (e.g., more frequent sexual intercourse than is true for males). The social criticism and praise is likely to be negatively and positively reinforcing, respectively. To the degree to which the social feedback comes

from important peers, such as close friends, the power of the feedback as either negative or positive reinforcement increases. The nature of the social network from which an individual receives the same feedback also affects the power of punishment or reinforcement. Thus, the young male who reports to his closest buddies that he successfully persuaded his girlfriend to engage in sexual intercourse is likely to receive praise. As the rumors spread, he may receive additional praise from even distant male friends. This can add greatly to the reinforcing effects of the actual experience and serve as a model for imitation by his close friends.

Although peers provide reinforcement, the most powerful influences of sexual behavior are likely those involved in the social relationship and sexual pleasures obtained from a sexual dyad. Boyfriends and girlfriends provide one another with extremely powerful prompts and reinforcement for their intimate relationship. Initially, the young man may play an assertive role in persuading the young woman to comply with his interest in having sexual intercourse. Once she complies and has experienced sexual intercourse, especially if the experience was pleasurable, she comes under the influence of the reinforcing effects of the behavior. Subsequent instances of sexual intercourse may be prompted by the young woman, rather than the young man. Once the pair has had intercourse and enjoyed it, chances are they will do it many times again and eventually will come to describe their relationship as love. When the pair defines their relationship as love, the expectations for behavior change, and intercourse, is more likely.

Even if the initial experiment with sexual intercourse does not provide the young woman with a sexual climax or even was somewhat painful and distasteful (i.e., not reinforcing and somewhat punishing), the persuasive power of the young man may sustain the relationship and set the stage for additional instances of sexual intercourse. This is especially likely if the woman is trying to please the young man in order to maintain the relationship or if she is testing herself to see if she is "normal" and can achieve sexual pleasure. Conversely, this same "self-testing" might apply to the young man. It may take a number of instances of sexual intercourse for the pair to learn how to please one another, or to learn that they are not likely to do so. In the latter instance the relationship is likely to dissipate, with each member looking for a new potential partner.

The hypothetical sequence above probably depicts most adolescents' sexual development. The process of acquiring experience and competence at sexual intercourse requires some practice and good fortune. For most adolescents this practice entails having multiple sequential partners. Most do not marry their first boyfriend or girlfriend, nor would that be likely to work out as an optimal partnership. Thus, development of normal social/sexual competence requires (in most instances) multiple partners — one of the more serious risk factors for transmission of STDs and AIDS — and repeated practice in order to learn how to have pleasurable sexual intercourse.

This sequence of social/sexual competence development raises questions about the effects of truly effective suppressive procedures. The U.S. culture tends to promote abstinence until marriage as the official standard. If efforts to suppress sexual development were effective, they might inadvertently compromise the development of adult interpersonal skills with unknown compromises in quality of life.

Social Skills. Adolescents contend with the risks of STDs, pregnancy, and ensuing emotional pain and suffering as inherent components of the maturational process. With the advent of more effective and available contraceptives (e.g., "the pill"), the risk of pregnancy has been reduced but not eliminated. The risks for STDs and emotional pain (i.e., a "broken heart") have not been reduced, and may have increased as the pressure to have sexual intercourse increased. The effective management of these risks has required some assertiveness, especially on the part of women. However, if the woman failed to assert herself, but used "the pill," she could at a minimum avoid pregnancy. AIDS, at least, has increased the social and assertiveness requirements of adolescents well above those previously required.

To avoid pregnancy a young woman does not need to discuss the issues with her partner at all. She can take birth control pills or use a diaphragm, with little involvement from the young man. She is not dependent on him to perform in some particular way, nor is his permission required. However, the only two means of reliable prevention of HIV infection are abstinence and use of a condom. The male must remain abstinent or use a condom. For young women, typically trained to be somewhat submissive and less assertive than men, their responsibility now includes the initiation of a discussion on possible risks of AIDS, including a review of her potential partner's sexual and drug history and ultimately requiring her partner to use a condom without destroying the romantic and loving relationship. The assertive skills necessary to perform these discussion and negotiation tasks are not clearly established in the verbal repertoire of many adults, let alone most adolescents.

The social demands for the adolescent male are somewhat different than the female, but greater than prior to the AIDS epidemic. The traditional role for the male has been to be the assertive partner, persuading the female to comply with sexual desires. Indeed, most cultures teach men to play this type of role. Yet, in the context of AIDS, the young man now must be prepared to discuss the possible risk history of his girlfriend; he must consider the possibility of discontinuing the relationship if the young woman has had numerous sexual partners or a history of injection drug use. Finally, the male must be prepared to use condoms, even if the young woman is taking birth control pills, and even if the young man feels that sexual pleasure is reduced when using a condom. Thus, today the young man must have much greater social/assertive skills than might have been true prior to AIDS, but more importantly, the male is now called on to use these skills in a manner contrary to his typical social role and contrary to his personal reinforcement history for sexual behavior. Again, it is not clear whether many adult males can live up to these new standards.

Communication within the sexual dyad has been related to contraceptive use.[45] However, it is not clear how often contraception is discussed in sexual dyads and it may be relatively infrequent.[46] To make matters more complex, it appears that general assertiveness skills are not sufficient. Wills, Baker, and Botvin found that general assertiveness was not predictive of assertiveness needed for resistance of drug use and abuse, but the skills necessary for drug use resistance were related to the assertiveness required for control of sexual risks.[47] Thus, it appears the assertiveness required to prevent exposure to AIDS requires formal training over and above that sufficient to establish general assertiveness skills.

Alternatively, it is possible that some youth have advanced assertiveness skills, even for sexually sensitive issues, but do not employ them. Rather, they accept the risks of AIDS in order to obtain the reinforcement derived from sexual intercourse. Evidence of this type of motivational problem comes from the HIV testing programs. Over half of adults who tested positive for HIV did not tell their sexual partner(s) of their infection.[48] This demonstrates the difficulty in bringing individuals to act in a manner that could reduce the risk of AIDS for others when such communication could cost them in terms of relationships and sexual pleasures. In other words, the motivational processes may preclude the use of assertive skills, even when the adolescent (or adult) has acquired relatively advanced verbal abilities. Formal training programs aimed at social skills have demonstrated merit. Based largely on learning theory, the use of models and practiced imitations (role-playing) and shaping procedures in analogue situations has been effective for increasing the assertive skills for drug use resistance;[49] similar training has decreased cigarette use.[50] Kelly and colleagues have used an intensive version of the same training to teach gay males assertive skills to reduce their risk of probability in risk behavior for AIDS.[51] Gilchrist and Schinke have used these procedures with adolescent girls for pregnancy control and demonstrated an increase in contraception use at six-months follow-up.[52] These same skill training procedures are now being tested in a number of clinical trials to determine whether they can establish the necessary skills and reduce the risk of AIDS in adolescents (Project STARRT).[53]

Social skills training involves shaping procedures and use of both models and practice with feedback. These techniques are provided in the context of role-played exercise. Project STARRT (Skills Training for Aids Risk Reduction) uses the following procedures for training social skills for reduction of AIDS risk behavior. (See also chapters 9 and 13, and the description of Project SHOUT in chapter 16). First, training entails about two hours per session for nine sessions—once per week. This represents considerably more training time than most programs in public schools or community centers. The curriculum starts with an overview of anatomy and reproductive physiology at the most basic level, which is essential to understanding the transmission of AIDS viruses and their prevention. This is followed by an overview of common techniques of birth control, with emphasis placed on condom use, as the only reliable means of preventing HIV infection. At this time non-sensitive topics (e.g., inviting a best friend out after school) are role-played, followed by role-play instruction in how to: (1) say no, (2) say no to drugs or sexual overtures, (3) inquire about the sex and drug history of a potential partner, (4) discuss options and set limits regarding sexual behavior with a partner, (5) discuss sexual concerns with an adult adviser (possibly a parent), and (6) purchase condoms in a public store. In order to maintain the shaping procedures for overall training, these skills are introduced in the order of least invasive or sensitive to the most intimate issues.

Shaping procedures are used in the role-plays as well. Each role-play is between thirty seconds and three minutes long, depending on the teachers judgment and the student's ability. First, the teacher provides a model to illustrate how to say no (or some other verbal skill). This is followed by a formal rationale, which emphasizes the benefits to be realized by the adolescent. The rationale is followed by the adolescent practicing the skill illustrated by the teacher in a role-play with another peer or the teacher. The role-played performance is critiqued by the teacher with emphasis on the features of the practice that were performed well and assertively. This is followed by an additional demonstration by the teacher, emphasizing features of the same skill which needs improvement and a request to the adolescent to repractice the skill in another role-play. The students in the audience benefit from watching the whole process until they have an opportunity to engage in role-played exercises with the teacher or with each other. The process repeats with changes in the scenario and with continued attention to refinement of quality and assertiveness in verbal exchange. Attention is also given to non-verbal body language, especially active listening skills.

Education.   Knowledge of sexual risks and risk avoidance procedures can make risk reduction possible. Education about condoms, for instance, can be an important prerequisite for risk reduction. However, as noted earlier, the acquisition of knowledge about disease or risk conditions and their means of reduction is not likely to be sufficient to alter high probability behavior. This is most evident in the recent data that show that over 95 percent of the U.S. population is aware of AIDS and knows that the virus can be spread by sexual contact, but no where near 95 percent have discontinued risky sexual behavior.[54] Even more recent efforts at social skills training are not sufficient. If the use of assertive skills to effect use of condoms or other risk reduction behavior endangers the loss of sexual reinforcement, most adolescents (and probably most adults) will avoid the use of condoms, and take the risk. Thus, education alone is not likely to effect much reduction in the AIDS epidemic.

Drug Use and Abuse.   As noted earlier, drug use and abuse is a risk factor for HIV infection. The most obvious is IV narcotic use, where the virus can be inadvertently injected into the bloodstream in the course of taking a narcotic. Drugs can lower one's resistance to infection, such as through alcohol's immune-compromising effects. However, for most people who are not addicted to drugs or using narcotics by injection, the most subtle risk of HIV infection is derived from behaviors occurring while intoxicated and the conditions under which drugs are consumed. A young man who has had a few drinks at a party may be more likely to make advances for sexual intercourse than when free of alcohol. He is also less likely to use a condom under these same conditions. Similarly, the young woman who has had a few drinks is less likely to resist overtures for sexual intercourse and even less likely to request that a condom be used. All drugs tend to reduce the probability of responsible behavior.

From two million to seven million American high school students have used various kinds of illegal drugs, not counting alcohol.[55] As many as 6 percent have injected cocaine, heroin, or other illegal substances.[56] Over 80 percent of adolescents have used alcohol. Clearly the opportunity to "lose control" due to drug use is common among adolescents and could increase the chance of engaging in HIV risk behavior. Evidence to date suggests that sexual activity and drug use co-occur and that intoxicated adolescents are less likely to use condoms.[57]

Figure 19–4 shows the use of drugs near the far right of the antecedent side. This is to depict its occurrence, in part, as a function of previous variables and to show that drug use is likely to com-

promise assertiveness for condom use. It is important to note that drug use can alter the consequences of sexual behavior, as well. The use of some drugs heighten the pleasure or enable the male to sustain an erection longer or more frequently; others make erection more difficult to obtain. Thus, drug use immediately prior to and during sexual behavior can increase the probability of risks for HIV.

Reinforcement History.   The final box on the far right of the antecedent side of Figure 19–4 depicts reinforcement history. This is to represent the individual's previous experience practicing the target behavior—condom use—and the degree to which he/she has been reinforced or punished for that behavior. The right side of the figure depicts a series of boxes representing various possible consequences following a given instance of condom use. Again, these are arranged along a temporal continuum, representing relatively immediate to long-term consequences. The combination of consequences actually experienced and the cumulative experience over multiple instances of condom use combine to define an individual's reinforcement history. Presumably, the more reinforcing the history, the more firmly established the pattern of condom use.

As discussed earlier, the immediate pleasure obtained in the course of sexual intercourse in the context of using a condom will have profound influence on future use of condoms. Similarly, the partners sexual and social reactions will have an important impact on future condom use. Perhaps less obvious is the potential impact of peers, family, and the general community. The feedback from these sources is likely to be delayed and obtuse. Ordinarily, an individual's immediate social network knows very little about one's sexual behavior and such things as use of a condom. However, adolescents will confide in their closest friends. In this process peer friends have an opportunity to praise or criticize the use of condoms or other protective behavior as reported. This feedback can have substantial influence over future condom use, although such feedback is somewhat weaker than immediate consequences. Family members are even less likely to learn of sexual behavior, such as the use of a condom. However, exceptions can be important influences on future condom use. For instance, if a mother discovers a condom in the clothing of her son or daughter, a discussion about its use might follow. The parent who understands and encourages the use of condoms, even in the context of encouraging the avoidance of sexual intercourse as much as possible, will probably serve to reinforce future use. Parents who realize that their child is now sexually active and not likely to give up sex, no matter what action they take, can adopt a supportive role regarding safe sex. This is likely to lead to greater probability of condom use. Conversely, parents who attempt to suppress all sexual behavior, forbid the adolescent to date, or take other restrictive actions have lost an opportunity to strengthen the adolescent's likelihood of using a condom during inevitable sexual behavior.

The general community can support condom use. The degree to which TV and other media provide illustrations similar to a given adolescent's experience and depict the use of condoms as a valued behavior important to the community can serve as incidental reinforcement for the adolescent who sees such models shortly after using a condom. These theoretical relationships between safe sex behavior and the communities opportunity to support such behavior raise implications for designing programs of parental training and community support systems.

The bottom right portion of Figure 19–4 shows a box describing the balance of consequences as defining the overall reinforcing function for a given instance of condom use. Clearly, some consequences will be reinforcing, others punishing, and still others essentially neutral. The exact combination and relative strength of these consequences will determine the future probability of condom use. The absence of information regarding which consequences work in what ways decreases researchers' abilities to predict condom use or related behavior. However, this does not eliminate the utility of the model. The model can guide interventions that attempt to provide as much reinforcement for condom use as possible. Because the incidental reinforcement for sexual behavior in the absence of a condom is likely to be great, the need to program as much community support for condom use at all levels (from peers, through family and general community) is critical if such protective behavior is ever to become the norm.

Implications for Interventions. Interventions for safe sex and suppression of HIV infection could

be established more completely and in a more precise manner if planned systematically. This can be accomplished on a number of levels concurrently — neighborhood or special group, city, state and countrywide campaigns. To do so will change the specific targets of "educational" efforts from that of providing general information about AIDS risks to explicit promotion of social action on the part of all people when they encounter friends or acquaintances for whom it becomes apparent that they are engaging in risky or safe sex. Members of the community should be prompted and reinforced for criticizing risky sex and for praising or applauding safe sex practices. The process of asking would-be dating partners about their HIV status and risk history should become commonplace. Indeed, models on TV and in other media should illustrate it as a normal and desirable part of the dating process. The formal targeting of the community's reactions to an individual when that individual's sexual practices become apparent to members of the community should be added to the public health agenda for prevention of AIDS.

Teenagers are a good target population with whom to develop techniques useful for the larger society. Because most youth attend schools and because they are audiences for TV and other media, it should be possible to access youth and target a shift in the social pressure applied to one another for a given type of behavior, in effect to change norms. Social marketing and many other interventions should be in place concurrently. Youth could be taught formal responses to peers when they are discovered engaging in safe or unsafe sexual behavior, drug use, or other risk factors. Media could provide models and instructions to catch a friend "being good," and let them know what you think of them. Media could offer incentive programs to reinforce youth who have counseled a friend or acquaintance regarding safe sexual behavior. The range of potential interventions for targeting the general adolescent populations is tremendous (actually overwhelming). Experience from application and evaluation will demonstrate which interventions are most cost effective in particular situations.

One comprehensive intervention plan involves the implementation of medical and family planning clinics directly associated with schools. Few have been established to date, but those which have been initiated suggest promise. Pregnancy rates have been decreased, and contraception use rates have increased in association with school clinics.[58] One program used a store-front office situated between two inner-city schools and offered medical and contraceptive services. Classroom lectures and counseling services were offered in conjunction with the medical components. The program was associated with a 30 percent decrease in pregnancy rates at the target school, while pregnancy at the control school increased by 50 percent. Perhaps even more important for its AIDS prevention potential was that those girls in the program for at least three years postponed sexual intercourse by an average of seven months.[59] These programs were introduced before efforts to prevent AIDS were well underway and did not concentrate on condom use or safe sex per se. Yet, the results for contraception in general and pregnancy prevention in particular are quite promising for application to AIDS prevention.

A South Carolina program took a somewhat different approach. School teachers were formally trained and then provided sex education in the schools. Parents and clergy were asked to be involved in the training program and attended classes as well. The media were asked to promote the same sex education messages presented in class. This program was a good example of bringing a number of different community resources to bear on the same issue and as such approached the development of a comprehensive, multiple-level intervention. Results indicated a lowered teen pregnancy rate compared to control communities.[60] Hingson and associates reported changes in both knowledge and condom use that might be attributed to the statewide and national education programs concerning AIDS.[61]

Thus, there are early indications that communitywide programs can have a beneficial effect on AIDS prevention, but greater effects are certainly possible. However, no intervention program to date has targeted the adolescent social response to others as a contingent reinforcer or punisher for safe and unsafe sexual behavior, respectively. The relative success of both the operant and social learning models of health behavior, along with these community programs' partial success, suggest that formal tests of "metacontingencies" for AIDS prevention are warranted.

Kelly and colleagues have approximated the use of social contingencies with a gay male popu-

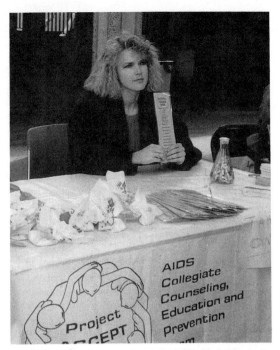

FIGURE 19–5. AIDS prevention interventions have combined education, training, motivation, and marketing techniques for reaching sexually active young adults. *Photo courtesy of Betsy Clapp.*

lation.[62] Gay males were taught assertive skills to resist peer pressure for "unsafe sex," and later were contracted (reinforced) for practicing with a set number of friends not in the training program. In addition, opinion leaders (e.g., bartenders) in the gay community were identified and taught social skills to promote safe sex and were instructed to talk frequently with friends and acquaintances to promote safer sex. Results showed a decrease in risk behavior, including increased condom use and decreased number of sexual partners, relative to a control community. This study was unique in that it provided a community-wide approach and used formal reinforcement contingencies in order to increase the social contingencies applied by members of the community regarding safe sexual behavior. This is the most direct attempt to establish metacontingencies in the literature to date. Its generalization to the larger population, or even to that of adolescents, remains to be demonstrated, but it offers strong encouragement for this approach.

Learning Theory Models. Figure 19–4 depicts the basics of an operant and social learning theory model to "explain" condom use. It should be just as applicable to general sexual behavior or to drug use and other health-related performance. The figure, however, does not provide the whole story. Concepts of ever changing conditions resulting in ever changing behavior, shaping, or the gradual acquisition of increasingly complex skills, are not depicted in Figure 19–4 and yet are critical influences on behavior. Given these qualifications, this model seems the most likely to serve as a practical prototype for the design of effective interventions for AIDS prevention. Additional correlational evidence of this comes from two sources. Kastner has explored a somewhat simpler model of contraception behavior and found that similar social variables accounted for about 55 percent of the variance in contraception use.[63] Among the variables most strongly related to contraception was strong "boyfriend support."

More recent data exploring variants of the model depicted in Figure 19–4 have produced significant multiple correlations and "verified"

that family, school, peers, and the other major concepts in the model contribute significantly to the total variance in sexual behavior among Hispanic and Anglo adolescents.[64] For instance, Figure 19–6 shows the amount of variance explained by this type of model when sexual behavior was regressed on these concepts. Hillman and colleagues demonstrated that as much as 60 percent of the variance in sexual behavior could be explained by the model, and all key concepts in the model remained significant contributors to the variance explained.[65] These results demonstrate that a multivariate model is required to explain and probably to control AIDS risk behavior. This model suggests that education is useful, but not a major contributor; that family variables are more important than often described in the literature; that social skills are important, but probably not as important as peer pressure or the influences from public schools.

Although these results do not speak to change in behavior, the model suggests that behavior will change as conditions change. To establish a steady reliable pattern of behavior may require an

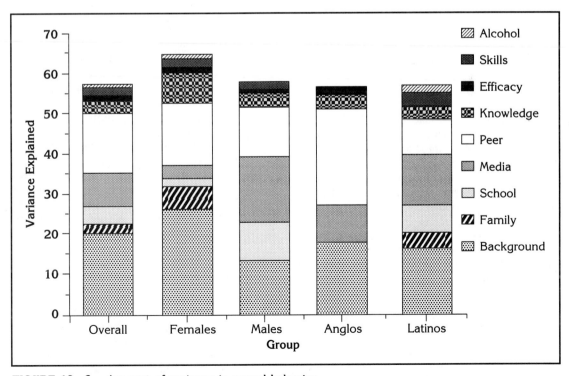

FIGURE 19–6. Amount of variance in sexual behavior

on-going and changing multivariate intervention program with formal contingencies of reinforcement at least for changing social reactions to unsafe sexual behavior. Such programs will be expensive and difficult to carry out, but they may be the only realistic means of controlling the AIDS epidemic. Additional behavioral epidemiology and intervention research is needed to test and refine this model.

SUMMARY

There may be a small silver lining in the terrible tragedy of the AIDS epidemic. The nature of the AIDS disease requires that much more be learned about the immune system, viruses, and the opportunistic diseases that are common in HIV-infected individuals. This new knowledge might eventually lead to an immunization for the AIDS viruses, and in so doing it will shed light on the development of immunizations for other viral diseases. The medical treatment of AIDS patients will teach us a great deal about pathology and normal neurology and the aging process in general. It is not exactly clear in what ways this new information will benefit the community, but improvements in medicine and public health technology are likely.

The spin-off benefits of the AIDS epidemic within medicine are obvious. However, there are likely to be even greater additions to knowledge in the behavioral and social sciences as applied to issues of relatively private behavior. We will learn much about sexual relations, with a better understanding of intimacy and love relationships. Greater knowledge in these areas will contribute to control of AIDS, other STDs, and teen pregnancy epidemics. The same information and resulting technologies will contribute to the control of the run-away world population growth, and this, in turn, could contribute to the salvation of both human kind and life in general. Enroute to such great breakthroughs, our better understanding of relationships could contribute to the control of violence, child abuse, spouse abuse, homicide, suicide, marriage discord, etc. In short, the AIDS epidemic has required the aggressive advance in behavioral science and behavior modification technology on a population-wide scale, and this may result in both the improvement in quality of life as well as make the continuation of life possible.

ADDITIONAL READINGS

These sources will maintain your awareness of issues related to teen sexuality and AIDS:

1. CDC HIV/AIDS, special reports, CDC, PHS, U.S. Dept. of Health and Human Services, Atlanta, GA.
2. The Alan Guttmacher Institute, 2010 Massachusetts Ave., NW, Washington, D.C. 20036
3. *Journal of Acquired Immune Deficiency Syndromes,* Raven Press, N.Y.
4. AIDS Education and Prevention, Guilford Publishers, Inc., 72 Spring Street, New York, NY 10012

ENDNOTES

1. This chapter was prepared, in large part, based on the ongoing efforts of Dr. Hovell, Ms. Sipan and Blumberg, Drs. Atkins, Elder, and Hofstetter, and Ms. Kreitner in the course of conducting Project STARRT. Many of the ideas expressed here evolved as a function of our team effort.
2. Jones, E., Forrest, J., Goldman, N., Henshaw, S., Lincoln, R., Rosoff, J., et al. (1985). Teenage pregnancy in developed countries: Determinants and policy implications. *Family Planning Perspectives, 17,* 53–63.
3. Hayes, C. (Ed.). (1987). *Risking the future: Adolescent sexuality, pregnancy, and childbearing.* Washington, D.C.: National Academy Press.
4. Primary and secondary syphilis—United States, 1981–1990. *Morbidity & Mortality Weekly Report, 40*(19), 314–323, 1990.
5. Progress toward achieving the 1990 objectives for the nation for sexually transmitted diseases. *Mortality & Morbidity Weekly Report, 39,* 53–57, 1990.
6. WHO predicts up to 30 million world AIDS cases by year 2000. *Nation's Health,* pp. 1–8, January 1991.
7. Centers for Disease Control. (1991). *HIV/AIDS Prevention: Special Report on Evaluation.* Atlanta, GA: Public Health Service, U.S. Department of Health & Human Services.
8. Molgaard, C., Nakamura, C., Hovell, M., & Elder, J. (1988). Assessing alcoholism as a risk factor for acquired immunodeficiency syndrome (AIDS). *Social Science & Medicine, 27,* 1147–1152.
9. Stall, R., McKusic, K., Wiley, J., Coates, T., & Ostrow, D. (1986). Alcohol and drug use during sexual activity and compliance with safe sex guidelines for AIDS: The AIDS Behavioral Research Project. *Health Education Quarterly, 13,* 359–371.

10. Padian, N., Shiboski, S., & Jewell, N. (1991). Female to male transmission of Human Immunodeficiency Virus. *Journal of the American Medical Association, 261,* 2501–2502.

11. Levine, C. & Nolan, K. (1989). Counseling and antibody testing to prevent HIV infection. *Journal of the American Medical Association, 261,* 2501–2502.

12. Farthing, C., Jesson, W., Taylor, H., Lawrence, A., & Gazzard, B. (1987, June). *The HIV antibody test: Influence on sexual behavior of homosexual men.* Proceedings of the Third National Conference on AIDS, Washington, D.C.

13. Landis, S., Earp. J., & Koch, G. (1992). Impact of HIV testing and counseling on subsequent sexual behavior. *AIDS Education & Prevention, 4,* 71–83.

14. U.S. Department of Health and Human Services. (1991). *Healthy People 2000.* Washington, D.C.: Government Printing Office.

15. Basch, P. (1990). Three diseases: Smallpox, malaria, and AIDS. In *Textbook of International Health* (pp. 355–376). New York: Oxford University Press.

16. Hayes, C. (Ed.). (1987). *Risking the future: Adolescent sexuality, pregnancy and childbearing.* Washington, D.C.: National Research Council, National Academy Press.

17. Centers for Disease Control. *HIV/AIDS prevention;* and Forrest, J. & Singh, S. (1990). The sexual and reproductive behavior of American women, 1982–1988. *Family Planning Perspectives, 22,* 206–214.

18. Sexual behavior among high school students— United States, 1990. *Morbidity & Mortality Weekly Report, 40,* 005–008, 1992.

19. Centers for Disease Control. *HIV/AIDS Prevention.*

20. Forest & Singh, Sexual and reproductive behavior of American women.

21. *Morbidity & Mortality Weekly Report.* Sexual behavior among high school students.

22. Hingson, R., Strunin, L., & Berlin, B. (1990). Acquired immune deficiency syndrome transmission: Changes in knowledge and behaviors among teenagers, Massachusetts statewide surveys, 1986–88. *Pediatrics, 85,* 24–29.

23. Nelson, C. & Keith, J. (1990). Comparison of female and male adolescent sex role, attitude and behavior development. *Adolescence, 25,* 183–204; and Strahle, W. (1983). A model of premarital coitus and contraceptive behavior among female adolescents. *Archives of Sexual Behavior, 12,* 67–95.

24. Ajzen, I. & Fishbein, M. (1980). *Understanding attitudes and predicting social behavior: Illustrations of applied social research.* Englewood Cliffs, NJ: Prentice-Hall; and Fishbein, M. (1972). Toward an understanding of family planning behaviors. *Journal of Social Psychology, 4,* 37–51.

25. McCarty, D. (1981). Changing contraceptive usage intentions: A test of the Fishbein model of intention. *Journal of Social Psychology, 11,* 192–211.

26. Jorgensen, S. & Sonstegard, J. (1984). Predicting adolescent sexual and contraceptive behavior: An application and test of the Fishbein model. *Journal of Marriage & the Family, 46,* 43–55.

27. Morrison, D. (1985). Adolescent contraceptive behavior: A review. *Psychological Bulletin, 98,* 538–568.

28. Furstenberg, F., Moore, K., & Peterson, J. (1985). Sex education and sexual experience among adolescents. *American Journal of Public Health, 75,* 1331–1332.

29. Hillman, E., Hovell, M., Williams, L., Burdyshaw, C., Rugg, D., Atkins, C., et al. (1991). Pregnancy, STDs and AIDS prevention: Evaluation of New Image Teen Theatre. *AIDS Education & Prevention, 3,* 328–340.

30. Wenger, N., Linn, L., Epstein, M., & Shapiro, M. (1991). Reduction of high risk behaviors among heterosexuals undergoing HIV antibody testing: A randomized trial. *American Journal of Public Health, 81,* 1580–1585.

31. Brown, L., Fritz, G., & Barone, V. (1989). The impact of AIDS education on junior and senior high students. *Journal of Adolescent Health Care, 10,* 386–392.

32. Bandura, A. & Walter, R. (1963). *Social learning and personality development.* New York: Holt, Rinehart & Winston.

33. Hagenhoff, C., Lowe, A., Hovell, M., & Rugg, D. (1987). Prevention of the teenage pregnancy epidemic: A social learning theory approach. *Education & Treatment of Children, 10,* 67–83; and Rugg, D., Hovell, M., & Frazini, L. (1989). Behavioral science and public health perspectives: Combining paradigms for the prevention and control of AIDS. In *Psychological perspectives on AIDS: Etiology, prevention, and treatment.* Hillsdale, NJ: Erlbaum.

34. Alternatively, the male may be negatively reinforced for condom use by a female who insists on it as a prerequisite for intercourse.

35. Hingson, R., Strunin, L., & Berlin, B. (1950). Acquired Immunodeficiency Syndrome transmission: Changes in knowledge and behaviors among teenagers, Massachusetts Statewide Surveys, 1986–1988. *Pediatrics, 85,* 24–29.

36. Jolly, D., Nolan, T., Moller, J., & Vimpani, G.

(1991). The impact of poverty and disadvantage on child health. *Journal of Pediatric Child Health, 27,* 203–217.

37. Mosher, W. & McNally, J. (1991). Contraceptive use at first premarital intercourse: United States, 1965–1988. *Family Planning Perspectives, 23,* 108–116.

38. Hayes, *Risking the future: Adolescent sexuality, pregnancy, and childbearing.*

39. Newcomber, S. & Udry, J. (1985). Parent-child communication and adolescent sexual behavior. *Family Planning Perspectives, 23,* 203–217.

40. Yarber, W. (1988). Evaluation of the health behavior approach to school STD education. *Journal of Sex Education Therapy, 14,* 33–38.

41. Stout, J. & Rivara, F. (1989). Schools and sex education: Does it work? *Pediatrics, 83,* 375–379.

42. Lowry, L. & Towles, D. (1989). Soap opera portrayals of sex, contraception, and sexually-transmitted diseases: A public health perspective. *Journal of Communication, 39,* 76–83; and Lowry, D. & Towles, D. (1989). Prime time TV portrayal of sex, contraception, and venereal disease. *Journalism Quarterly, 66,* 347–352.

43. Cvetkovich, B. & Grote, B. (1980). *Psychological development and the social problems of teenage illegitimacy in adolescent pregnancy and childbearing.* Washington, D.C.: U.S. Government Printing Office.

44. Sack, A., Billingham, R., & Howard, R. (1985). Premarital contraceptive use: A discriminant analysis approach. *Archives of Sexual Behavior, 14,* 165–182.

45. Polit-O'Hara, D. & Kahn, J. (1985). Communications and contraceptive practice in adolescent couples. *Adolescence, 20,* 33–43.

46. Welch-Cline, R., Johnson, S., & Freeman, K. (1989). *Talk among sexual partners: Interpersonal communication as an AIDS-prevention strategy.* Proceedings of the International Communication Association, San Francisco.

47. Wills, T., Baker, E., & Botvin, G. (1989). Dimensions of assertiveness: Differential relationships and substance use in early adolescence. *Journal of Consulting & Clinical Psychology, 57,* 473–478.

48. Marks, G., Richardson, J., & Maldonado, N. (1991). Self-disclosure of HIV infection to sexual partners. *American Journal of Public Health, 81,* 1321–1322.

49. Botvin, G., Baker, E., Botvin, E., Filazzola, A., & Millman, R. (1984). Prevention of alcohol misuse through the development of personal and social competence: A pilot study. *Journal of Studies on Alcohol, 45,* 550–552.

50. Schinke, S., Gilchrist, L., Snow, W., & Schilling, R. (1985). Skills-building methods to prevent smoking in adolescents. *Journal of Adolescent Health Care, 6,* 439–444.

51. Kelly, J., St. Lawrence, J., Hood, H., & Brasfield, T. (1989). Behavioral intervention to reduce AIDS risk activities. *Journal of Clinical Psychology, 57,* 60–67.

52. Gilchrist, L. & Schinke, S. (1983). Coping with contraception: Cognitive and behavioral methods with adolescents. *Cognitive Therapy & Research, 7,* 379–388.

53. Hovell, M., Hofstetter, R., Atkins, C., Sipan, C., Blumberg, E., & Felice, C. (1988–1993). Teaching youth skills: An AIDS prevention trial. Bethesda, MD: NICH-HD, NIH. No. 25021.

54. Hardy, A. (1990). *AIDS knowledge and attitudes for October–December, 1989.* Advanced Data from Vital and Health Statistics of the National Center for Health Statistics, Report No. 186, 1–4.

55. Quackenbush, M. & Sargeant, P. (1986). *Teaching AIDS: A resource guide on acquired immune deficiency syndrome.* Santa Cruz, CA: Network Publishers.

56. HIV-related beliefs, knowledge and behaviors among high school students. *Morbidity & Mortality Weekly Report, 37,* 717–721.

57. Donovan, J., Jessor, R., & Costa, F. (1988). Syndrome of problem behavior in adolescence: A replications. *Journal of Consulting & Clinical Psychology, 56,* 762–765; and Hingson, R., Strunin, L., Berlin, B., & Heeren, T. (1990). Beliefs about AIDS, use of alcohol and drugs, and unprotected sex among Massachusetts adolescents. *American Journal of Public Health, 80,* 295–299.

58. Dryfoos, J. (1988). School-based health clinics: Three years of experience. *Family Planning Perspectives, 20,* 193–200; and Zabin, L., Hirsch, M., Smith, E., Streett, R., & Hardy, J. (1986). Evaluation of a pregnancy prevention program for urban teenagers. *Family Planning Perspectives, 18,* 119–126.

59. Zabin, Hirsch, Smith, Streett, & Hardy. Ibid.

60. Vincent, M., Clearie, A., & Schiuchter, M. (1987). Reducing adolescent pregnancy through school and community-based education. *Journal of the American Medical Association, 257,* 3382–3386.

61. Hingson, Strunin, & Berlin. Acquired Immunodeficiency Syndrome transmission.

62. Kelly, J., St. Lawrence, J., Diaz, Y., Stevenson, L., Hauth, A., Brasfield, T., et al. (1991). HIV risk behavior reduction following intervention with key opinion leaders of population: An experimental analysis. *American Journal of Public Health, 81,* 168–171.

63. Kastner, L. (1984). Ecological factors predicting adolescent contraception use: Implications for intervention. *Journal of Adolescent Health Care, 5*, 79–86.

64. Hovell, M., Stoecklin, M., Blumberg, E., Atkins, C., Hofstetter, R., Sipan, C., Elder, J., & Felice, M. (1992). Family influences on Hispanic adolescents' sexual behavior: A test of social learning theory, under editorial review.

65. Hillman, E., Hovell, M., Hofstetter, R., Atkins, C., Sipan, C., Blumberg, E., et al. (1992, March). *Adolescent risk of pregnancy, STDs, and AIDS: A conceptual model*. Proceedings of the Annual Meeting of the Society for Behavioral Medicine. New York.

Chapter 20

Promoting Health and Child Survival in the Developing World

OBJECTIVES

By the end of this chapter, the reader should be able to:

1. Compare and contrast the concept of paternalism with the medical model, social planning, and locality development.
2. Discuss the role of social action in health promotion and development.
3. List major priorities for health in the developing world.
4. Operationalize major health priorities in terms of behavioral targets for health promotion.
5. Identify factors which may optimize success for development programs.
6. Describe the major assessment issues for child survival programs.

INTRODUCTION

As outlined in detail in chapter 3, the health status of any population is far more than a direct function of the provision of health services.[1] People benefit less from health services than from other critical indicators of health status, including the status of women, income distribution, education and literacy, and more general socio-environmental factors such as housing, sanitation, roads and transportation, political stability, and social security.[2] Close cooperation of a variety of health and other professionals and governmental bodies whose actions directly affect the health of the population is critical. More important still is the cooperation and involvement of the people in villages and communities who are targets of "development" efforts for health, agricultural, and economic advancement.

ORGANIZATIONAL ISSUES

Locality Development

In his compelling guide book for development in agriculture called *Two Ears of Corn,* Roland Bunch outlined procedures for the effective dissemination of farming innovations for better food production in underdeveloped nations. Very similar to the ONPRIME model, Bunch's approach is generalizable to health promotion and therefore referred to extensively in the present chapter.

In his discussion of principles of community organization, Bunch warns against "the paternalism of the give away." Food, services, or health products which are merely donated to a community will create dependency, rivalry or embarrassment. Not only do give-aways entail tremendous direct costs, they also subvert the efforts of existing or potential change agents and thereby destroy long-term possibilities for success. Bunch advocates instilling enthusiasm as the most viable substitute for paternalism, which can be accomplished through programs which:

1. meet perceived needs of the community;
2. are sufficiently simple and inexpensive;
3. use competent and committed personnel; and
4. involve the community in all aspects of planning and implementation.

Although such approaches may engender enthusiasm initially, Bunch warns that early and recognizable program successes will be necessary for program maintenance.

More than in the industrialized world, participation is a key element of community organization for developing countries. Staff and other change agents should be recruited from the target population, or co-ops can be organized in which a cadre of trained individuals share skills and resources among themselves and with neighbors. Participation, however, can be threatened by a variety of factors. First, one individual may attempt to dominate others. Second, a lack of visible success may convince villagers that a program is ineffective and that their participation is a waste of time.

Regardless of the specific organizational model or professional discipline serving as the context for a large-scale development effort, health and development programs will realize an optimal chance for success when:

1. Enthusiasm and commitment are promoted.
2. Programs are initially small and simple.
3. "Outsiders" are relatively invisible and are phased out as quickly as possible.
4. Personnel are taught to monitor, evaluate, and refine their programs.
5. A leadership "pyramid" is developed whereby the number of participants in a program can continue to accelerate.
6. The role of financial resources—especially donations—is minimized.
7. An attempt to meet everyone's needs is avoided.[3]

Social Action

The Nestlé Boycott. It is difficult to prescribe social action from afar. Although Bunch's approach offers an appealing alternative to social planning, social action may be culturally unsuitable in some societies or even meet with brutal suppression in others. The most appropriate social action is that which emanates from the population being affected by a problem. Many root causes of health problems are international in nature, however, as perhaps best exemplified by the multinational promotion of tobacco (chapter 16). In such cases, we all have a responsibility to consider participation in organizational activities under the social action banner.

One of the most effective blows ever struck for child survival was the renowned Nestlé boycott of the 1970s and 1980s. The call for action against the use of processed milk had been sounded decades earlier by notables such as British physician Cicely Williams, who stated in 1939 that "misguided propaganda on infant feeding should be punished as the most criminal form of sedition, and that these [infant] deaths should be regarded as murder.[3] Clement noted that industrialized countries could compensate for the unhealthy shift toward bottle feeding through improved nutrition and sanitation, but this was not the case in underdeveloped countries, where an estimated one million children die each year because they are not breastfed.[5] Nevertheless, Nestlé, Borden, and other multinationals expanded aggressively into international markets, with sinister yet imaginative broadcast, print, and display advertising. (In the Belgian Congo, Borden even promoted a song which was entitled "Klim [their formula] has saved a baby," and contained the lyrics "the child is going to die because the mother's breast has given out. Mama, O Mama, the child cries! If you want your child to get well, give it Klim milk.")[6]

Finally, in 1972, the United Nations began pressuring the formula industry to pull in its marketing claws. Concurrently, a Swiss social action group began domestic and international agitation against the practices of Swiss-based Nestlé through a document called "The Baby Killer." Although they were taken to court by Nestlé and found guilty of libel, their actions fomented international actions against Nestlé. One year later, in 1977, a coalition of U.S. groups launched the Nestlé boycott.

Although supported by U.S. and many international groups, the boycott was resisted by Nestlé and their friends in the U.S. government and elsewhere. This resistance further strengthened the resolve of the grassroots organizations involved and stimulated an increasingly broader economic offensive. Nestlé slowly began to modify its marketing practices. Finally, in 1984, they agreed to: (1) limit their gift-giving to health professionals; (2) revise their product labels in accord with the international code; and (3) work within a strict definition of what infants could be given free formula samples. After the suspension of the boycott for a ten-month "observational" period, the international organizations of grassroots groups called it off. However, surveillance continues.[7]

NEEDS AND RESOURCES ASSESSMENT (N/RA)

The selection of needs and resources assessment approaches will, of course, depend on the organizational background from which this effort is initiated. Major issues in N/RA include the following:

1. Who in the Community Represent the Best Candidates for Selection as Change Agents? Naturally, we first look to the formal health care system and its doctors, nurses, and nurse auxiliaries. In many cases, however, these individuals do not represent the best interpersonal channel for health promotion intervention.

Much of the developing world receives at least some health care from traditional healers and opinion leaders, human resources which have enormous potential for health promotion. Careful assessment is needed of the care which healers are currently providing and are capable of providing.[8]

Deciding what health promotion efforts should be implemented outside of the formal health care system involves sensitive social issues. By working with volunteers and traditional healers, a faulty but repairable system can be fatally subverted. The reduction in staff morale and other negative side effects resulting from well-meaning "outside" efforts can leave a community with worse health care than it had previously.

2. Training and Supervision. Assuming that a decision is reached to work at least in part within the formal primary care system, the next step in the N/RA is to look at the training and supervision received by health workers, both in clinical techniques and health education/promotion. Opportunities for incorporating health promotion techniques into regular training and supervision should be noted and taken advantage of.

3. What Are the Existing Influences of Other Social Sectors on Health? Since health is far more than simply a product of the health care system, it is necessary to determine methods of liaison with religious leaders, educators, and others at each level of society. School teachers, priests, mullahs, and monks, for example, should be encouraged to advocate health promotion as a part of their various role behaviors.[9] They can also be useful in helping select appropriate personnel for auxiliary staff roles. Private employers, food vendors, and others should be encouraged to adopt a pro-health stance.

4. What Existing Community and Primary Health Care Resources Exist? Clinic supplies, transportation, and the availability of a variety of reasonably priced nutritional foodstuffs at the local markets are all factors that influence program outcomes. Also, many countries have very lax controls on pharmaceutical products; the availability and sales of "self-prescribed" drugs also needs to be examined.

Needs and Resources Assessment Techniques

Bunch listed the following methods for needs and resources assessment: (a) reading about an issue, community, or culture; (b) observations of villages and their environments; (c) conversations, open-ended interviews, and formal surveys; (d) group interviews; and (e) participant observation by living among the villagers.[10] He noted that hiring program leaders from among the target population will lessen the need for N/RA efforts.

Other Needs and Resources Assessment Issues

A variety of other considerations should be addressed for effective implementation of any program, including local cultural practices, technological limitations, material and personnel resources, influences of other social sectors on health, and a curative rather than preventive orientation.[11] Many developing countries have heterogeneous populations among which many languages and dialects are spoken, different power structures and social systems are found, and knowledge about health is limited. One N/RA issue is to what extent do clinic and rural health center staff know and understand the culture and language of the population they are serving.

Beyond the utility of involving the people themselves, it is necessary to incorporate existing cultural practices into an intervention. For instance, nutritional programs should focus on the slight variations in current food preparation and consuming patterns rather than on supplanting current practices with totally different ones. The value of traditional medicines must be investigated carefully and used to advantage whenever possible.[12]

PRIORITIES

Women's Work

Putting today's essential health knowledge into practice will be seen by many as "women's work." But women already have work. They already grow most of the developing world's food, market most of its crops, fetch most of its water, collect most of its fuel, feed most of its animals, weed most of its fields. And when their work outside the home is done, they light the third world's fires, cook its meals, clean its compounds, wash its clothes, shop for its needs, and look after its old and its ill. And they bear and care for its children. The multiple burdens of womanhood are too much. And the greatest communications challenge of all is the challenge of communicating the idea that the time has come, in all countries, for men to share more

fully in that most difficult and important of all tasks—protecting the lives and the health and the growth of their children.[13]

The above words introduce *Facts for Life,* a concise summary of the behavioral issues relevant to family planners and child survival specialists working in the underdeveloped world. In the context of this philosophy and the morbidity and mortality profiles of the bulk of the world, *Facts for Life* presents priorities for health promotion and specific targets within each priority category. These are summarized in Table 20–1. Clearly, each of these priorities directly or implicitly specifies behavioral targets.

RESEARCH

Targeting Behaviors

As with any health promotion effort, the first step in developing an intervention is to target specific behaviors related to a health problem or goal. This targeting begins with a breakdown of a broad health/illness area into specific dimensions of interest (e.g., prevention and control), followed by a delineation of the behaviors relevant to these dimensions. An example of this breakdown as

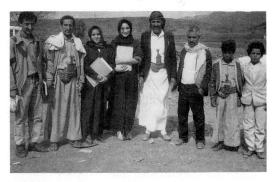

FIGURE 20–1. Health promotion efforts in developing as well as industrialized countries must transcend barriers to female-male communication. Above, two women working on a national maternal and child health promotion campaign in Yemen work with regional and village health workers—all of whom are male. *Photo courtesy of John Elder.*

TABLE 20–1
Health Priorities of the Developing World

A. Birth Timing: 3 million children and 200,000 women die per year
   1. Pregnancies between ages 18 and 35
   2. Spacing between births > 2 years
   3. Having four or fewer children
   4. Use of family planning
B. Safe Motherhood: 1,000 women die per day
   1. Regular prenatal checkups
   2. Trained birth attendants present at birth
   3. Know warning signs of pregnancy dangers
   4. More food and rest during pregnancy
   5. Spacing and timing pregnancies (A1 & A2)
   6. Healthier female children and adolescents have healthier pregnancies as adults
C. Breastfeeding
   1. Breast milk alone for 4–6 months
   2. Start breastfeeding as soon as possible after birth
   3. Frequent sucking is needed to stimulate production of breast milk
   4. Bottle-feeding can lead to illness or death
   5. Continue some breastfeeding into second year or beyond
D. Child Growth
   1. Monthly weighing between ages of 6 months and 3 years; no weight gain for two consecutive months indicates problem.
   2. Breast milk alone for 4–6 months
   3. Add other foods after this period
   4. Children under 3 need food 5–6 times per day
   5. Children under 3 need small amounts of additional fat/oil added to food
   6. Children need foods rich in Vitamin A
   7. Children need extra meals to catch up after an illness
   8. Conversation, affection and play time are all important
E. Immunization: Without it, 3%, 2% and 1% of children will die from measles, whooping cough, and polio.
   1. Immunizations protect against dangerous diseases, malnourishment, disability and death
   2. All immunizations should be completed in child's first year
   3. It is safe to immunize a sick child
   4. Women from 15 to 44 should be immunized against tetanus
F. Diarrhea: 3.5 million children die per year
   1. Diarrhea kills through dehydration: children with it need plenty of liquids and possibly oral rehydration solution
   2. Continue breastfeeding or regular feeding through a bout of diarrhea
   3. Professional attention is needed for severe diarrhea
   4. During the week of recovery, one extra meal per day is needed
   5. Medicines should be used only upon medical advice
   6. Prevent diarrhea by breastfeeding, washing hands, using latrines, and keeping food/water clean
G. Respiratory Infections: 2–3 million children die per year
   1. Pneumonia can be prevented through proper breastfeeding, other nourishment and immunizations
   2. Children with coughs or colds should be helped to eat and drink plenty of liquids

3. Children with coughs or colds should be kept warm and protected from smokey or contaminated air
4. If a sick child starts breathing rapidly, he/she should be taken to the clinic

H. Hygiene
1. Hands should be washed with soap and water before handling food and after contact with feces
2. Latrines should be used
3. Clean water prevents illness; it should be boiled if it does not come from a safe supply
4. Food should be clean
5. Garbage should be buried

I. Malaria: 100 million cases + hundreds of thousands of deaths/year
1. Children should be protected from mosquito bites
2. Breeding sites & larvae should be destroyed
3. Where malaria is endemic, pregnant women should take anti-malaria tablets
4. Children with a fever and suspected malaria should receive professional attention and anti-malaria drugs
5. Children with fevers should be kept cool
6. Children recovering from malaria need plenty of food and liquids

J. AIDS: 5–10 million are already HIV positive
1. AIDS is incurable, and is transmitted by sexual intercourse, infected blood and from infected mothers pre- or neonatally
2. "Safe sex" includes monogamous relationships and using a condom when in doubt
3. Unsterilized needles/syringes are dangerous
4. HIV positive women should avoid pregnancy
5. Parents should teach their children how to avoid AIDS

applied to diarrhea control is provided in Table 20–2.

As illustrated in Table 20–2, diarrhea-related illnesses owe their existence largely to human behavior. This should not diminish the importance of non-behavioral factors, for example, people without access to clean water or fire fuels to boil it are likely to get sick from contaminated water and food, and children malnourished in the first place are far more likely to suffer and die from this extra loss of nutrients and fluids. Nevertheless, this major illness of the underdeveloped world could be substantially controlled through strengthening the behaviors in the first, third, and fourth columns of Table 20–2 and eliminating those in the second. Research efforts may help determine the appropriate target behaviors for interventions in each priority area.

INTERVENTIONS

Family Planning and Population Control

Population growth is among the most threatening of all world problems. Whereas technologies for birth control are widely applied in industrialized countries, the developing world continues to suffer from high levels of wasteful fertility. Nevertheless, the development of many innovative and effective behavior change programs for promoting family planning have somewhat brightened the prospects for improvement.

In a review of the family planning and behavior change literature, Elder and Estey outlined three dimensions for consideration in the development and implementation of motivational procedures: the incentive, the recipient, and the behavior.[14]

TABLE 20-2

Behaviors Which Contribute to Health and the Causes, Prevention, and Control of Diarrhea

General Preventive Measures	Causes of Diarrhea	Prevention of Diarrhea	Control of Diarrhea
• Washing hands and kitchen utensils • Using mosquito nets and insect sprays • Keeping poisons out of the reach of children • Maintaining barriers to cooking fires	• Bottle feeding, esp. with unclean bottles • Drinking unpurified water • Eating with dirty hands • Eating with improperly cleaned utensils • Toileting in inappropriate places • Leaving garbage in the open • Leaving food uncovered • Cooking food only partially (and not killing bacteria) • Eating spoiled leftovers	• Breastfeeding all infants • Filtering/boiling drinking water • Obtaining drinking water from uncontaminated sources • Washing hands before and after eating • Washing utensils in clean water and soap • Toileting in latrines and washing hands afterwards • Covering food to protect it • Disposing of waste properly • Washing all food • Washing hands before handling food • Cooking vegetables in boiling water	• Giving child plenty of liquids • Continuing breastfeeding • Administering oral rehydration fluids • Continuing regular feeding • Going to clinic if diarrhea persists

SOURCE: World Health Organization. (1988). *Education for health.* Geneva: World Health Organization, pp. 3–6.

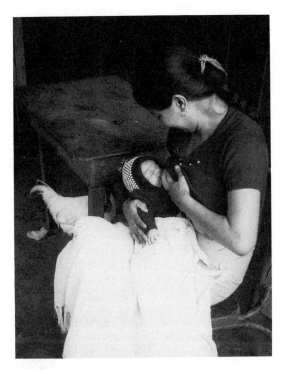

FIGURE 20–2. Breast feeding continues to be an important factor in infant and child health and survival. *Photo courtesy of John Elder.*

Family planning incentives have included monetary, material, social, and activity reinforcers. Reinforcement has targeted individuals, groups, early adopters, diffusers, and providers. Target behaviors have included both contraception and procreation.

Monetary incentives have been used widely, especially for promoting sterilization. These incentive systems have often been graduated. For example, one program in India offered seventy-five rupees for sterilization after three children, forty-five rupees after four, and 25 rupees after five or more.[15] Elsewhere in India, transistor radios, buckets of grain, clothing, and umbrellas have increased sterilization rates.[16] For exceeding their family planning targets, officials in Maharashtra, India, received activity reinforcers, including participation in foreign tours.[17]

Incentives typically target individual adopters or their families. In the latter category, a common behavior modification approach in East Asia is to offer free education for children of couples with only one or two offspring, whereas such privileges can be lost for all children if more than the target number are born. Early adopters may be reinforced for promoting family planning to their more reluctant neighbors. For instance, local men who had already undergone vasectomy operations in India were far more credible sources than project staff in promoting the benefits of the operation.[18] In South Korea, "diffusers" such as housewives, beauticians, and church deacons earned money for every acceptor recruited.[19]

Family planning programs can target either contraception or procreation (or conversely, "non-birth"). The former is behavior-specific: a prescribed procedure is promoted and reinforcers are administered contingent upon the behavior change. When non-birth is targeted, couples typically receive some sort of social security bonus or other deferred payment for periods of non-fertility. The advantages of the latter approach are that (1) couples can make their own choices among

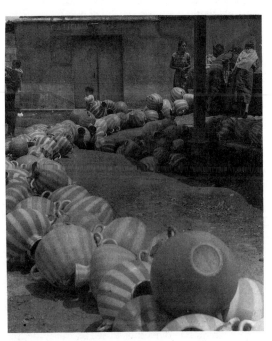

FIGURE 20–3. Clean and accessible water, taken for granted in industrialized countries, is a luxury in many underdeveloped ones. Here, these Guatemalan women wait in line all day with their pots to fill them at a village tap. *Photo courtesy of John Elder.*

family planning techniques, and (2) the social security function directly offsets the competing motivation for having large families, in that many offspring can help provide for aging parents.

Reinforcement for non-birth can also be categorized as "differential reinforcement of other behaviors" (DRO). That is, individuals are motivated to accomplish lower rates of reproduction through later marriages, longer child spacing, and later first births.[20] For example, socioeconomic and policy changes which would result in the delay of marriages would include the provision of marriage benefits to parents of women who marry after the age of twenty-one, governmentally-funded marriage ceremonies for brides of this age or older, and first marriage grants to couples who marry beyond their twenty-fifth birthday.[21] Promotion of female participation in the labor force outside of the home and the provision of a variety of extra familial distractions for promoting outside interests (e.g., additional cultural, athletic, and other programs), are also examples of DRO. Many of these techniques emulate social changes which have evidently reduced population growth in industrialized countries.

Aversive procedures also play a significant role in motivating family planning. For instance, withdrawing maternity benefits or other governmental allowances after a certain number of children are born, and levying taxes on births after a certain number represent examples of negatively reinforcing the practice of birth control. Response cost approaches include the use of governmentally-vended licenses to have children, assessment of larger fees for marriage licenses, and the withdrawal of previously awarded maternity benefits and other governmental allowances after a certain number of children.

China's One-Child Policy. Perhaps the best known (and most controversial) of all systematic behavioral approaches to family planning is found in the People's Republic of China. The One-Child Policy has been developed in response to China's rapidly growing population, which is now over one billion. China has over four times as many people as does the U.S. — with only about 20 percent of the arable land. In response to this problem, the Chinese leadership has determined that each family should set a goal of no more than one child per family. This policy has been in effect for over a decade and has been relatively successful.[22] The

One-Child Policy uses virtually every type of motivational procedure at all levels of intervention, as well as sophisticated educational, social marketing, and training techniques. It is perhaps one of the most comprehensive health-related behavior change programs to date.

Chinese officials use both "persuasion" and "mobilization" to get couples to accept these reproductive goals. Their "persuasion" may be defined as social marketing and the use of positive reinforcement techniques, while "mobilization" involves coercing individuals to accept goals for the (ostensibly) greater good of the group or community. The Chinese health system offers convenient access to oral contraceptives, IUDs, condoms, sterilization, and abortion.[23] Chinese policy allows for local variation and innovation, but successful techniques developed at the local level are often promoted to the entire country. Birth planning units at all levels of societal organization help ensure that adequate family planning materials are available and that people make use of family planning procedures.

The birth control delivery system is built into the entire health care system, including at the "barefoot doctor" level. This ensures that in every medical center at least one of the barefoot doctors will be a female. Her activities in patient counseling and medical interventions are closely supervised by a management cadre which, in turn, is responsible for ensuring that a particular region or community reaches its family planning targets. Birth planning delegations in each community use a variety of positive and negative reinforcement techniques, including frequent follow-up visits to any woman or couple who is not attending a family planning meeting on a regular basis or has otherwise indicated resistance to family planning.

A variety of positive reinforcement procedures are used for accepting family planning practices and sterilization. Unlike other medical services, sterilization operations or IUD insertions can be free of charge and are even offered to individuals on a home service basis.[24] Individuals who accept sterilization are given extra leave and work points (which, in turn, have a monetary value in the marketplace). Individuals also receive greater travel freedom and other benefits for participation in the program. Family planning cadres, factories, and other units of society also receive special recognition or even financial remuneration for achieving pre-set quotas.

In addition to the longer established incentives described above, the One-Child Policy was bolstered in 1980 with the addition of benefits like the following:

1. Parents with only one child can receive a monthly stipend amounting to 5 to 8 percent of the average worker's wage.
2. Grain and other food ration supplements for parents with only one child are given, as well as the allocation of extra private farming space to individuals in agricultural areas.
3. Living space equivalent to that for a two-child family is given to parents with only one child.
4. The waiting list for public housing is shorter for one-child families.
5. Two weeks of extra maternity leave may be given to mothers having only one child.
6. Only-children receive highest priority for health care.
7. Retired people who had only one child receive a supplementary pension (to compensate for less "social security" from having only one child).
8. Only-children receive highest priority in admission to nurseries, kindergartens, and other school programs.
9. Tuition may be waived for only children in primary and secondary schools.[25]

In contrast, families with more than two children do not receive subsidies or loans when they have financial difficulties; may be charged for extra health care and food needed for the extra child; may be ineligible for job promotions, raises, or worker competitions; and may be criticized publicly.[26] In summary, the couple deciding to have only one child may do so for any of a variety of consequences, whereas decisions to have more than two children are punished.

Clearly, the Chinese One-Child Policy is a very controversial one, especially given the use of "coercion" or clearly aversive techniques in addition to non-aversive ones. Such controversy has resulted in a variety of international reactions to the policy. Among these responses was the cutting off of funds to the United Nations family planning efforts, largely due to the efforts of pro-life legislators in Washington. One-Child detractors have found further vindication for their action with the recent suppression of the democracy movement

in China. However, most demographic projections are at very best modestly optimistic with respect to the potential for controlling the population growth in China. Should the problem not be dealt with and the population continue to increase to 1.5 billion or more, the people of China will face consequences surely more drastic than those applied in the One-Child program.

Malnutrition and Diarrhea Control

Deficiencies in protein and calorie intake and other forms of malnutrition constitute a major threat to the health of the populations of developing countries, especially to that of infants and young children. Malnutrition is both causally and dependently related to rapid population growth, as more and more children must share the limited foodstuffs available, while parents have excessive numbers of children as part of their "social security." An additional major killer of young children in the developing world is diarrhea, which is exacerbated by malnutrition and causes more malnutrition. Oral rehydration therapy and other measures administered by mothers or health workers could save a high percentage of children who currently die from dehydration subsequent to diarrhea (see Table 20–2).

Working in the Philippines, Guthrie and his colleagues applied positive reinforcement to improve the feeding patterns of young mothers.[27] These mothers were reinforced for (a) maintaining breast feeding until at least the age of 12 to 15 months, (b) supplementing breast milk adequately beginning about the fourth month, (c) planting green, leafy vegetables near the home, (d) attaining weight gain each month, and (e) returning to the Health Center for regular medical checks and growth monitoring. Mothers received reward coupons were used for lottery drawings every three months with prizes being sacks of corn or rice provided by the government. Following an initial demonstration of success, these researchers broadened their approach to three villages, randomly assigned to the lottery reinforcement condition, reinforcement with the use of a photograph of the mother and baby, or a control condition in which health education and weight monitoring was used. Evaluation results indicated that children from the ages of twelve months to thirty months in special reinforcement conditions evi-

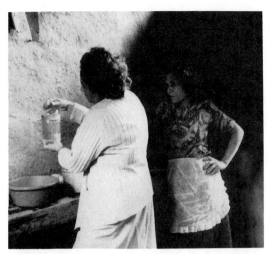

FIGURE 20-4. This Honduran health worker models the mixing of oral rehydration solution, a major vehicle for preventing the deaths of tens of thousands of children annually due to diarrhea-related dehydration. *Photo courtesy of John Elder.*

denced substantial weight gains and other health advantages.

The authors concluded their report with a few qualifications and recommendations. First, "reinforcement sampling" was necessary in order to determine acceptable and effective reinforcement approaches. Many mothers in this study objected to the initial lottery because those with a larger number of coupons often did not win, whereas women with smaller numbers sometimes did win. They also encountered problems in using foodstuffs as reinforcers, since these materials were at times provided free of charge by the government and international relief organizations. This could explain, in part, why the photos were effective.

Control of Dehydration in Gambia. In the early 1980s, a combination of social marketing, educational, and motivational approaches to treating dehydration secondary to diarrhea was evaluated in Gambia. Since Gambia's population is largely illiterate and has limited access to mass media or transportation, the national campaign for controlling dehydration due to diarrhea had to overcome a variety of barriers. In Gambia, a flyer

visually depicting how to mix sugar, water, and salt and treat dehydration was the focal point of the health promotion intervention. Village women who had been trained by health workers to champion the oral rehydration program received a bright colored flag to display over their homes. Additionally, mixing contests were held around the country over a five-week period whereby women could earn a small prize by showing that they knew how to mix the water-sugar-salt solution correctly. Moreover, villages which had a high percentage of mothers who were able to demonstrate mastery of the oral rehydration technique received additional communal prizes such as radios. Not only did this result in a gain in knowledge throughout the country, but maladaptive customs like purging or withholding food during episodes of diarrhea decreased substantially.[28]

Not all behavior change interventions for child survival have relied on lotteries and prizes. Elder, Louis and their colleagues combined training and organizational behavior management (chapter 14) to improve the quality of the face-to-face communication about diarrhea control between Indonesian health volunteers and mothers.[29] Indonesia uses these health volunteers (called *kader*) to carry out primary health care responsibilities in this heavily populated country. As part of the HEALTHCOM project in West Java, it was decided that the complexity of counseling for diarrhea control was such that additional assistance was needed for the volunteers. Therefore, a training program was developed whereby the volunteers received diarrhea "counseling cards," a tool to assist in the diagnosis and treatment of diarrhea. The cards, in essence, represented a portable supervision and prompting system, with a step-by-step algorithm for diagnosing the severity of the illness and telling the mother what to do accordingly. In an evaluation, the teaching impact of volunteers who received the counseling cards and training in how to use them was compared with that of volunteers in a control condition who received only training on diarrhea control. Not only did the counseling cards result in fewer mistakes in role-play situations, the mothers counseled by the volunteers with counseling cards demonstrated much more competence in rehydration knowledge and skills than did mothers counseled by control volunteers (i.e., no counseling cards).

Communicable Diseases

Comprehensive approaches to any form of communicable disease control must cover all phases of the communicable disease cycle. Behavior modification technologies can serve as adjuncts or primary approaches at each phase of the cycle. For example, procedures can be established for reinforcing appropriate disposal of human waste; keeping water clean and/or cleaning it before use; controlling rodents, insects, and other vectors; inoculating children and others against various diseases; and detecting early symptoms of diseases in infected individuals.

Operation Smallpox Zero in India. One of the greatest triumphs in the annals of public health involves the worldwide control of smallpox. The control of smallpox in India was accomplished, in part, through incentive systems attached to general community surveillance.[30] Surveillance teams and allied health workers were trained to visit villages and (a) report fever cases with rashes; (b) conduct special searches in high risk and/or remote areas; (c) conduct searches at public markets where relatively large numbers of people can be found in a small period of time; and (d) to "multiply" their effectiveness by "soliciting" government employees, teachers, postal workers, and others to assist in the surveillance.[31] (To help promote the surveillance, each worker could earn up to 1,000 rupees (more than U.S. $50) for the detection of smallpox). Citizens at large apparently were eligible for a variety of reinforcers as well, which "greatly improved all forms of surveillance."

Although the reward publicity included the use of wall markings, posters, media advertisements, and loudspeakers, the most effective form of publicizing the reinforcer itself was word-of-mouth information from health workers or others. Loudspeakers were the second most effective approach, especially in open areas, markets, and other crowded locations. To improve the discriminability of the surveillance, citizens and workers were provided with "recognition cards" depicting people stricken with smallpox and not chickenpox or related illnesses. Apparently the use of both rewards and marketplace targets was effective,[32] although no component analysis of the contributions of these two techniques is available.

Acute Respiratory Infection (ARI) Management in Honduras. An interesting combination of communication and behavioral management techniques is provided by studies which have shown the effectiveness of the use of radio in training populations or professionals in various adaptive behaviors. These target populations are often in areas which are very difficult to access. Media-based education therefore may supplement educational techniques that health workers or others are using. Health workers can be made aware of a particular time for a radio broadcast, and can organize a group of mothers or others to listen to the broadcast together. Subsequently, the health workers may decide to lead a discussion of the information and perhaps even practice the skills prescribed during the broadcast with the group.

Other organizational behavior management (OBM) procedures can be combined with training to develop more adequate skills among health workers. For instance, the acute respiratory infection (ARI) intervention recently conducted in Honduras emphasized health worker skills in promoting behavior change among mothers who learned how to detect and manage acute respiratory infections in their children. The ultimate target behaviors included recognizing the symptoms of ARI, keeping the nasal passage clear and the baby fed, and taking the child to the health center immediately if symptoms worsened. The specific skills promoted among the health workers involved their getting mothers to practice ARI management skills and receive positive recognition in clinic charlas (health talks). Mothers who attended these charlas were encouraged to share the health information with their neighbors. In turn, knowledge sharing was reinforced with village-wide lotteries, whereby mothers who could respond to three ARI-management questions received small prizes. Following the success of this intervention in four pilot regions, health workers throughout the nation were taught how to implement similar training and motivational procedures for ARI control in their catchment areas.[33]

Acceptance of Immunization in Ecuador. Relative to many behaviors, immunization represents a straightforward target. It is highly effective, observable, and non-controversial in medical and political circles. Nevertheless, three factors contribute to an underutilization of immunizations:[34] (1) the punishment and avoidance created by fear of injections and the negative side effects (e.g., fever, swelling) of vaccinations; (2) the competing priorities mothers have which may preclude taking their children in to be immunized; and (3) the lack of immediate reinforcement inherent in this or any prophylactic procedure. Health promotion interventions need to address not only lack of knowledge related to immunizations, but they also need to reduce barriers to bringing children to health centers for immunization.

In 1986, the PREMI vaccination campaign in Ecuador sought to address these three factors in order to increase diptheria, pertussis, and tetanus (DPT) coverage throughout the country. Comic books, radio spots (with time donated by the stations), and modeling by highly recognizable personalities promoted an increase in knowledge and reduction of fears concerning vaccinations. Actual immunization efforts were channeled into periodic campaigns (jornadas) in which the primary health care system focused its energies and resources into making immunizations as convenient as possible for a few specific days. High school students posted over 250,000 awareness/announcement posters and delivered calendars with dates of the vaccinations marked to mothers' homes. The Ministry of Health, National Institute for the Child and Family, armed forces, Ministry of Education, oil companies, foreign donors, and others all contributed to the mobilization of the campaign. Diplomas were given to mothers whose children were completely vaccinated, with additional gold stars affixed to them when vaccinations were completed before the age of one. In all, these efforts resulted in vaccinations for over a half million children.[35]

FACTORS TO OPTIMIZE SUCCESS IN DEVELOPMENTAL PROGRAMS

Monitoring

As in any monitoring system, sensitive and yet easily measured indicators of health or health worker activity must be measured on a frequent basis, with continual feedback provided to health personnel and the communities they serve. Two barriers to effective monitoring common in under-

developed countries must be overcome, however. First, even very simple time-series measurement can become extraordinarily complicated when faced with a lack of transportation, telephone or radio communication, or other methods by which to collect information. This situation is rendered even more difficult when combined with a weakened primary health care system that has not proven capable of providing even basic services. Demoralized or poorly trained frontline staff are unlikely to be effective monitors of the fruits of their own and their colleagues' labor.

The second barrier to monitoring was labeled by Bunch as the "conspiracy of courtesy."[36] Many societies regard publicizing someone's shortcomings as the height of rudeness: flattery is often the only acceptable form of feedback. Developing a monitoring system which breaks through or outflanks this barrier is unlikely to be appreciated. This presents a major professional challenge.

The best method for developing a monitoring system is to work with an existing one. For example, most child survival programs incorporate some form of patient-retained records including a growth monitoring card for regular recording and charting of growth progress for children under five. This visual feedback system can be expanded to include other information (e.g., immunization history, oral rehydration therapy (ORT) training, family planning practices) which prompts the health worker to interact with the parent regarding various health-related behaviors. Additionally, this information can be extracted by the health worker or an external evaluator who visits homes directly to determine the prevalence of selected target behaviors. Like much of health promotion, the key to effective monitoring is to start small and work with existing (measurement) practices.

Evaluation

Bunch indicated that "there is something basically paternalistic in assuming that villagers capable of learning to manage a program are incapable of learning to evaluate it well."[37] He described "aided self-evaluation" as a process by which an external evaluation "expert" acts as an adviser rather than the head of an evaluation effort. Clearly, Bunch embraced a philosophy emphasizing the decentralization of such authority, giving it to each community. All planning, intervention, and evaluation activities must be undertaken within the realization that communities will soon have to "go it alone" (i.e., without external funding); therefore, the greater the skill level and sense of responsibility left in the community, the better the chance of long-term program success.

SUMMARY

Although burdened with excessive poverty and socio-political upheavals, the world's underdeveloped people could realize important health gains if progress were achieved in several areas. Birth spacing, safe motherhood, and breastfeeding protect the health of both mothers and children. Growth monitoring and promotion, immunizations, and diarrhea and respiratory infection control would help abate the extremely high rates of illness and mortality among young children. Hygiene, malaria control, and the prevention of HIV infection protect the health of all segments of a population. Yet, among all health promotion measures, protecting the rights of women and promoting their status and welfare in society is arguably the most effective.

Health promotion efforts in underdeveloped countries often are sponsored by international donors or private, voluntary organizations. These development programs run the risk of offering assistance in paternalistic fashion, which by either patronizing the recipient community or making it dependent, have limited long-term effects. Such assistance efforts must leave behind both an enhanced skill level and increased sense of local responsibility.

Recent years have witnessed a surge in the appreciation of the technology of changing behavior for enhancing health in underdeveloped countries. This appreciation has been even slower to develop in the area of environmental protection, described in the next chapter.

EXERCISE

Do research on a country of your selection, and determine what a family in that country can spend on food on a typical day. (Depending on the country, this will probably range from $0.75 to $3.)

Multiply this amount by five, and "give yourself an allowance" of this resulting amount to go shopping. See if you can personally last from a Monday to the following Friday on the amount of food purchased. What did you buy? For how long did it last? What conclusions can you draw?

ADDITIONAL READINGS

These references travel widely and well:

1. R. Bunch. *Two ears of corn: A guide to people-centered agricultural improvement*. 2nd ed. Oklahoma City: World Neighbors.
2. D. Jelliffe & E. P. Jelliffe. *Programmes to promote breastfeeding*. Oxford: Oxford University Press, 1988.
3. W. B. Johnson, F. Wilder, D. Bogue, et al. *Information, education and communication in population and family planning*. Chicago: University of Chicago Press, 1973.
4. B. Pillsbury (Series Coordinator). *Behavioral issues in child survival programs*. A series of monographs and bibliographies. Malibu, CA: International Health and Development Associates, 1990.
5. M. Rasmuson, R. Seidel, W. Smith, & E. Booth. *Communication for child survival*. Washington, D.C.: Academy for Educational Development, 1988.
6. UNICEF/WHO/UNESCO. *Facts for life: A communication challenge*. Oxfordshire, UK: P&LA, 1990.
7. D. Werner. *Where there is no doctor*. Palo Alto, CA: Hesperian Foundation, 1982.
8. D. Werner & B. Bower. *Helping health workers learn*. Palo Alto, CA: Hesperian Foundation, 1982.
9. World Health Organization. *Education for health: A manual on health education in primary health care*. Geneva, Switzerland: World Health Organization, 1988.

ENDNOTES

1. Kristien, M., Arnold, C., & Wynder, E. (1977). Health economics and preventive care. *Science, 195*.
2. Fendall, N. (1972). *Auxiliaries in health care*. Baltimore: Johns Hopkins Press.
3. Bunch, R. (1982). Paternalism, enthusiasm and participation. In R. Bunch, *Two ears of corn*. Oklahoma City: World Neighbors.
4. Cited by Clement, D. (1988). Commerciogenic malnutrition in the 1980s. In D. Jelliffe & E. Jelliffe

(Eds.). *Programmes to promote breastfeeding.* Oxford: Oxford University Press.

5. Ibid.

6. Ibid., p. 351.

7. Ibid.

8. Elder, J. P. (1987). Applications of behavior modification to health promotion in the developing world. *Social Science & Medicine, 24,* 335–349.

9. Hathirat, S. (1983). Buddhist monks as community health workers in Thailand. *Social Science & Medicine, 17,* 1485–1487.

10. Ibid., pp. 52–53.

11. Fendall, N. (1972). *Auxiliaries in health care.* Baltimore: Johns Hopkins Press.

12. Caragay, R. (1982). Training indigenous health workers: A Philippine experience. *World Health Forum, 3,* 159–163.

13. UNICEF/UNESCO/WHO. (1991). *Facts for life.* New York: UNICEF House, p. xii.

14. Elder, J. & Estey, J. (1992). Behavior change strategies for family planning and population control in developing countries. *Social Science and Medicine, 35,* 1065–1076.

15. Veatch, R. (1977). Governmental planning incentives: Ethical issues at stake. *Studies in Family Planning, 8,* 100–108.

16. Jacobsen, J. (1983). Promoting population stabilization: Incentives for small families. *World Watch Paper, 54.*

17. Satia, J. & Rushikesh, M. (1986). Incentives and disincentives in the Indian family welfare program. *Studies in Family Planning, 17,* 136–145.

18. Rogers, E. (1973). *Communication strategies for family planning.* Glencoe, IL: Free Press.

19. Kwon, K. H. (1971). Use of the agent system in Seoul. *Studies in Family Planning, 2,* 237–240.

20. Elder, 1987. Applications of behavior modification to health promotion in the developing world.

21. Berelson, B. (1969). Beyond family planning. *Studies in Family Planning, 38,* 17–27.

22. This is admittedly a challengeable assertion. This policy has apparently been less successful in rural areas, and at a minimum has not extinguished the practice of female infanticide.

23. Chen, P. & Kols, A. (1982). Population and birth planning in the People's Republic of China. *Population Reports, 10,* 1, J–577, J–618.

24. Ibid., p. 589.

25. Ibid., p. 603.

26. Ibid., p. 603.

27. Guthrie, G., Guthrie, H., Fernandez, T., & Estrera, N. (1982). Cultural influences and reinforcement strategies. *Behavior Therapy, 13,* 624–637.

28. Meyer, A., Foote, D., & Smith, W. (1985). Communication works across cultures: Hard data on ORT. *Development Communication Report, 49,* 3–4.

29. Elder, J., Sutisnaputra, D., Elaeiman, N., Ware, L., Shaw, W., de Moor, C., & Graeff, J. (1992). The use of diarrhoeal management counselling cards for community health volunteer training in Indonesia: The Healthcom Project. *Journal of Tropical Medicine and Hygiene, 95,* 301–308.

30. Basu, R. & Jezek, Z. (1978). Operation Smallpox Zero. *Indian Journal of Public Health, 22,* 1, 38–54.

31. Ibid.

32. Ibid.

33. Pan American Health Organization/World Health Organization. (1986). *Guide for planning, implementing, and evaluating programs to control acute respiratory infection as part of primary health care.* WHO/RSD 186.29. Washington, D.C.: PAHO/WHO.

34. Pillsbury, B. (1990). *Immunization: The behavioral issues.* Washington, D.C.: USAID Office of Health/International Health and Development Associates.

35. Rasmuson, M., Seidel, R., Smith, W., & Booth, E. (1988). *Communication for child survival.* Washington, D.C.: Academy for Educational Development.

36. Ibid., p. 68.

37. Ibid., p. 190.

Chapter 21

Protecting and Preserving the Environment

OBJECTIVES

After reading this chapter, the reader should be able to:

1. State current problems threatening the environment and Planet Earth.
2. Design a behavior-based intervention program to prevent environmental problems or improve environmental quality.
3. Develop an evaluation scheme for assessing the behavioral or environmental impact of a community-based program targeting environmental protection.
4. Distinguish between physical and behavioral engineering approaches to environmental protection.
5. Describe a comprehensive, community-wide process for large-scale environmental protection.
6. Distinguish between antecedent and consequence interventions for environmental protection.

INTRODUCTION

If present trends continue, the world in 2000 will be more crowded, more polluted, less stable ecologically, and more vulnerable to disruption than the world we live in now. Serious stresses involving population, resources, and environment are clearly visible ahead. Despite greater material output, the world's people will be more poor in many ways than they are today.[1]

In its *Global 2000 Report to the President,* the U.S. Council on Environmental Quality (USCEQ) offered rather pessimistic projections for environmental conditions through the end of this century. Indeed, similar concerns for the environment and its resources have been voiced by others.[2] Oskamp and Stern categorized such warnings about current and future ecological stresses into eight target areas: (1) population, (2) food, (3) land, (4) water, (5) energy, (6) solid wastes, (7) minerals, and (8) atmosphere.[3] Obviously, the health of the planet's population will be directly threatened without substantial progress in protecting the environment. For such progress to be realized, the present chapter argues that the field of health promotion and the technology of behavior modification must play a central role.

The world's population is expected to increase by 50 percent over the next two decades, reaching 6-1/3 billion in the year 2000, and 90 percent of this growth will occur in the less developed countries.[4] About half a billion people in the poorest countries are estimated to be currently below the United Nations standard of adequate **food** intake, and by 2000 as many as 1.3 billion people could be in this situation.[5] Food productivity continues to fall behind population growth which spurted in the 1970s. It has been projected, for example, that the worldwide availability of ocean fish will decrease 30 percent by the year 2000.[6] The worldwide availability of fish, mutton, beef, and grains has already decreased by 10 percent after reaching peak levels in the 1970s.[7] Yet, demand continues to increase for beef and other inefficient sources of nutrition: it takes sixteen pounds of feed grain to produce one pound of beef.[8] The analogous pounds of feed grain for other protein sources are: six pounds for pork, four pounds for turkey, and three pounds for poultry and eggs.[9]

Contributing to reduced food production is the overuse and misuse of **land.** Urban sprawl in the U.S. has been destroying a million acres of farmland every year, and the intensive cultivation of the remaining U.S. farmland has led to severe losses of topsoil.[10] Deforestation (i.e., the cutting down of trees for building materials or firewood or for increasing pasture land), has been increasing critically and has led to devastating consequences, including life-threatening floods, soil erosion, water pollution, and the extinction of certain biological species.[11]

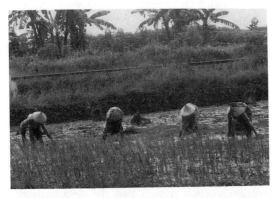

FIGURE 21–1. Rice and other grains can meet many of the world's nutritional needs. But many crop lands are being converted to production of less efficient livestock, while others are being eaten up by urban sprawl. *Photo courtesy of John Elder.*

Land misuse presents problems for another critical environmental resource — **water.** Fertilizing with nitrogen and phosphate, for example, causes water pollution, resulting in the eutrophication of lakes which causes massive growth of algae, and the extinction of certain fish species.[12] Water pollution is a major health threat in many countries, carrying bacteria which cause various diseases, including cholera, typhoid, and dysentery.[13] Although these diseases have been virtually eliminated in the U.S., insufficient sewage treatment in many U.S. communities spreads such diseases as hepatitis, and the waste products from U.S. industries are major sources of toxic chemicals in rivers, lakes, and residential drinking water.[14]

Thus, the pollution, overuse, and misuse of water threatens the availability of a prime necessity for life. In several areas (e.g., California's San Joaquin Valley and the Ogallala Aquifer region of Nebraska), more water is taken from underground reservoirs than is being replenished, resulting in falling water tables and dried-up wells.[15] In fact, some have predicted global water shortages by the year 2000 if the world's population growth and water consumption continue at their current rate.[16]

The whole world is dependent upon supplies of gas and oil for energy, as dramatically shown by the threats posed by the Arab oil embargo in 1973, the Iranian revolution in 1979, and the Gulf War in 1991. While progress in developing renewable sources of energy has actually slowed, a long-term decrease in petroleum supplies has already set in.[17]

Appropriate solid waste management (including litter control, waste reduction, and recycling) can result in substantial energy savings, as well as preserve increasingly scarce minerals. Processing recycled aluminum, for example, uses only 4 percent of the energy required to smelt the virgin ore.[18] Litter pollution not only defaces the environment (resulting in nationwide clean-up costs exceeding $1 billion per year) and presents safety, fire, and health hazards,[19] but littering often represents the loss of natural resources which could have been recycled.[20]

The average American discards three to five pounds of trash daily, and the annual cost for managing this waste is nearly $6 billion per year.[21] Most urban areas are out of landfill sites for disposing solid wastes and must use substantial energy to transport their solid waste to rural areas, at

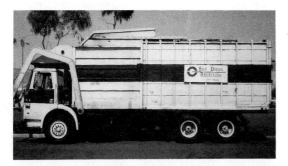
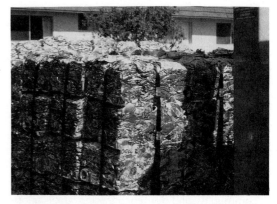

FIGURE 21–2. Municipal recycling efforts keep tremendous amounts of cans and other recyclable materials out of rapidly filling landfills. *Photo courtesy of Betsy Clapp.*

costs second only to education expenditures in most city budgets.[22] Further environmental problems occur when leachate (the liquid produced when water seeps through soil wastes) pollutes underground resources.[23] When the discarded waste is toxic (like the 20,000 tons of chemicals dumped in the Love Canal disposal site in Niagara Falls), the outcome can have catastrophic health effects.[24]

Pollution of the earth's atmosphere has potentially disastrous consequences worldwide. For example, the burning of fossil fuels, especially coal, produces sulphur oxides, which combine with water to make "acid rain" pollution. Recently it has killed fish life in thousands of lakes in the U.S., Canada, Scandinavia, and other countries.[25] We are only beginning to discover the damage done to former Eastern Bloc countries, yet all indications point to drastic ecological problems in that part of the world. Atmospheric pollution from chlorofluorocarbons released from spray cans and jet planes threatens to weaken the ozone layer which protects humans from skin cancer and plants and animals from serious injury by absorbing ultraviolet radiation.[26] Even more potentially catastrophic is the "greenhouse effect," or the warming of the earth, as a result of the carbon dioxide pollution from extensive use of fossil fuels.[27] A temperature increase of only a few degrees Fahrenheit could severely alter the earth's climatic zones for centuries, changing farmlands to deserts and melting the polar ice caps which, in turn, would cause flooding throughout the earth's coastal areas.[28]

Finally, the developing countries in the world, in their scramble to catch up economically with the West, have converted more and more land from forests and wild areas to cash-producing ventures. This conversion is often short-lived. Unstable terrain without trees quickly becomes eroded and useless, while overgrazed pastures turn into deserts. Cutting the forests also reduces the amount of oxygen given off by plants and needed by animals and humans for respiration. The undesirable human health consequences are obvious.

COMMUNITY ORGANIZING FOR ENVIRONMENTAL PROTECTION

The idea of preserving the environment has actually been an integral part of U.S. history. Theodore Roosevelt, for instance, was an environmentalist well before he was president or even a Rough Rider. Yet the rapid acceleration in ecological problems described above has presented us with an urgency not known to early environmentalists. A century ago, environmental problems went unnoticed among an American public who worshipped heroes like Buffalo Bill (known for slaughtering bison and letting tens of thousands of carcasses rot). Modern environmentalists are much more aggressive, working through national and international organizations such as the Sierra Club and Greenpeace. The Sierra Club for the most part practices social planning with a touch of locality development, flexing its financial muscle especially around election time. Greenpeace, in contrast, is a relatively pure example of a social action organization, promoting the public's awareness of eco-enemies by tangling fishing nets, disrupting businesses of toxic waste dumpers, and otherwise engaging in activities which invite retaliation (and, of course, media coverage).

Depending on whether we are attacking the "bad guys" or mobilizing the "good guys," social action, social planning, or locality development can be appropriate places to start in environmental protection. One of the authors (ESG) developed a locality development strategy for disseminating energy conservation strategies throughout a community and for encouraging their adoption.[29] This plan, termed an Energy Conserving Community (ECC) System, was influenced by the organizational scheme of the Clean Community System (CCS) of Keep America Beautiful, Inc. (KAB), which has been quite successful in promoting practical collaborations between local governments, businesses, and civic organizations for cooperative community action toward solving waste management problems.[30]

Strategies for motivating individual and group action are important aspects of both the CCS and ECC processes and are largely based on principles of positive reinforcement, with social approval and public recognition being primary rewarding consequences. Indeed, anticipated local and national commendation are major potential motivators for becoming a "certified clean community" under the CCS. The ECC proposal is a two-stage plan, whereby communities first initiate conservation action in order to earn eligibility as a "certified energy conserving community" (ECC), and then specific criteria are developed for qualification as a "certified energy efficient community" (EEC).

Completing each stage of the ECC process results in local, state, and national acknowledgement and special financial rewards through government grants. Throughout an ECC system, local incentive/reward tactics must be implemented to encourage the accomplishment of successive approximations toward reaching EEC status. After becoming an EEC, local incentive/reward systems are essential to motivate maintenance activities.

Figure 21–3 outlines the basic components of the ECC process—from initial application as an ECC to eventually earning certification as an EEC. A community initiates ECC application with a letter of endorsement from the mayor (or similar high-ranking official), and a commitment to send a ten-member work team to an ECC training conference and to allocate sufficient funds for the first year of operation.

The training conferences are organized through state extension systems and/or state energy offices who, in turn, are accountable to a national coordinating agency. The ten-member ECC work team includes one representative for each cell of the factorial array of two basic intervention approaches (physical engineering vs. behavioral science) $\times$ five targets for energy conservation intervention (heating/cooling, solid waste management, transportation, equipment efficiency, and water).

At the training conference the community work teams learn the ECC plan for coordinating, motivating, and evaluating a community-wide program for energy conservation. Some workshops are specialized according to the five conservation targets and two basic intervention approaches, and on these occasions the work teams split up according to individual areas of expertise. As a group, the teams are given the background, techniques, and materials for presenting local workshops to three community sectors (i.e., residential/consumer, governmental/institutional, and commercial/industrial). These local workshops are designed to inform citizens of practical conservation strategies for their particular situations, and to collaborate with the work teams on the design of local incentive/reward programs for stimulating and maintaining conservation activities in the five target areas within three community sectors.

After the week-long training conference, the ten-member work teams return home to initiate large-scale conservation programs. The participating community is considered a certified ECC, and local progress toward becoming a certified EEC community is continually monitored and rewarded by local, state, and federal intervention. Major initial tasks of the ECC work team include: (1) establishment of a local headquarters; (2) allocation of financial support; (3) administration of ECC workshops to key leaders in government institutions, commercial enterprises, industrial complexes, and community agencies; (4) implementation of an overall community analysis of energy consumption in the five target areas of the three major community sectors; (5) selection of

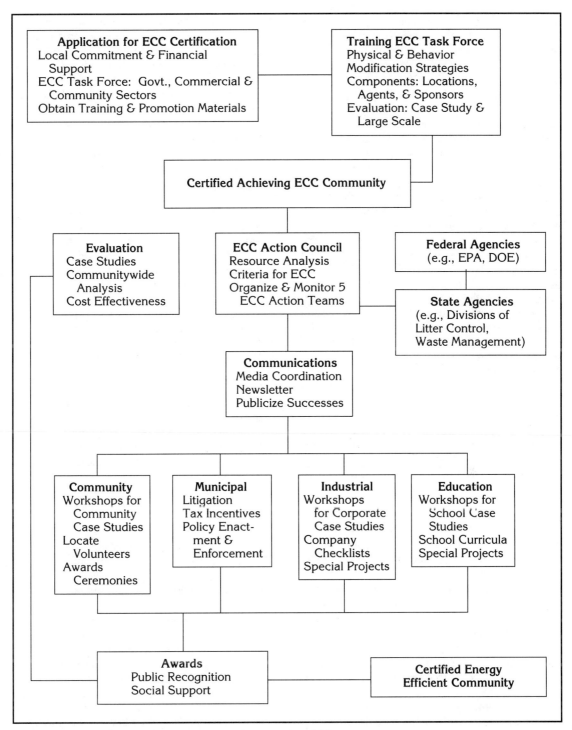

FIGURE 21–3.   The Energy Conserving Community (ECC) process

demonstration projects, representing each target area within each sector; and (6) organization of an ECC Action Council.

The ECC Action Council is the key organizational component and work force of the ECC process. This thirty-member council includes influential leaders from the three community sectors, experts in the five target areas, and professionals from disciplines related to both the physical and behavioral science approaches to energy conservation (e.g., architecture, economics, education, engineering, physics, psychology, and sociology). Important responsibilities of this committee include: (1) maintaining a library of resources relevant to energy conservation; (2) maintaining communications with local extension agents and with the energy conservation specialists who ran the ECC training conference, certified the community as an ECC, and is responsible for certifying communities as energy efficient (i.e., an EEC); (3) organizing and monitoring the five ECC action teams (described below) which carry out energy conservation education, promotion, and demonstration projects; (4) evaluating progress of the ECC action teams, including comparisons of baseline, treatment and follow-up data; and (5) developing criteria for an energy efficient community (EEC).

The success of a local ECC program is largely determined by the activities of five ECC action teams coordinated and monitored by the ECC Action Council. The following five components of the comprehensive ECC process outline briefly the primary responsibilities of the five concomitant action teams.

- The *Communication Team* is responsible for communicating the activities of an ECC, thereby publicly commending individual and group efforts toward energy conservation and showing others specific techniques for reducing energy consumption. All communication media are used (TV, radio, newspaper) and an in-house newsletter is developed.
- The *Education Team* is responsible for keeping all other teams informed of relevant techniques for conserving energy and for promoting increases in energy education in public schools. This committee may sponsor public education programs for teaching energy concepts or special school projects which demonstrate principles of energy use and energy savings.

- The *Community Team* is responsible for locating and coordinating local civic organizations for energy conservation activities. The located volunteer groups are taught to administer mini-workshops, implement neighborhood conservation projects, assist in community-wide analysis of energy use, and to run special award programs among individuals and groups for motivating action toward conservation goals.
- The *Government Team* is responsible for applying governmental policy to encourage energy conservation and for planning strategies to meet long-range energy needs. For example, such a team would formulate policies, ordinances, and tax-rebate programs for motivating energy education and conservation techniques. Municipal agencies and institutions could establish simple conservation programs in any of the five target areas, and thus establish themselves as public examples for the appropriate application of conservation strategies. This team also sponsors the administration of energy conservation workshops for government personnel.
- The *Industrial Team* is responsible for promoting energy conservation in the commercial/industrial sector of the community, and for establishing visible examples of the successful application of energy conserving procedures in corporations and business enterprises. An attempt is made to demonstrate publicly the application of conservation strategies in all five target areas. This committee promotes the ECC by administering energy conservation workshops to special work groups in commercial and industrial settings.

This ECC process for coordinating community activities toward energy and environmental protection was proposed only as a general framework within which specific policies and action plans might be developed, implemented, and tested.[31] The essential contribution of this ECC process is a scheme for coordinating the numerous facets of environmental protection among the citizens of communities where major program control should be focused. State environmental offices, university extension services, local community agencies, and even the U.S. Department of Energy and the U.S. Environmental Protection Agency have implemented various environmental programs which relate to particular components of the ECC process. Now it is time to coordinate the most cost-effective strategies and schemes under a nation-wide program to protect the environment. Such a program should emphasize interdisciplinary and comprehensive input, large-scale and long-term intervention, integration of the physical and behavioral sciences, immediate reinforcers and punishers to motivate behavior change, cost-effectiveness evaluations of physical (high technology) vs. behavior modification (low technology) strategies, local participation in planning community programs and policies, and the mutual contribution of as many individuals and groups as possible in as many different situations as possible.

NEEDS ASSESSMENT AND RESEARCH ISSUES

Defining Target Behaviors

Whether it be the area of energy conservation or other categories of environmental protection, the variety of relevant human behaviors occur daily in almost every setting (e.g., at home, at work, at school, at a commercial location, or in transition between settings). Assessing, defining, and researching environmentally relevant behaviors, and making recommendations regarding desirable change requires interdisciplinary input. For example, engineers can advise which vehicle or appliance is most energy efficient or polluting; architects are helpful in defining optimal insulation techniques and landscape designs for conserving energy in home heating and cooling; biologists can prescribe desirable procedures for composting and for disposing of hazardous waste; and information from physics and human factors engineering is relevant for defining ways to conserve when using home appliances, vehicles, industrial machinery, and heating, cooling, resource recovery or water-management systems.

To categorize the potential target behaviors of a comprehensive community needs assessment approach for environmental protection, the three dimensional matrix defined above for the ECC process should be considered: (a) two basic intervention *approaches* (physical vs. behavioral engineering); (b) three community *sectors* requiring direct intervention (the residential/consumer sector, governmental/institutional sector, and commercial/industrial sector); and (c) various *targets* or domains for intervention within each sector

(i.e., heating/cooling, solid waste management, transportation, equipment efficiency, and water).

Repetitive vs. One-Shot Behaviors. Some procedures for preventing environmental problems require repetitive action, whereas others involve only a one-time behavior modification. In other words, one class of behaviors requires repeated occurrences in order to effect significant environmental protection. Examples in this category include: setting back room thermostats each night; using contraceptives consistently; following antipollution guidelines regularly; driving 55 mph or less; taking shorter and cooler showers; purchasing low-phosphate detergents, white toilet paper, and returnable bottles; using separate containers for recyclable paper, metal, glass, and biodegradable trash; maintaining a compost pile for food and yard wastes; and wearing more clothes in order to withstand lower room temperatures. On the other hand, a particular strategy to preserve the environment may require only one occurrence of a particular response such as: installing a thermostat capable of automatically changing room temperature settings to preprogrammed levels; undergoing surgical sterilization; purchasing an energy-efficient vehicle with optimal emission controls; wrapping insulation around a water heater; inserting a shower-flow limiter in a showerhead; installing a solar heating system; adding insulation to a building; purchasing longer-lasting equipment; applying appropriate irrigation technology; and constructing a high technology waste separation system.

It is noteworthy that for "one-shot" behaviors, the user usually pays an initially high cost in time and money for the subsequent convenience of not having to make continued response input. However, several strategies for environmental protection involve both a one-shot investment and repeated actions. Thus, one can purchase a window fan to substitute for an air conditioner or a moped to substitute for an automobile, but energy conservation does not occur unless the individual makes repeated decisions to use the more energy-efficient machine. Likewise, energy-saving or antipollution settings on new energy-efficient and environment-protective equipment and appliances are not worth much unless they are used regularly. Furthermore, innovative engineering devices for separating, transporting, and reprocessing recyclable trash are not preventing environmental problems unless they are used appropriately on a daily basis by various individuals (e.g., from residents who initiate the redistribution process to retailers who promote the purchase of recyclable and recycled commodities).

Peak Shift Behaviors. In the domain of energy conservation, there is an additional category of potential target behaviors. These have been termed "peak shift behaviors," referring to changing the time when individuals emit energy consumptive behaviors. Reducing peak demands for energy decreases the need for power companies to build or borrow supplementary generators or other energy sources (e.g., nuclear reactors). Indeed, electricity suppliers have been willing to vary their rates according to peak demand (termed peak-load pricing), although residents have found it difficult to shift various energy-consuming tasks.[32]

Peak shifting is usually associated with residential energy use (e.g., changing times for cooking, showering, or sleeping), but it could be much more cost-effective as a large-scale conservation strategy for the corporate and municipal sectors of a community. Consider, for example, the peak shift advantages of altering the scheduling and/or length of work shifts at industrial complexes and government agencies (e.g., through the adoption of flexible work schedules or a four-day work week). Certain large-scale changes in work schedules could result in peak shifts (and energy savings) at the work setting, at home, and during commuting. For example, even the most fuel-efficient vehicles become gas hogs when creeping through hours of stop-and-go traffic. The major function of urban transit systems is to serve people going to and from work, and since most of such commuting occurs during two short rush periods per weekday, numerous bus drivers make non-productive runs or actually sit idle most of the day.[33] Before instituting large-scale shifts in work schedules, however, it is necessary to do pilot research in order to define the most energy-efficient schedules which do not disrupt family life, leisure activity, and other functions of a "healthy" community.[34]

SETTING PRIORITIES

There are some who claim it is too late to protect the environment from inevitable destruc-

tion[35] or insist that recent efforts to decrease environmental destructive responses are basically insufficient with regard to finding practical large-scale solutions to environmental problems.[36] Others, perhaps, have been overly optimistic when describing the potential for wide-scale behavior modification to preserve the environment.[37] A compromising and actually realistic position is that many solutions to environmental problems require changes in human behavior, and behavioral science can offer suggestions for attacking the behavioral aspects of environmental protection.[38] In the case of litter control, for example, it is desirable both to decrease the frequency of behaviors that produce litter and to increase the occurrence of behaviors that reduce litter. Tactics for decelerating littering are typically referred to as "antilitter" techniques, whereas approaches to accelerate litter pick-up behavior might be termed "unlittering" procedures. Note that an antilitter goal usually requires a different behavior modification strategy than does an unlitter goal. Furthermore, the target audience would likely be different for an antilittering versus an unlittering goal.

Antilitter campaigns or PSAs should target the litterbug (i.e., people who litter the environment regularly or intermittently), whereas unlittering PSAs should probably aim their message at those who are already concerned about litter control (e.g., members of local environmental groups) and perhaps have already picked up environmental litter (e.g., as a contributor to a community unlitter program). Thus, when designing a PSA for litter control, it may be constructive to consider at least five categories of individuals: (1) the habitual litterbug (who is probably uninfluenced by an environmental PSA); (2) the intermittent litterbug (who might be influenced by an antilitter PSA if the PSA is supported by local action strategies); (3) the uninvolved non-litterer (who does not litter the environment but considers litter control a relatively unimportant problem and never gets involved in environmental projects); (4) the concerned non-litterer (who is somewhat concerned about environmental degradation and might therefore be affected by an "unlittering" PSA if the promotion is supported by community action groups); and (5) the involved unlitterer (who has already shown personal commitment to environmental issues through intermittent or daily behaviors and, thus, would be likely to volunteer in a litter control campaign aimed at either antilittering or unlittering).

It would be worthwhile to know the individual and situational characteristics of the habitual litterbug, the intermittent litterbug, the uninvolved non-litterer, the concerned non-litterer, and the involved unlitterer and to obtain an estimate of the proportion of people per category. At this point, it is only safe to estimate that the extreme audience types (i.e., habitual litterbug and involved unlitterer) are in the minority, each accounting for no more than 5 to 10 percent of the population, and that most U.S. citizens could probably be considered "uninvolved non-litterers" (e.g., perhaps 60 percent to 70 percent of the population). It is likely that an antilitter or unlitter PSA (with supportive community programming) will change most persons to an adjacent category (i.e., a habitual litterbug might become an intermittent litterbug, an intermittent litterbug might become an uninvolved non-litterer, and so on). However, the particular category shifts are dependent upon the nature of the PSA (e.g., antilitter versus unlitter approach) and the local community action strategies.

For each target area (i.e., population, land, water, food, energy, solid waste, minerals, and

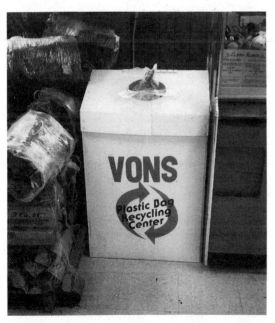

FIGURE 21–4. Although this supermarket chain promotes the recycling of plastic shopping bags, it also sells firewood wrapped in several layers of (presumably non-recyclable) plastic. *Photo courtesy of Betsy Clapp.*

atmosphere), goals should be specified and target behaviors related to each goal identified. Subsequently, before developing a behavior modification intervention, it would probably be useful to match particular audiences and situations with target behaviors. Such an analysis would undoubtedly be more complex than it was for litter control, but note that litter control is only a subcategory of the solid waste category. Other areas within the solid waste category with their own environmental goals and target behaviors include waste reduction, resource recovery, waste treatment and disposal, hazardous waste transportation and dumping, and toxic waste clean-up. Moreover, extensions of these approaches can alleviate problems in the other seven target areas of environmental protection. Likewise, each of the categories for environmental concern should be sliced into target subareas in order to develop a feasible prevention program.

Table 21–1 gives examples of individual-level target behaviors for environmental protection programs.

INTERVENTIONS

Marketing and Education

Messages for promoting environment preservation have been delivered through television commercials, pamphlets, films, verbal instructions, and demonstrations (e.g., from peers, parents, teachers, or public officials), and through environmental displays (such as speed limit signs, feedback meters, beautified trash receptacles, and "energy saving" settings on appliance controls). Some basic characteristics of effective messages include: (1) messages should refer to specific behaviors (desirable or undesirable); (2) when the avoidance of undesirable behaviors is prompted (e.g., antilittering), it is best to specify an alternative desirable behavior that is relatively convenient; (3) messages should be stated in polite language which do not threaten an individual's perceived freedom; and (4) to be most effective, behavior modification messages should occur in close proximity to the desired target behavior.[39]

Research has shown at least some success in prompting occupants of public buildings to turn off room lights when they placed messages at light switches stating the lights should be turned off when leaving the room.[40] On the other hand,

TABLE 21-1
Example of Individual-Level Target Behaviors for Environmental Protection

Food	Transportation	Residential Energy	Solid Waste Disposal
1. Eat more grains and vegetables and less meat (especially beef).	1. Use carpools or public transportation.	1. Use efficient fluorescent lighting and appliances.	1. Recycle newspapers, cans, bottles, etc.
2. Buy organically grown food.	2. Walk or ride a bike whenever possible.	2. Insulate/weatherproof home.	2. Bring your own bag or basket when you shop.
3. Share food with the hungry.	3. Buy a high gas mileage car or one that uses alternative energy sources.	3. Limit use of heating or cooling; wear warmer or cooler clothes.	3. Avoid purchasing products which produce waste; buy in bulk or buy reusable products (e.g., rechargeable batteries).
	4. Keep engine tuned, tires inflated and air filter clean.	4. Use low energy settings on dishwasher, water heater, etc.	5. Avoid polystyrene foam.
	5. Drive at 55 mph and limit use of air conditioners.	5. Consider solar energy.	

356

educational awareness sessions and informational packages (without special incentive provisions) have been unsuccessful in motivating the occurrence of relatively inconvenient and/or time-consuming energy conservation strategies.[41] Furthermore, flyers with a general plea and specific instructions regarding a campus paper recycling program were not sufficient to get residents of university dormitories to bring recyclable paper to a particular collection room,[42] even when these handbills were given personally to dorm residents and accompanied by verbal exhortation.[43]

Contingency Contracting

Researchers have only recently studied the behavior modification potential of contingency contracting strategies, but so far the results are quite encouraging. For example, two studies found markedly increased participation in a neighborhood recycling program after residents signed pledges that requested participation.[44] More research is needed on the application of contingency contracting to change environmentally-related behaviors, especially given the feasibility and inexpensiveness of this tactic for a large number of target behaviors in a variety of settings. Geller and Lehman,[45] for example, reviewed a series of similar contingency contracting inventions that were remarkably effective at increasing the use of vehicle safety belts (see also chapter 12).

Response Facilitation Strategies

Engineering or design approaches to prevent environmental problems involve the design or redesign of devices, machinery, or environmental settings which either provide for environment protection behaviors or facilitate such behaviors. For example, litter control strategies vary from the application of engineering technology to increasing the number and availability of more "user friendly" trash cans.

Simple modifications in the design of a milieu or litter collection device can reduce the response cost (i.e., increase the convenience) of litter control or resource recovery (e.g., by increasing the availability or size of trash cans or providing large, obtrusive, partitioned receptacles for depositing different types of recyclables). Alternatively, such response facilitation interventions can actually help to motivate antilittering or unlittering (e.g., by adding specific response messages to trash receptacles or environmental settings). Demonstrations of litter control have been achieved through simple modifications in the appearance, positioning, and availability of trash receptacles,[46] and each of these design interventions could be readily combined with other behavior modification tactics to produce a greater and longer-term impact.

Consequence Techniques

Generally, behavior modification interventions for preserving the environment have been much more effective when pleasant or unpleasant consequences were contingent upon the target behavior or upon the outcome of one or more target behaviors. Such consequences can be an extrinsic stimulus (e.g., a monetary rebate, a self-photograph, a speeding ticket, a verbal commendation or condemnation), or an opportunity to engage in a particular behavior (e.g., the privilege to use a preferred parking space, add one's name to an "Energy Efficient" honor roll, or attend a special litter control workshop). Punishment and negative reinforcement procedures to promote environmental protection usually take the form of policy enactment through laws or ordinances (e.g., fines for littering, illegal dumping, excessive water use, or for polluting air or water). To be effective, punishment and reinforcement to protect the environment require extensive enforcement and litigation.

Response-Contingent Vs. Outcome-Contingent Consequences. The positive reinforcement consequences applied toward environmental protection have varied widely. Some consequences have been given contingent upon the performance of a certain desired response, whereas other consequence strategies did not specify a desired behavior, but were contingent upon a given outcome (e.g., on the basis of environmental cleanliness, energy consumption, or water savings). The following response-contingent consequences were successful in significantly increasing the frequency of the environment-related behavior indicated: (1) raffle tickets per specified amounts of paper delivered to a recycling center;[47] (2) a merchandise token (redeemable for goods and services at local businesses) for riding a particular bus;[48] (3) a coupon redeemable for a soft drink following litter deposits in a particular trash receptacle;[49] (4) $1 and a posted self-photograph for collecting a specially-marked item of litter;[50] and (5) points exchangeable for family outings and special favors following reduced use of designated home appliances.[51]

Examples of outcome-contingent consequences (i.e., those based on "permanent products," see chapter 3) which were effective at increasing the frequency of environment-beneficial behaviors include: (1) 10¢ for cleaning a littered yard; (2) $5 for averaging a 10 percent reduction in miles of travel over 28 days and $2.50 for each additional 10 percent reduction up to 30 percent;[52] (3) $2 per week for a 5 percent to 10 percent reduction in home-heating energy, $3 for a 11 percent to 20 percent reduction, and $5 per week for reductions greater than 20 percent;[53] and (4) 75 percent of energy savings from expected costs returned to the residents of a master-metered apartment complex.[54]

Feedback Interventions. The variety of energy conservation studies which showed beneficial effects of giving residents frequent and specific feedback regarding energy consumption can also be considered outcome consequences.[55] Feedback consequences are an indication of energy consumption in terms of kilowatt hours, cubic feet of gas, and/or monetary cost, and such consequences can be pleasant or rewarding (if the feedback implies a savings in energy costs) or they can be unpleasant or punishing (if the feedback indicates an increase in consumption or costs).

Successful methods of giving residential energy consumption feedback have included: (1) a special feedback card delivered to the home on a monthly,[56] weekly,[57] or daily[58] basis; (2) a mechanical apparatus which illuminated a light whenever current electricity use exceeded 90 percent of the peak level for the household;[59] (3) an electronic feedback meter with digital display of electricity cost per hour;[60] (4) the use of a hygrothermograph to give readings of room temperature and humidity;[61] and (5) training packages for teaching and motivating residents to read their own electric meters regularly and record energy consumption.[62]

Some feedback studies have targeted transportation conservation, demonstrating reduction of vehicular miles of travel (vmt) with public display of vmt per individual,[63] and increases in vehicular miles per gallon (mpg) with a fuel flow meter indicating continuous mpg or gallons-per-hour consumption,[64] or with a public display of mpg for short-run and long-haul truck drivers.[65] In addition, one feedback intervention targeted litter control, demonstrating a 35 percent average reduction in ground litter following daily displays of litter counts on the front page of a community newspaper.[66]

Comprehensive plans have been proposed for implementing community-wide behavior modification programs for environment protection and preservation,[67] but systematic behavior-based evaluations of large-scale programs are rare. There are a few exceptions and these are worth noting, especially since each illustrates a successive progression from small-scale demonstration experiments to community-wide intervention.

Bachman and Katzev,[68] for example, evaluated community-level reward and commitment strategies for promoting bus ridership which were modeled after the earlier small-scale research by Everett and his students at Penn State University.[69] Similarly, Hake and Zane[70] tested a community-wide gasoline conservation project which was an extension of prior reward-based campus programs designed to motivate reductions in the use of personal vehicles.[71] McNees et al.[72] assessed the environmental impact of a community-based litter control system for youth that incorporated many of the litter control strategies which had been developed from a variety of small-scale field experiments, including an innovative technique for motivating the collection of small litter items.[73] This technique, termed "the marked item technique," involves the marking of certain litter (including small pieces of litter) and rewarding litter collectors for finding the marked items. For one variation,[74] certain litter was marked with a "clue spray" that got on a litter-collector's hands when touching the item and could only be detected when the litter on the collector's hands was held under an ultraviolet light. In addition, Winett and his students[75] have shown how to implement community-wide the communication and feedback strategies for promoting residential energy conservation which developed from the case studies of a few residences.[76]

SUMMARY

Behavior modification principles were first applied to environmental problems in the early 1970s, following the first Earth Day. During this period, numerous behavior modification studies focused on the development and evaluation of interventions to reduce environment-destructive behaviors such as littering, lawn trampling, vehicle miles of travel, and the purchase of beverages in throwaway containers. Other behavioral studies showed how to increase such environment-preserving behaviors as picking up litter, collecting and delivering recyclables, composting, car pooling, and practicing a number of low-cost conservation techniques (e.g., installing insulation and shower-flow limiters, adjusting thermostat settings and wearing appropriate clothing, reducing the use of air conditioners, adjusting for peak-load demands, and increasing the use of mass transit). Several innovative behavior modification techniques emerged from this research, many proving to be cost-effective for community-wide application. Although the results from this domain of behavior modification research were encouraging, large-scale applications of the practical intervention programs were not to be. The textbooks[77] that reviewed this work were read by very few individuals besides students at the relatively few colleges or universities offering courses in environmental psychology. The failure to apply this knowledge is unfortunate, especially in light of the profound intensification of environmental destruction occurring since the first Earth Day.

There are many possible reasons for the lack of governmental, corporate, and societal interests in the behavioral environmental research of the 1970s, including ineffective dissemination of the practical research findings to agencies and audiences who were more intrigued with high technology and quick-fix approaches to solving environmental problems. Indeed, the theme of this behavior modification research—conservation through low technology community-based intervention—has been typically viewed as incompatible with big business and consumer convenience. This viewpoint was summarized succinctly by Clive Seligman, one of the behavior modification researchers of the 70s:

Unless business can make money from environmental products or politicians can get elected

on environmental issues, or individuals can get personal satisfaction from experiencing environmental concern, then individuals and organizations will simply do whatever competes with environmentalism if they see the payoff as greater.[78]

National, state, and local governments have seemed content to pass environmental control legislation and then penalize individual, group, or corporate infractions of such policy. This is partly because laws, policies, and ordinances are relatively quick and easy to implement and monitor; they represent the traditional governmental approach to behavior modification, and the monetary fines from infractions provide funds for the mandating government, organization, or community.

This chapter has summarized a number of behavior modification approaches to environmental protection and preservation that did not incorporate mandates, disincentives, or punishment— the techniques which should actually be used only as a last resort if public acceptance and positive attitude change are desired. Although this applied research focused on individuals in the residential/consumer sector, many of the lessons learned can be applied to the governmental/institutional and commercial/industrial sectors. Hopefully, Earth Day 1990 has begun an era of corporate and government concern and community empowerment for addressing environmental issues in sharp contrast to the corporate and individual greed of the 1980s, which occurred at the expense of community and environmental enhancement.

Unlike twenty years ago, it is now fashionable and profitable for companies to promote their products as being environmentally protective. Public health professionals can play an important role in increasing corporations' environmentally protective behavior by helping them develop more effective environmental programs with the low-technology behavior modification interventions reviewed in this chapter. Along these same lines, the government should provide incentives and reinforcers (e.g., tax breaks) for companies demonstrating environment preserving practices, and should establish funding for researchers interested in studying the human element of environmental issues. Such research support was essentially nonexistent for the behavioral environmental psychologists of the 1970s, and thus most of these researchers and teachers abandoned the field in the early 1980s.[79] There is cause for optimism, however, given the increased amount of media attention to environmental issues and the overwhelming expression of environmental concern by the public. These are promising signs that the culture is beginning to change toward a concern for environmental protection. Clearly, the *Zeitgeist* is ripe for governments, scientists, public health officials, corporations, environmental groups, and citizens to work together to preserve the quality of environment we now enjoy. The future of our Planet Earth is indeed in our hands!

EXERCISES

1. Select an environmentally-relevant personal behavior which you could modify. Using some of the techniques of behavior change described in the previous three sections, design a self-change project for making you a more environmentally-friendly person.
2. With a pair of heavy gloves and permission from a responsible person, sort through some household garbage in an apartment complex or some single-family dwellings. What could have been mulched? Recycled? At what personal or material costs to the individual residents?

ADDITIONAL READINGS

Keep your skies blue and your water clear with these resources:

1. Council on Economic Priorities. *Shopping for a Better World.* (30 Irving Place, New York, NY 10003).
2. E. S. Geller, R. A. Winett, & P. B. Everett. (1982). *Preserving the environment: New strategies for behavior change.* New York: Pergamon Press.
3. Hollender, J. (1991). *How to Make the World a Better Place.* New York: Quill William Morrow.
4. Earth Works Project Staff. (1990). *50 Simple Things You Can Do to Save the Earth.* Earthworks Press, Box 25, 1400 Shattuck Avenue, Berkeley, CA 94709.

ENDNOTES

1. U.S. Council on Environmental Quality and U.S. Department of State. (1980). *The global 2000 report to the president: Entering the twenty-first century.* Washington, D.C.: Government Printing Office, p. 1.
2. For example, Davis, W. J. (1979). *The seventh year: Industrial civilization in transition.* New York: Norton; Erlich, P. R., Erlich, A. H., & Holdren, J. P. (1977). *Ecoscience: Population, resources, environment.* San Francisco: Freeman; Humphrey, C., & Buttle, F. (1981). *Environment, energy, and society.* Belmont, CA: Wadsworth; Watt, K. (1982). *Understanding the environment.* Newton, MA: Allyn & Bacon; and Welch, S. & Miewald, R. (Eds.). (1983). *Scarce natural resources: The challenge to public policymaking.* Beverly Hills, CA: Sage.
3. Stern, P. & Oskamp, S. (1987). Managing scarce environmental resources. In D. Stokols & I. Altman (Eds.), *Handbook of environmental psychology* (pp. 1043–1088). New York: John Wiley.
4. U.S. Council on Environmental Quality and U.S. Department of State.
5. Ibid.
6. Brown, L. R. (1980). *Building a sustainable society.* New York: Norton; and U.S. Council on Environmental Quality and U.S. Department of State.
7. Stern & Oskamp, Managing scarce environmental resources.
8. U.S. Council on Environmental Quality and U.S. Department of State.
9. Ibid.
10. Brown, L. R. (1981). *Building a sustainable society;* and U.S. Council on Environmental Quality and U.S. Council on Environmental Quality and U.S. Department of State.
11. U.S. Council on Environmental Quality and U.S. Department of State.
12. Erlich, P. R., Erlich, A. H., & Holdren, J. P. (1977). *Ecoscience: Population, resources, environment.* San Francisco: Freeman.
13. Hayes, D. (1979). *Pollution: The neglected dimensions.* (Worldwatch Paper 27). Washington, D.C.: Worldwatch Institute.
14. Stern & Oskamp, Managing scarce environmental resources.
15. Brown, *Building a sustainable society.*
16. Kalenin, G. P. & Bykov, V. C. (1969). The world's water resources present and future. *Impact of science on society, 19,* 135–150; and Simmons, I. G. (1974). *The ecology of natural resources.* London: Edward Arnold.
17. *National Geographic.* (1981, February). An atlas of America's energy resources, pp. 58–69; Stern & Oskamp, Managing scarce environmental resources.
18. Hayes, D. (1978). *Repairs, reuse, recycling—First steps toward a sustainable society.* (World-

watch Paper 23). Washington, D.C.: Worldwatch Institute.

19. Geller, E. S. (1980). Applications of behavioral analysis for litter control. In D. Glenwick & L. Jason (Eds.), *Behavioral community psychology: Progress and prospects* (pp. 254–283). New York: Praeger.

20. Geller, E. S. (1980). Saving environmental resources through waste reduction and recycling: How the behavioral community psychologist can help. In G. L. Martin & J. G. Osborne (Eds.), *Helping in the community: Behavioral applications* (pp. 55–102). New York: Plenum.

21. Purcell, A. H. (1981, February). The world's trashiest people: Will they clean up their act or throw away their future? *Futurist*, 51–59.

22. Geller, E. S. (1981). Waste reduction and resource recovery: Strategies for energy conservation. In A. Baum & J. E. Singer (Eds.), *Advances in environmental psychology, Vol. III. Energy conservation: Psychological perspectives* (pp. 115–154). Hillsdale, NJ: Erlbaum; and Hayes, Pollution: The neglected dimensions.

23. Weddle, B. & Garland, G. (1974, October). Dumps: A potential threat to our groundwater supplies. *Nation's Cities*, 21–26.

24. Epstein, S. S., Brown, L. O., & Pope, C. (1982). *Hazardous waste in America.* San Francisco: Sierra Club Books; Levine, A. G. (1982). *Love canal: Science, politics, and people.* Lexington, MA: Lexington Books.

25. Boyle, R. H. & Boyle, R. A. (1983). Acid rain. *American Journal, 4,* 22–37; Marshall, E. (1982). Air pollution clouds U.S.-Canadian relations. *Science, 217,* 1118–1119; and U.S. Council on Environmental Quality and U.S. Department of State.

26. National Academy of Sciences, Committee on the Atmosphere and the Biosphere. *Atmosphere-biosphere interactions: Toward a better understanding of the ecological consequences of fossil fuel combustion.* Washington, D.C.: National Academy Press, 1981; and U.S. Council on Environmental Quality and U.S. Department of State.

27. Bernard, Jr., H. W. (1981). *The greenhouse effect;* and U.S. Council on Environmental Quality and U.S. Department of State.

28. Erlich, Erlich, & Holdren, *Ecoscience: Population, resources, environment;* and Lovins, A. B., Lovins, L. H., Krause, F., & Bach, W. (1981). *Least-cost energy: Solving the CO_2 problem.* Andover, MA: Brick House.

29. Geller, E. S. (1983). The energy crisis and behavioral science: A conceptual framework for large-scale intervention. In A. W. Childs & G. B. Melton (Eds.), *Rural psychology.* New York: Plenum.

30. Keep America Beautiful, Inc. (1977). *Clean community system: Photometric index instructions.* 99 Park Avenue, New York, NY 10016.

31. Geller, The energy crisis and behavioral science.

32. Kohlenberg, R. J., Phillips, T., & Proctor, W. (1976). A behavioral analysis of peaking in residential electricity energy consumption. *Journal of Applied Behavior Analysis, 9,* 13–18.

33. Zerega, A. M. (1981). Transportation energy conservation policy: Implications for social science research. *Journal of Social Issues, 37,* 31–50.

34. Winett, R. A., Neale, M. S., & Grier, H. C. (1979). The effects of self-monitoring and feedback on residential electricity consumption. *Journal of Applied Behavior Analysis, 12.*

35. Erlich, Erlich, & Holdren. *Ecoscience: Population, resources, environment;* and Rifkin, J. (1980). *Entropy: A new world view.* New York: Viking Press.

36. Stern, P. C. & Gardner, G. T. (1981). The place of behavior change in the management of environmental problems. *Journal of Environmental Policy, 2,* 213–239; and Willems, E. P. & McIntire, J. D. (1983). A review of preserving the environment: New strategies for behavior change. *Behavior Analyst, 5,* 191–197.

37. Cone, J. D. & Hayes, S. C. (1980). *Environmental problems/behavioral solutions.* Monterey, CA: Brooks/Cole; and Geller, E. S., Winett, R. A., & Everett, P. B. (1982). *Preserving the environment: New strategies for behavior change.* Elmsford, NY: Pergamon.

38. Oskamp, S. (1984). Psychology's role in the conserving society. *Population & Environment, 6,* 255–293; and Geller, E. S. (1987). Environmental psychology and applied behavior analysis: From strange bedfellows to a productive marriage. In D. Stokols & I. Altman (Eds.), *Handbook of environmental psychology* (pp. 361–388). New York: Wiley.

39. Geller, Applications of behavioral analysis for litter control, 1980; Geller, Winett, & Everett, *Preserving the environment: New strategies for behavior change.*

40. Delprata, D. J. (1977). Prompting electrical energy conservation in commercial users. *Environment & Behavior, 9,* 433–440; and Winett, R. A. (1978). Prompting turning-out lights in unoccupied rooms. *Journal of Environmental Systems, 6,* 237–241.

41. Hayes, S. C. & Cone, J. D. (1977). Reducing residential electrical use: Payments, information and feedback. *Journal of Applied Behavior Analysis, 14,* 81–88; Heberlein, T. A. (1975). Conservation information: The energy crisis and electricity consumption in an apartment complex. *Energy Systems & Policy, 1,* 105–117; Winett, R. A., Kagel,

J. H., Battalio, R. C., & Winkler, R. C. (1978). Effects of monetary rebates, feedback and information on residential electricity conservation. *Journal of Applied Psychology, 63,* 73–78; and Kohlenberg, Phillips, & Proctor, A behavioral analysis of peaking in residential electricity energy consumption.

42. Geller, E. S., Chaffee, J. L., & Ingram, R. E. (1975). Prompting paper recycling on a university campus. *Journal of Environmental Systems, 5,* 39–57; and Witmer, J. F. & Geller, E. S. (1976). Facilitating paper recycling: Effects of prompts, raffles, and contests. *Journal of Applied Behavior Analysis, 9,* 315–322.

43. Ingram, R. E. & Geller, E. S. (1976). A community-integrated, behavior modification approach to facilitating paper recycling. *JSAS Catalog of Selected Documents in Psychology, 5,* 327 (Ms. No. 1097).

44. Pardini, A. U. & Katzev, R. A. (1983). The effect of strength of commitment on newspaper recycling. *Journal of Environmental Systems, 13,* 245–254; and Burn, S. M. & Oskamp, S. (1986). Increasing community recycling with persuasive communication and public commitment. *Journal of Applied Social Psychology, 16,* 29–41.

45. Geller, E. S. & Lehman, G. R. (1991). The buckle-up promise card: A versatile intervention for large-scale behavior change. *Journal of Applied Behavior Analysis, 24,* 91–94.

46. Finnie, W. C. (1973). Field experiments in litter control. *Environment and Behavior, 5,* 123–144; and Geller, E. S., Brasted, W., & Mann, M. (1979–80). Waste receptacle designs as interventions for litter control. *Journal of Environmental Systems, 9,* 145–160.

47. Witmer & Geller, Facilitating paper recycling: Effects of prompts, raffles, and contests; and Davis, *The seventh year: Industrial civilization in transition.*

48. Everett, P. B., Hayward, S. C., & Meyers, A. W. (1974). Effects of a token reinforcement procedure on bus ridership. *Journal of Applied Behavior Analysis, 7,* 1–9; and Erlich, Erlich, & Holdren, *Ecoscience: Population, resources, environment.*

49. Kohlenberg, R. & Phillips, T. (1973). Reinforcement and rate of litter depositing. *Journal of Applied Behavior Analysis, 6,* 391–396.

50. Bacon-Prue, A., Blount, R., Pickering, D., & Drabman, R. (1980). An evaluation of three litter control procedures—trash receptacles, paid workers, and the marked item technique. *Journal of Applied Behavior Analysis, 13,* 165–170.

51. Wodarski, J. S. (1976). The reduction of electrical energy consumption: The application of behavior analysis. *Behavior Therapy, 8,* 347–353.

52. Hake, D. F. & Foxx, R. M. (1978). Promoting gasoline conservation: The effects of reinforcement schedules, a leader and self-recording. *Behavior Modification, 2,* 339–369.

53. Winett, R. A. & Nietzel, M. (1975). Behavioral ecology: Contingency management of residential use. *American Journal of Community Psychology, 3,* 123–133.

54. Slavin, R. E., Wodarski, J. S., & Blackburn, E. L. (1981). A group contingency for electricity conservation in master-metered apartments. *Journal of Applied Behavior Analysis, 14,* 357–363.

55. Shippee, G. (1980). Energy consumption and conservation psychology: A review and conceptual analysis. *Environmental Management, 4,* 297–314; Winett, R. A. (1980). An emerging approach to energy conservation. In D. Glenwick & L. Jason (Eds.), *Behavioral community psychology.* New York: Praeger; and Winett, R. A. & Neale, M. S. (1979). Psychological framework for energy conservation in buildings: Strategies, outcomes, directions. *Energy & Buildings, 2,* 101–116.

56. Seaver, W. B. & Patterson, A. H. (1976). Decreasing fuel oil consumption through feedback and social commendation. *Journal of Applied Behavior Analysis, 9,* 147–152.

57. Kohlenberg, Phillips, & Proctor, A behavioral analysis of peaking in residential electrical energy consumption.

58. Seligman, C. & Darley, J. M. (1977). Feedback as a means of decreasing residential energy consumption. *Journal of Applied Psychology, 62,* 363–368.

59. Blakely, E. Q., Lloyd, K. E., & Alferink, L. A. (1977). *The effects of feedback on residential electrical peaking and hourly kilowatt consumption.* Unpublished manuscript, Department of Psychology, Drake University, Des Moines, IA.

60. McClelland, L. & Cook, S. W. (1979–80). Energy conservation effects of continuous in-home feedback in all-electric homes. *Journal of Environmental Systems, 9,* 169–173.

61. Winett, R. A., Hatcher, J. W., Fort, T. R., Leckliter, I. N., Love, S. Q., Riley, A. W., & Fishback, J. F. (1982). The effects of videotape modeling and daily feedback on residential electricity conservation, home temperature and humidity, perceived comfort, and clothing worn: Winter and summer. *Journal of Applied Behavior Analysis, 15,* 381–402.

62. Winett, R. A., Love, S. Q., & Kidd, C. (1982–83). The effectiveness of an energy specialist and extension agents in promoting summer energy conservation by home visits. *Journal of Environmental Systems, 12,* 61–70.

63. Reichel, D. A. & Geller, E. S. (1980, March). *Group*

versus individual contingencies to conserve transportation energy. Paper presented at the 26th Annual Meeting of the Southeastern Psychological Association, Washington, D.C.

64. Lauridsen, P. K. (1977). *Decreasing gasoline consumption in fleet-owned automobiles through feedback and feedback-plus-lottery.* Unpublished master's thesis, Drake University, Des Moines, IA.

65. Runnion, A., Watson, J. D., & McWhorter, J. (1978). Energy savings in interstate transportation through feedback and reinforcement. *Journal of Organizational Behavior Management, 1,* 180–191.

66. Schnelle, J. G., Gendrich, J. G., Beegle, G. P., Thomas, M. M., & McNees, M. P. (1980). Mass media techniques for prompting behavior change in the community. *Environment and Behavior, 12,* 157–166.

67. Geller, Winett, & Everett. *Preserving the environment: New strategies for behavior change;* Geller, E. S. The energy crisis and behavioral science: A conceptual framework for large-scale intervention; Keep America Beautiful; and Johnson, R. P. & Geller, E. S. (1980). Engineering technology and behavior analysis for interdisciplinary environmental protection. *Behavior Analyst, 3,* 23–29.

68. Bachman, W. & Katzev, R. (1982). The effects of non-contingent free bus tickets and personal commitment on urban bus ridership. *Transportation Research, 16A,* 103–108.

69. Everett, P. B. (1973). The use of the reinforcement procedure to increase bus ridership. *Proceedings of the 81st Annual Convention of the American Psychological Association, 8,* 891–892. (Summary); and Everett, Hayward, & Meyers, Effects of a token reinforcement procedure on bus ridership.

70. Hake, D. F. & Zane, T. (1981). A community-based gasoline conservation project: Practical and methodological considerations. *Behavior Modification, 5,* 435–458.

71. Hake, D. F. & Foxx, R. M. Promoting gasoline conservation: The effects of reinforcement schedules, a leader and self-recording; Winett & Nietzel,

Behavioral ecology: Contingency management of residential use; and Reichel & Geller, *Group versus individual contingencies to conserve transportation energy.*

72. McNees, M. P., Schnelle, J. F., Gendrich, J., Thomas, M. M., & Beegle, G. P. (1979). McDonald's litter hunt: A community litter control system for youth. *Environment and Behavior, 11,* 131–138.

73. Hayes, S. C., Johnson, V. S., & Cone, J. D. (1975). The market item technique: A practical procedure for litter control. *Journal of Applied Behavior Analysis, 8,* 381–386.

74. Bacon-Prue, A., Blount, R., Pickering, D., & Drabman, R. (1980). An evaluation of three litter control procedures—trash receptacles, paid workers, and the marked item technique. *Journal of Applied Behavior Analysis, 13,* 165–170.

75. Winett, R. A., Hatcher, J. W., Fort, T. R., Leckliter, I. N., Love, S. Q., Riley, A. W., & Fishback, J. F. (1982). The effects of videotape modeling and daily feedback on residential electricity conservation, home temperature and humidity, perceived comfort, and clothing worn: Winter and summer. *Journal of Applied Behavior Analysis, 15,* 381–402; and Winett & Neale, Psychological framework for energy conservation in buildings: Strategies, outcomes, directions.

76. Hayes & Cone, Reducing residential electrical use: Payments, information, and feedback; and Winett & Neale, Psychological framework for energy conservation in buildings: Strategies, outcomes, directions.

77. Cone & Hayes, Environmental problems/behavioral solutions; and Geller, Winett, & Everett, Preserving the environment: New strategies for behavior change.

78. Seligman, C. (March 8, 1990). Personal communication to E. S. Geller.

79. Geller, E. S. (1990). Behavior analysis and environmental protection: Where have all the flowers gone? *Journal of Applied Behavior Analysis, 23,* 269–273.

Chapter 22

The Future of Health Promotion

OBJECTIVES

By the end of this chapter, the reader should be able to:

1. Discuss resource-generating (and -conserving) strategies for health promotion programs.
2. Describe skills to make health promotion professionals more marketable in the future.
3. List ethical safeguards for health promotion programs from the ONPRIME perspective.
4. Apply these safeguards to health promotion programs.

INTRODUCTION

Motivating Health Behavior has addressed relatively typical areas of health promotion, such as chronic disease prevention and the use of motivational and educational techniques to improve the health and safety of people and to protect their environment. Clearly, this focus is appropriate. Techniques for cancer and heart disease prevention approaches have by no means been perfected, whereas drug and alcohol abuse is on the increase. Sexually transmitted diseases have been on the rampage, both in developed and underdeveloped countries.

The promotion of child survival and reproductive health in the underdeveloped world is largely in the formative research stage. Those newly entering the field of health promotion should find plenty of work to keep them going until retirement.

In this final section, however, we transcended these typical boundaries somewhat, especially with the chapter on preservation of the environment. The future of health promotion is difficult to predict, given (a) its extraordinarily rapid growth and expansion in the past two decades, and (b) correspondingly rapid changes in society as the Cold War ends and a "baby boomer" takes over the leadership of the U.S. Perhaps the course health promotion's future takes will depend on factors similar to those which got it going in the first place (chapter 1):

- a recognition that existing models and technologies are ineffective for growing world problems (e.g., starvation, deforestation, ozone depletion, forced migration, racism);

- an acknowledgement of the role of human behavior in these problems and their solutions; and
- a reawakening of individuals and communities to their ability to make a difference through autonomous or professionally-facilitated actions.

As we approach the end of a millennium, there is an increasing tendency to wax philosophical about where we have been and where we are going. In this chapter we do some of that, as well, but we hope to go beyond simple prognostication and wishful thinking. In addition, we outline some practical steps we can all consider which at a minimum may make health promotion more effective. In the best case scenario, the technology of behavior change as outlined in this book can be applied to ever broader areas to "make the world a better place."

FUNDING AND SUSTAINING HEALTH PROMOTION EFFORTS

As numerous chapters in this text have pointed out, behavior must be reinforced to be maintained. Health behavior is especially difficult to establish and maintain because it often is in competition with health damaging behavior, for which immediate and powerful reinforcement is routinely available. Eating high fat or high sugar diets, sedentary life styles, and sexual behavior, to name just a few risk behaviors for which reinforcement is virtually immediate, compete with health promoting life styles. In contrast, eating low fat diets and exercising do not provide immediate reinforcement, but, in the case of exercise, performance may generate mildly aversive consequences (e.g., work). Much of this text has been devoted to descriptions of contingencies of reinforcement which were designed to establish and maintain health promoting and protective behavior, for which immediate reinforcement is not usually present. Examples in this text document that when such contingencies have been employed, substantial gains in health promotion can be achieved. However, how can these interventions be afforded?

The California Tobacco Initiative serves as an important health promotion model in that it provides for explicit financing for anti-tobacco health promotion programs. It also uses a peer reviewed system of competitive grant awards, similar to the National Institutes of Health (NIH). The combination provides liberal funding for the "best" research and demonstration (R&D) programs. The same type of financing could be used to support all types of health promoting life styles and the R&D necessary to identify target behaviors and intervention programs to establish them. Although federal entitlement legislation has been established for funding medical care of the indigent, no parallel legislation provides ongoing funding for behavioral prevention programs.

Neither the California Tobacco Tax nor NIH serve as a particularly good funding model in one respect. They both provide only short-term funding. To effect and sustain health behavior, funding is necessary for periods longer than three to five years. Yet, it is important that a new entitlement program not come to represent non-contingent support for a whole profession by accident. Funds should be guaranteed for health promotion and preventive medicine purposes, but only for those interventions shown to be effective in changing objectively measured outcomes (e.g., behavior or health status). Periodic review of outcomes should be the basis for sustaining program support. No funding should be delegated to health education or any other particular service. Rather, funding should be tied to ethical means of changing target health behavior—whether by education or social engineering. Legislation at state or federal levels to affect funding is critical for the rapid expansion of a behavioral health promotion technology. Perhaps a self-initiated tax, with stipulations that all new revenues be used exclusively for health promotion purposes, can provide the needed funds to support the establishment of healthy life styles and an ongoing behavioral science and technology aimed at enhancing the welfare of the community.

RESOURCE-GENERATING STRATEGIES FOR HEALTH PROMOTION PROGRAMS

With decreases in tax support for health agencies and health promotion activities projected to continue or accelerate, innovative and effective revenue raising schemes are more important than ever. Here are a few of the directions future resource generation efforts might take:

1. As the California "Prop 99" experience showed, voters and health-oriented politicians can raise taxes and earmark them for specific health promotion efforts. The political feasibility of such campaigns can be enhanced by making a connection between the tax and the health behavior being changed, as best exemplified by taxing the "sins" of alcohol and tobacco use and directing these funds toward health education in these areas.

2. Increasingly, health promotion programs must (at least in part) "pay for themselves." For example, Project Salsa charges a minimal fee for cholesterol checks, which offset nearly half of the actual expenses. Staff compiled a heart healthy, Spanish/English cookbook which presents delicious Mexican and other recipes. Their hope is to market the cookbook throughout the Southwest, offering it at cost to residents of their target community of San Ysidro and using profits from other sales to fund non-paying programs (e.g., breast feeding promotion to indigent mothers).

3. Partnerships with the private sector are expanding in depth and breadth. Abilities of health professionals to attract corporate contributions to or sponsorships of health promotion programs have gained greater prominence. This trend is related to three factors: (a) governmental resources for health promotion are diminishing; (b) conservative political trends in the past one and a half decades in the U.S. and other Western nations have been accompanied by generally cozier relations between government and business; and (c) the private sector can enhance the beneficial effects of a health promotion effort by offering access to its consumer markets and distribution systems.

   Nevertheless, health professionals must consider the reputation and mission of the potential private sector partner carefully before striking any deals. For example, it is best to avoid having breweries promote healthy eating.

4. In any case, future health promotion programs will have to make do with fewer resources. Using volunteers and other community change agents, contributed advertising and media, and

other inexpensive resources will help conserve what precious few funds are available for changing health behavior.

COMMUNICATION SKILLS MAKE THE HEALTH PROFESSIONAL

How should the health professional, especially the health promotion specialist, prepare for the future of the field? The answer is simple enough: through some very new and very old forms of communication. Let's begin with the latter.

Speaking in Several Tongues

In few fields is it so important to be able to speak with our consumers. But this seemingly straightforward task is becoming increasingly difficult for an elementary reason: we frequently do not speak in the same tongue as our audience. The most rapidly growing segments of the U.S. population have their roots in Latin America and Asia, and include individuals who may speak limited English. On the international scene, economic and military power made English a language that "traveled well"; however, with new economic powers emerging in Japan, Germany, and elsewhere, this may prove less true in the future. The breakdown of the former Soviet Union and the Communist Bloc has brought about the potential for true world peace, but the corresponding reawakening of ethnic identities in these regions, and uprooting of large numbers of people, makes it increasingly important to be familiar with several tongues. In the future, employability in all but the most highly technical health professions may be predicated on language skills.

Knowledge of Computers and Other Electronic Technology

At the other end of the communication spectrum are electronic media and technology. Barely a decade ago secretaries balked at giving up their electric typewriters for word processors, and photojournalists carried fifty pounds of equipment with them on assignments. Today's hand-sized cameras, scanners, color laser printers, notebook computers, and increasingly sophisticated software packages make us forget the last time we selected our own lens aperture setting or used typewriters (or for that matter, mainframe computers). Marketability in the health promotion field will continue to rely on high levels of sophistication in the use of electronic technology and communication.

A Technological Revolution

We have not yet seen the extent to which behavior change technology can be perfected. Our guess as to the directions the field will take may be less than accurate, but by sharing them we may increase their likelihood. We see behavior change technology combining with numerous computer, communication and micro-electronics technologies in a manner that will make greater behavior change possible.

Personal computer-assisted diagnosis and prevention advice is already available. The future will see a marked increase of such tools, and they will be more accurate in diagnosing problems and better at suggesting courses of preventive action. Linking personal computer systems to medical facilities is already feasible. The better trained preventive medicine physician is taught to take extensive personal histories to differentially diagnose diseases and to plan the best course of preventive intervention. Imagine how much more accurate these histories could be if the patient were to bring in his/her personal computer disk on which their routinely measured vital signs had been recorded since birth! Or, imagine that the home computer is electronically linked with the physician's computer and automatically relays vital signs. The home machine alerts the patient to simple preventive and urgent care needs; the physician's machine alerts the physician to ask the patient to come in for more elaborate diagnostic and/or treatment services. In each case, the machine system will have effects on individuals' behavior and that of health care professionals.

It takes little imagination to see a new home in which the appliances are automated for convenience. The home of tomorrow will include a personal computer that can be programmed to control the T.V. set, the exercycle, the refrigerator, and the cooking, as well as the humidity, temperature, and general ventilation. The physical environment can be arranged to make exercise more

likely (e.g., decrease the humidity and temperature). The T.V. will remind us to begin dinner, and the "stove" will prepare a nutritious meal based on our recent history of eating and exercise. In short, the personal machine-based programming of the near future will provide frequent prompts and reinforcement for healthy behavior and will decrease environmental support for "unhealthy" behavior. With portable computers and communication devices, these "programs" will be transportable to work and recreation sites. The limits of the integration of behavioral and electronic technologies for behavior change and health promotion are unimaginable. Even today, computer and communication technologies have created equipment which the community is ill prepared to use; we don't know how to make the best use of new tools.

An example of a potentially important technological breakthrough is provided by Norris Communications, who recently created a new telephone that fits inside the ear. Imagine emergency medical teams in the field connected to an emergency room physician with the new phone in the ear and full telecommunications links. A technician will be able to assist an accident victim while the physician observes and gives ongoing directions for emergency care. Think of the workers at risk of attack when they leave their workplace after dark. With the phone in the ear, they are never more than seconds away from 911 emergency help.

Similar electronic telemetry and physiological monitoring devices available in the home now will enable the individual to record his/her own heart rate, blood pressure, blood sugar, blood cholesterol, and other vital and physiological signs and automatically record them on their personal computer. The computer will automatically summarize these data and provide directive feedback for changes as needed. The potential good to come from the integration of electronic and behavior change technologies is limited only by the imagination of the health promotion specialists in the field.

Media and Advocacy

Lawrence Wallack[1,2] is among those who urge us to look beyond the way we think of communications and social marketing, and look instead at media as a tool for advocacy and community organization. He noted that social marketing, based in psychology and other behavioral sciences, considers the individual as part of the audience that will change his or her health behavior given our (hopefully effective) health messages. "Media advocacy," in contrast, is based in political science, considers the individual as a citizen who will participate in community organization or policy development given appropriate prompts to do so. The focus of media advocacy is therefore to change the sociopolitical environment in ways which support healthy behavior and protect the vulnerable segments of society. As health promotion moves toward an emphasis on empowerment rather than individual behavior change, we can expect to see more use of the media as a tool of community organization.

THE CITIZEN-PROFESSIONAL

Many professionals with formal training in health promotion will continue to apply for and obtain positions in public health offices, school systems, worksites, clinics, and research programs. These positions will probably be titled "health promoter," "health educator," "preventive medicine specialist," etc. A second group of individuals will continue to learn about health promotion because it is interesting. Hopefully, they will apply this knowledge at home and at work and in some way create a healthier environment for themselves, their supervisees, and their patients, clients, students, or children.

But all of us are citizens and neighbors as well as professionals. We write letters to editors. Some of us buy products from one company and not another, and some eat vegetables and chicken instead of beef. We contribute to campaigns and vote, and give testimony at city council meetings. We invest in certain stocks, and pay dues or donate to certain organizations. We car-pool. We recycle. We encourage others to do the same. People receive training in health promotion because they want to learn how to help others. *Motivating Health Behavior* emphasizes ways in which this can be accomplished as part of one's job. Indeed, it is nice to earn a living while doing something personally and professionally fulfilling. As health professionals, however, we don't just "give at the office." Much of everything we do is a

health behavior. Whether through our professional work, as a role model for friends and others, or by being a good citizen of our neighborhood and planet, the field of health promotion offers rich rewards for all.

THE ETHICS OF CHANGING HEALTH BEHAVIOR

"Free Will" and "Coercion"

The field of behavior modification has frequently been attacked because of its potential for "mind control" and its ability to force people into behaving against their natural inclinations. Although our detractors are sometimes overly impressed with the power of behavior modification, the authors of this book admit that motivational procedures can be abused when not accompanied by appropriate checks and balances. But regardless of how other health promotion technologies and targets are labeled—such as "self-help groups," "decision-making skills," "positive choices," etc.—educational, training, marketing and organizational procedures *all* seek changes in human behavior. They might be more effective than direct behavior modification procedures, given their subtle invocation of self determination, which in turn is less likely to raise defenses against "manipulation." But just as teachers and educational institutions would not be around too long if students' academic skills were not changed, health promotion professionals will eventually fade into history if we fail to document behavior change. We will continue to discover and apply ever more effective behavior change technologies. Given this inevitability, adherence to ethical safeguards is a must.

Behavioral scientists have defined "coercion" as the use of excessively aversive or attractive consequences to modify behavior. Yet, how are these types of consequences defined? Clearly, those of us in the field would not dream of using physical punishment in a health promotion campaign. Yet, would we embarrass smokers by asking them to put out their cigarettes while they are sitting in a restaurant enjoying dinner with their families? On the positive reinforcement side, giving a diploma or raffle ticket to a child who has done well in our school heart health program seems innocuous enough. But what if this child

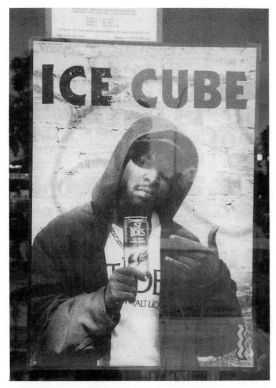

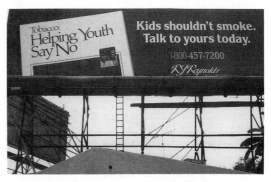

FIGURE 22-1.   The "Illness Industries" place a heavy emphasis on marketing their products in both aggressive and subtle ways. A well known African-American media personality promotes a high alcohol content malt liquor. R. J. Reynolds attempts to deflect criticism by suggesting that they don't want youth to smoke. *Photo courtesy of Betsy Clapp.*

has never had the chance to earn recognition for anything? Is this recognition now "excessive" or "manipulative," at least in terms of this child's baseline of reinforcement?

Individual Rights vs. The Common Good

> For the strength of the pack is the wolf
> and the strength of the wolf is the pack.
> from *The Jungle Book*
> —Rudyard Kipling

Like Kipling's wolves, humans are interdependent, communal beings. We rely on neighbors both in our community and throughout the world for social and material needs, and in turn contribute to the community through our own and our families' efforts. But the small town or rural "gemeinschaft" society, with its emphasis on mutu-

ally understood roles and rules, has largely been replaced by a more anonymous, insulated urban existence where people from substantially different cultural origins abide side by side. Individuals who live together in today's cities and nations probably do not share nor, in many cases, understand one another's rules by which to live, and therefore rely on written law to define acceptable social, including health-related, behavior.

Society looks at one's health-related decisions as a matter of "personal" (generally, culturally-based) choice, even if the decisions are bad ones. Lines are drawn only when these choices prove harmful to others. But in practice, these lines are indistinct. If you live and work in a smoke-free environment, my lighting up a cigarette next to you in an airport waiting area will likely annoy you, but it is unlikely to cause you lasting physical harm. Should there be statutes protecting you

20% of USA's Kids Live in Want, Group Says

A report released today by the Children's Defense Fund shows that children are twice as likely to be poor than people of any other age, including the elderly. Who the poor children are:

Number of poor children

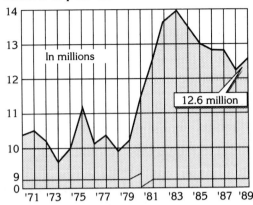

In millions

12.6 million

'71 '73 '75 '77 '79 '81 '83 '85 '87 '89

Race/ethnic group

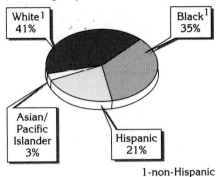

White[1]
41%

Black[1]
35%

Asian/
Pacific
Islander
3%

Hispanic
21%

1-non-Hispanic

Changes 1979 to 1989:

Percentage increase in poor children
from 1979 to 1989:

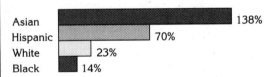

Asian   138%
Hispanic   70%
White   23%
Black   14%

Where poor children live [2]

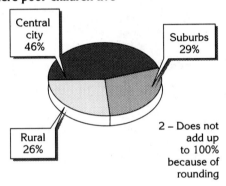

Central
city
46%

Suburbs
29%

Rural
26%

2 – Does not
add up
to 100%
because of
rounding

Downward trend in numbers aided

Percentage of poor children who benefit from
Aid to Families with Dependent Children:

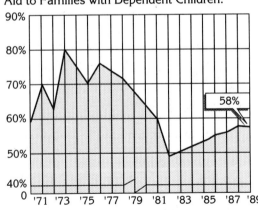

90%

80%

70%

58%

60%

50%

40%

0   '71 '73 '75 '77 '79 '81 '83 '85 '87 '89

Family Structure

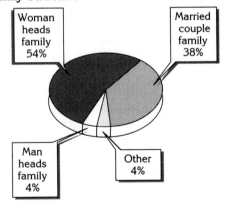

Woman
heads
family
54%

Married
couple
family
38%

Man
heads
family
4%

Other
4%

Source: The Children's Defense Fund; U.S. Census Bureau; Ways and Means Committee Green Book, 1991
By Marty Baumann, USA TODAY, June 3, 1991

from my smoke in all public situations, as many have suggested? Many states recently defined the common good to include ridding the roadways of drinking drivers through random sobriety checks. But to what extent are we violating the individual's (especially non-drinker's) rights through this behavior change procedure, as the Michigan courts have recently asserted? Do parents have the right not to seek medical treatment, immunizations, and other potentially life-saving actions for their children if their personal religious beliefs prescribe such procedures? Do they have the right to expose their children to their own smoking or alcohol abuse? Do health officials have the right to inform sexual contacts of people diagnosed with sexually transmitted diseases — including HIV — that they may have been infected? At an economic level, should a government close a polluting factory even if it costs a community half of its employment?

As society becomes more technically complicated and economically and culturally diverse, balancing individual rights with the common good will become even more complicated. On the one hand, health and political leaders will need to be continually reminded of the former, while the complementary promotion of community responsibility should be imbedded in all health initiatives.

Any of a variety of standards may be applied to determining whether any given health promotion program is "ethical." The authors of this text conclude it by referring back to the ONPRIME model as a system for ethical safeguards. This system is presented in the form of a series of questions for which the responsible health professional and governing body should have suitable responses:

1. Does the community participate in defining the need for, planning, and directing the health promotion program? Do the professional staff make a sincere effort to involve and empower the community?
2. Is the health promotion program truly addressing the community's health-related needs, and is it effectively using existing resources?
3. Are the health promotion priorities important for and to the community?
4. Is the health promotion program based in adequate scientific and formative research?
5. Is the intervention sufficiently powerful to be effective, yet at the same time non-coercive? Does it empower the community or make it more dependent on outside or professional help? If aversive measures are employed, for what reasons are they selected? By whom?
6. Are adequate program monitoring and evaluation mechanisms in place? Are program revisions made based on monitoring data?

SUMMARY

The reader of this section may have noted a surplus of question marks in the preceding paragraphs. This should not be interpreted as an indication that the authors do not have firm opinions on these issues — we do. However, there are no right or wrong answers to the many questions raised in this chapter. Nor can health promoters develop ethical or effective procedures and policies insulated from others in their community. Most importantly, individuals who represent the target population to be served in the program should be represented at all stages of planning, implementation, evaluation and dissemination. This representation should include board membership, respondents in needs assessment and formative research efforts, key staff positions, volunteers, and evaluators. In short, community participation and empowerment in all steps of the ONPRIME sequence will assure us of responsible — and hopefully effective — health promotion.

FIGURE 22-2. There is a substantial amount of political and philosophical debate as to whether adults are "responsible" for their own illness and misery. Few would argue, however, that children should not be blamed for being poor. Nevertheless, the last decade and a half has seen nearly a 25% increase in the number of children living in poverty in the United States. (Copyright 1991, USA Today. Reprinted with permission.)

EXERCISE

Review your progress on your self-change project. Share your results with the class, including which aspects worked well, what should be changed, and what plans for maintenance or additional efforts you have.

ENDNOTES

1. Wallack, L. (1990). Two approaches to health promotion in the mass media. *World Health Forum, 11,* 143–154.

2. Wallack, L. & Sciandra, R. (1991). Media advocacy and public education in the community intervention trial to reduce heavy smoking (COMMIT). *International Quarterly of Community Health Education, 11,* 205–222.

Glossary

AB research design — *see* baseline intervention.

ABC recording — an observer writes a narrative or a "story" describing in sequence all behaviors observed. These observations can be organized in a three-column chart — an ABC chart — consisting of the events occurring prior to the behavior (Antecedents), the subject's responses (Behaviors) following these antecedents, and the events following the behavior (Consequences). It is also called "narrative recording."

acquired immune deficiency syndrome (AIDS) — a disease, first recognized and reported in 1981, caused by the human immunodeficiency viruses (HIV) which attack the immune system of the body. The condition is an acquired deficiency of certain leukocytes, especially T cells, which results in a variety of opportunistic infections that ultimately result in death. AIDS is transmitted via body fluids, especially sexual secretions, and blood.

advertisements — paid messages that allow the marketer to select the time and duration of the announcement rather than having that controlled by the station.

Alma-Ata declaration — the International Conference on Primary Health Care held in 1978 at Alma Ata, capital of Kazakhstan. The declaration produced there, which was addressed to the world community, had the purposes of protecting and promoting the health of the world's population.

analytic data — data which allow the objective determination of kinds of program inputs (people, money, or other resources), using what techniques (marketing, face-to-face education, etc.) are effective with a given problem or target.

applied behavior analysis — the technology of behavioral modification which focuses primarily on observable behaviors of individuals and communities in their natural settings.

archival research — research involving existing sources of data or "archives," extracting relevant information, and presenting these data to the people governing the program.

association — two variables "co-vary" or change together in some way (although not necessarily in the same direction). This concept is known as covariance.

aversive control — the use of unpleasant consequences to control or modify behavior.

373

baseline data — information about how often and under what conditions the consumer is currently performing the target behavior.

baseline-intervention (AB research design) — a simple baseline to an intervention analysis of behavior change between phases.

behavior — the observable actions of people. We can see, hear, or sense what people do or do not do, i.e., their actions or inactions.

behavior analysis — a subdiscipline within psychology closely associated with the work of B. F. Skinner and others, which emphasizes the direct observation of behavior-environment relationships.

behavior assessment — the process of identifying, specifying, and quantifying health behaviors relevant to health promotion efforts.

behavior modification — (1) the identification and change of "functional determinants" of behavior in order to increase, decrease, or maintain such behaviors toward adaptive levels." (2) As used in this text behavior modification is the systematic application of principles derived from learning theory to alter environment-behavior relationships in order to strengthen adaptive and weaken maladaptive behaviors.

behavioral asset — a health-promotive or other adaptive consumer behavior.

behavioral deficit — a class of responses which are considered problematic by someone because of failure to occur (1) with sufficient frequency, (2) with adequate intensity, (3) in appropriate form, or (4) in appropriate situations.

behavioral excess — a class of related behaviors described as problematic by the consumer or an informant because of excess. They are (1) frequency, (2) intensity, (3) duration, or (4) situations.

biofeedback — provides physiological data to patients in order for them to monitor and change a physical or physiological condition.

Bloom's taxonomy of educational objectives — three major areas are defined by B. Bloom as cognitive, affective, and psychomotor. The cognitive domain emphasizes specific intellectual processes and tasks typically referred to as "knowledge," "understanding," "memorization," etc. The affective domain includes a person's feelings and attitudes with respect to certain information, other people, etc. The psychomotor domain consists of specific behavioral skills, whether they are related to athletic performance, technical ability, or the ease and efficiency by which one performs a task.

broadcast media — forms of mass communication: radio and television.

case control study — individuals with a disease or health problem are tracked backwards in time to find causal agents or risk factors; also called a retrogressive case control study.

case-fatality ratio — the number of people who have a disease compared to the number who die from it.

$$\text{Case Fatality Ratio} = \frac{\text{No. of people who die from a disease}}{\text{No. of people who have the disease}}$$

channel — the means by which a message is sent. The major channels are broadcast media, print media, display media, and face-to-face communication.

checklist — a recording procedure in which observers are simply interested in whether a specific behavior occurred. Observers often use a binary (i.e., "yes or no") recording format to indicate whether a certain behavior occurred. Also called binary recording.

cohort study — individuals with exposure to a disease or health problem are tracked forward in time to determine whether they develop the disease or health problem; also called a prospective cohort study.

communications-persuasion model — it considers how mass media and other forms of public communication can be used to change attitudes and behaviors; developed by William McGuire and others.

community forum — a forum in which individuals from a community can represent themselves and speak publicly regarding health or civic priorities.

community organization model — a model which advocates that individuals and entire populations need to take charge of their own lives in order to deal with not only the problem(s) at hand, but also with the root causes related to this and future problems.

community-level intervention — an intervention

which involves changes in the community's social and/or physical environment in such ways as to promote individual, group, and/or organizational health.

comparative data—whereas descriptive data give the "what" of program evaluation, comparisons with other programs or techniques put the "what" into a context.

contingency contract—a written contract on which a client agrees to a specific behavior change or health outcome by a given date. The contract also specifies consequences of completing (or not completing) the contract.

covariance—see association.

cross-sectional study—a study in which a sample of many people is looked at in a given point in time.

determinism—the doctrine which says that human behavior is controlled by one's physical environment, genetic predisposition, and physiological and physical functioning.

differential reinforcement—any procedure that has the characteristics: (1) two or more different behaviors can occur in one situation, (2) one behavior is reinforced, and (3) the other maladaptive behavior, often the primary target of the program, is extinguished.

duration recording—a type of recording procedure in which the observer measures the total length of time the behavior occurs during a predefined observational period.

epidemiology—the study of the distribution and determinants (causes) of disease frequency in human populations.

explanatory data—data which allows the streamlining of the program to its essential components, or the projection of types of target populations or problems it might be appropriate for in the future.

external validity—the generalizability of the results of a study to other populations, settings, points of time, etc.

extinction—the discontinuation of positive reinforcement or the imposition of a barrier to receiving that reinforcement, which in turn weakens the previously reinforced behavior.

facilitation—same as response facilitation.

false negative—a test indicates a person does not have a disease when, in fact, they do.

false positive—a test indicates a person has a disease when, in fact, they do not.

Field theory—a type of research which explains behavior in terms of the situation in which people find themselves as well as the needs they bring to those situations.

focus group—a type of research in which a moderator leads about eight to ten people to talk freely about a topic.

format—the varied forms of media the promotional message can take.

formative research—evaluative research conducted during program development. It includes the pretesting of programs, products, and materials through in-depth studies of small numbers of people.

frequency recording—a type of recording procedure in which the observer counts each occurrence of the target behavior during a predefined time period. Frequency recording gives an accurate record of response occurrence within designated time periods, thus allowing for an estimate of the rate at which the behavior occurs.

functional determinants—any of a variety of environmental stimuli including people, things, and situations.

generalization training—training to promote the spread of a specific behavior from one situation to another.

goal—a general criterion toward which progress can hopefully be made.

group-level intervention—one which emphasizes the interpersonal process, which is a material part of everyone's daily interactions with friends, relatives, and others as part of the health promotion effort.

health belief model—states that health behavior is a function of both knowledge and motivation. Specifically, the model emphasizes the role of perceptions of vulnerabilty to an illness and the potential effectiveness of treatment in decisions regarding whether to seek medical attention.

health prevention—one of three areas for health enhancement in *Healthy People 2000* which is for the health services sector. The five priority services are: maternal and infant care, HIV infection control, heart disease and stroke, cancer, and diabetes and other chronic disabling conditions.

health promotion — the modification of human behavior and environmental factors related to that behavior which directly or indirectly promote health, prevent illness, or protect individuals from harm.

health protection — emphasizes decreasing or eliminating health hazards in our physical environment. One of three categories for health enhancement in *Healthy People 2000*.

Healthy People 2000 — a volume published by the U.S. Department of Health and Human Services which sets out the health prospects and problems in the United States until the year 2000. It establishes three goals for the 1990s: (1) to increase the span of healthy life for Americans, (2) to reduce health disparities among Americans, and (3) to achieve access to preventive services for all Americans.

human immunodeficiency virus (HIV) — *see* acquired immune deficiency syndrome (AIDS).

impact evaluation — research designed to identify whether and to what extent a program contributed to accomplishing its stated goals (here, more global than outcome evaluation).

in-depth interview — a form of research consisting of an intensive interview to find out how a person thinks and feels about a given topic. It is a hybrid of focus group and survey techniques, combining the qualitative nature of the former with the one-to-one format of the latter.

incidence — the number of new cases with a specific problem divided by the number of people in the population.

individual health promotion — the modification of health behavior and related factors through motivational procedures, skills training, communication strategies, and educational techniques delivered on a one-to-one basis.

informant — the person who makes the observations or fills out the self-report form in an objective assessment.

intercept interview — a form of marketing research in which people are approached and interviewed at the point they are most likely to have been exposed to promotional material or engage in a health-related behavior (e.g., near a cigarette machine, in a supermarket, in a clinic waiting room, etc.).

internal validity — whether the change observed in a dependent variable can actually be attributed to a specific causal factor.

interpersonal channel — face-to-face communication.

interpersonal skills — *see* social skills.

intervention — a health promotion aimed at a target audience which alters a preexisting condition related to that target audience's behavior. The purpose of the intervention is to create healthful behavior(s).

KARS — an acronym for Key informant interview, Archival research, Rates-under-treatment, and Surveys.

key informant interviews (KII) — interviews conducted with people "in the know" — individuals who are very familiar with a community and its people, its health behavior patterns, health needs, and intervention techniques appropriate or inappropriate for the community.

locality development — a process-oriented approach to community organization involving self-help and grass-roots efforts in solving problems.

longitudinal analyses — determine the temporal order of associated variables.

longitudinal study — a study dealing with a group or individual over a period of time.

market analysis — an investigation in marketing used to establish the market boundaries (i.e., who and what are targeted or excluded), the geographic area encompassed, and whether the market size is growing or declining. The market analysis also obtains information about the wants, needs, perceptions, attitudes, habits and readiness for change, as well as satisfaction levels of the potential market. It also obtains basic demographic information.

market creation — the promotion of a product in a new market, such as to minorities, a new state, or a new country.

market defense — the stand an organization or company makes to protect and advance their product and its legitimacy.

market offense — typical marketing of a product that one sees in magazines or on a billboard.

market segmentation — the partitioning of a potential market into homogeneous submarkets based on the common characteristics identified from the market analysis.

mass media—newspapers, magazines, radio, television, videos and the like. They use impersonal communication approaches to deliver to large numbers of people.

medical model—the passive compliance of a patient to clinical procedures which the physician or other clinician directs, as though it were neither necessary nor even possible for the patient to understand and participate in the treatment regimen. The model implies that illnesses need to be treated rather than prevented.

modeling—following instruction a trainer demonstrates or "models" the skill behavior that he wants the student to learn. Modeling is used to clarify the description of the behavior given in the instruction phase.

monitor—the person responsible for observing the consumer's behavior and delivering reinforcers when the consumer appropriately performs the target behavior.

monitoring—same as process evaluation.

motivation—the interaction between a behavior and the environment in such ways as to increase, decrease, or maintain that behavior.

multiple baseline design—a time-series design which tracks the effects of an intervention replicated in a staggered fashion across different individuals or groups, behaviors, or settings. This design has, ideally, two or three replications of baseline followed by intervention.

narrative recording—see "ABC recording."

needs and resources assessment (N/RA)—research and planning activities used to determine: (1) a community's health behavior patterns, (2) the extent and kind of health needs and priorities in the community, and (3) approaches and resources to deal with these needs.

negative association—it exists when the presence (or occurrence) of one variable predicts the absence of the second; for example, the absence of vitamin C predicts, and causes, scurvy.

negative reinforcement—the removal of an unpleasant consequence which results in the strengthening of a behavior. The type of behavior reinforced with this procedure is called either escape or avoidance behavior.

nomograph—graph with a set of three parallel lines, one for each of three variables. When a straight edge connects two of them, information from the third unknown variable can be obtained.

objective—see SMART.

ONPRIME—an acronym for Organizing, Needs/resources assessment, Priority setting, Research, Intervention, Monitoring, and Evaluation.

operational definition—the product of breaking down a broad concept into observable and measurable component behaviors. Operational definitions usually quantify a variable or characteristic rather than refer to it in general or subjective terms.

organizational behavioral management (OBM)—a set of techniques designed for changing the behavior of change agents, as well as employees. The change agents are typically employees or professional staff in the health care or health promotion setting (e.g., medical clinic, health department office, nonprofit health promotion agency). These techniques also apply to managing and supervising volunteers, students, or other people who may be seeking to prevent disease and promote health among other people.

organizational intervention—an intervention which emphasizes individual (and group) behavior in the context of membership or participation in an organization; e.g., an employee of a worksite, a member of a union, a member of a religious organization or a club, or similar entity.

outcome evaluation—research designed to account for a program's accomplishments and effectiveness; also called "impact evaluation."

outcome expectations—the beliefs that a person holds about how certain events will occur.

performance deficit—a term used by behaviorists to describe a person who has knowledge and skills about a subject but not motivation.

permanent product recording—a simple observation (or notation) of the physical product, outcome, or permanent record of a behavior (e.g., a person's weight, the number of clinic visits, etc.).

place—a marketing term which refers to providing adequate distribution and response channels whereby the product (social idea) can reach the relevant public.

position — a marketing term which refers to the selection of a niche in the marketplace for a product or behavior, taking into account both the needs and wants of the consumer and whatever competition may exist.

positive association — the presence of one variable predicts the presence or occurrence of the second variable; the absence of one variable predicts the absence of the second.

positive reinforcement — the application of a consequence following a behavior which strengthens (increases or maintains) that behavior. The consequence is generally perceived as pleasant.

potential for improving performance (PIP) — the ratio of the performance of a typical or target worker to that of the best worker or "exemplar."

price — a marketing term which is the buyer's cost of a product. Such costs may include monetary expenditure, or time and energy spent.

print media — forms of mass communication, usually newspapers, magazines, and other printed materials — although print can be displayed through broadcast channels. Print media can generally be read and reread at the reader's convenience.

process evaluation — the evaluation of the implementation of a program contemporaneous with that implementation, and the attainment of short term objectives related to program inputs. Also called monitoring.

product — a marketing term referring to the idea or item being sold. The products of health promotion programs generally comprise specific health-related behaviors.

program evaluation — the systematic process of collecting and analyzing reliable and valid information at different points and processes in a program. Its objectives are to improve effectiveness, reduce costs, and contribute to planning future actions.

Project Salsa — a nutritional health promotion program for the largely Latino population of San Ysidro, California.

promotion — a marketing term which refers to publicizing and advertising of a product so it will be purchased and used. In health promotion, this is also the communication strate-

gies and tactics that make the social idea familiar, acceptable, and desirable to the target audience.

Proposition 99 (Prop. 99) — a voter-initiated proposition passed in California in 1988 which raised the tax on cigarettes from 10 cents to 35 cents a pack. The proposition also mandated that one-fourth of the tax revenues realized in this increase would be spent on anti-tobacco education and tobacco-related disease research.

public service announcement (PSA) — free time provided by a station, or paid for by a third party for the broadcast of messages generally considered for the public benefit.

punishment — the application of a consequence following behavior which weakens (decreases or eliminates) that behavior. The consequence is generally perceived as unpleasant.

rate of behavior — the number of times a behavior occurs in a given time period.

rates-under-treatment (RUT) — an assessment that represents a special category of archival research which involves visiting local or regional hospitals and clinics and gaining access to reports, computer files, or individual patient records. The purpose of RUT is to assess the number of people receiving treatment for various afflictions.

reliability — the consistency of an observation or association.

response cost — the removal of a consequence which weakens a behavior. It is very similar to punishment, and is generally perceived to be unpleasant.

response facilitation — the reduction of barriers or the discontinuation of a punishment or response cost procedure which results in the strengthening or reappearance of a behavior. Same as facilitation.

reversal design (ABA design) — the reversal of an effect realized during the initial change from baseline to intervention.

scientific method — the collecting of data, testing it empirically, and then formulating a hypothesis.

screening — an attempt to identify the onset or existence of a health problem in an individual.

secondary research — same as archival research.

segmentation — same as market segmentation.

self-efficacy — self-confidence.

self-monitoring — teaching the consumer to observe and record the frequency, duration, or "permanent products" of his/her behavior.

sensitivity — the percentage of people who actually have the disease who test positive.

$$\text{Sensitivity} = \frac{\text{No. of true positives}}{\text{No. of true positives} + \text{No. of false negatives}} \times 100$$

setting — the place where data are collected as part of objective assessment.

sexually transmitted diseases (STDs) — diseases passed from one person to another through sexual contact. The most infamous are gonorrhea, syphilis, chlamydia, herpes, and genital warts.

shaping — new behaviors that did not previously exist in a person's repertoire can be developed and reinforced.

skills deficit — a term used by behaviorists to describe a person who does not have the capability to engage in a behavior, regardless of whether the knowledge or motivation is present.

SMART — an acronym for five characteristics of an objective. The objective needs to be (1) Specific, (2) Measurable, (3) Attainable, (4) Realistic, and (5) Timed (occur by what date?).

social action — the process in which people assume that whatever problems exist are largely a function of inequality in a given system, and therefore seek changes in the system.

social learning theory — a theory which stresses the interrelationships between people, their behavior, and their environment through a process called "reciprocal determinism." This means that although the environment largely determines or causes behavior, the person in turn can act in ways to change the environment.

social marketing — the application of communication and marketing concepts to the design, implementation, and management of social change programs, such as health and safety promotion.

social planning — an approach to specific problems and the attempt to determine appropriate solutions to them. Social planners are likely to be advocates of specific policies or legislation which will protect or facilitate the population's health.

social skills — also called interpersonal skills. They are those behaviors which persons engage in while interacting with members of their social network (or, on occasion, with casual acquaintances or strangers).

specificity — the percentage of people who actually do not have a disease who test negative.

$$\text{Specificity} = \frac{\text{No. of true negatives}}{\text{No. of true negatives} + \text{No. of false positives}} \times 100$$

STEM — an acronym for Skills Training, Education, Motivation, and social marketing.

stimulus control — the linking of responses to antecedent stimuli.

stimulus generalization training — the procedure in which a behavior is reinforced in a variety of related situations.

target behavior — a behavior the consumer wants to change.

test marketing — the introduction of a product into a carefully (and usually narrowly) defined market, with immediate tracking of audience reactions through intercept interviews, surveys, or other techniques.

theory of reasoned action — emphasizes the roll of personal volition in determining whether a behavior will occur.

time-series study — an examination of a behavior (or products of behavior) of interest over a period of time.

true negative — a person does not have a disease and the test indicates he/she does not have the disease.

true positive — a person has a disease and the test indicates he/she has the disease.

Index